T0407705

CANCER ETIOLOGY, DIAGNOSIS AND TREATMENTS

BONE TUMORS

SYMPTOMS, DIAGNOSIS AND TREATMENT

CANCER ETIOLOGY, DIAGNOSIS AND TREATMENTS

Additional books in this series can be found on Nova's website under the Series tab.

Additional e-books in this series can be found on Nova's website under the e-book tab.

CANCER ETIOLOGY, DIAGNOSIS AND TREATMENTS

BONE TUMORS

SYMPTOMS, DIAGNOSIS AND TREATMENT

MONCEF BERHOUMA
EDITOR

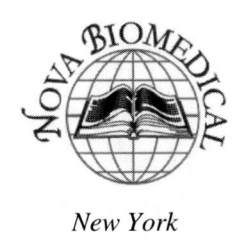

New York

For permission to use material from this book please contact us:
Telephone 631-231-7269; Fax 631-231-8175
Web Site: http://www.novapublishers.com

NOTICE TO THE READER

The Publisher has taken reasonable care in the preparation of this book, but makes no expressed or implied warranty of any kind and assumes no responsibility for any errors or omissions. No liability is assumed for incidental or consequential damages in connection with or arising out of information contained in this book. The Publisher shall not be liable for any special, consequential, or exemplary damages resulting, in whole or in part, from the readers' use of, or reliance upon, this material. Any parts of this book based on government reports are so indicated and copyright is claimed for those parts to the extent applicable to compilations of such works.

Independent verification should be sought for any data, advice or recommendations contained in this book. In addition, no responsibility is assumed by the publisher for any injury and/or damage to persons or property arising from any methods, products, instructions, ideas or otherwise contained in this publication.

This publication is designed to provide accurate and authoritative information with regard to the subject matter covered herein. It is sold with the clear understanding that the Publisher is not engaged in rendering legal or any other professional services. If legal or any other expert assistance is required, the services of a competent person should be sought. FROM A DECLARATION OF PARTICIPANTS JOINTLY ADOPTED BY A COMMITTEE OF THE AMERICAN BAR ASSOCIATION AND A COMMITTEE OF PUBLISHERS.

Additional color graphics may be available in the e-book version of this book.

Library of Congress Cataloging-in-Publication Data

ISBN: 978-1-62618-190-8

Library of Congress Control Number: 2013932901

Published by Nova Science Publishers, Inc. † New York

CONTENTS

PREFACE

Bone tumors are very rare, accounting for less than 0.2 % of all cancers. As our understanding of these tumors at the molecular level is improving, as well as recent advances in imaging and treatments, there was an obvious need for an update in this field. Our subject concerns mainly spinal neoplasms as these may compromise rapidly the neurological functions.

The first five chapters deal with spinal tumors, either primary or metastatic, giving the reader a clear clinical review of the disease and its pathophysiology, as well as therapeutic options. Following chapters are dedicated to new insights in the medical treatment of bone tumors, an overview on the mechanism of malignant transformation of benign bone tumors, the modern management of pain in bone metastases, and the modern therapeutics of bone tumors in prostate cancer patients.

The editor is grateful to the international panel of expert authors for their contributions, which aims to provide a comprehensive update of state-of-the-art management of bone tumors in general and spinal neoplasms in particular.

Moncef Berhouma, MD, PhD
Consultant Neurosurgeon
Associate Professor of Neurosurgery
Director of Minimally Invasive Neurosurgery Research Group (MINEUR)
Pierre Wertheimer Neurological and Neurosurgical Hospital
Lyon - France

In: Bone Tumors: Symptoms, Diagnosis and Treatment
Editor: Moncef Berhouma

ISBN: 978-1-62618-190-8
© 2013 Nova Science Publishers, Inc.

Chapter 1

PRIMARY TUMORS OF THE AXIAL SPINE

Paul E. Kaloostian, Patricia Zadnik and Daniel M. Sciubba
The Johns Hopkins Hospital, Baltimore, MD, US

ABSTRACT

Primary tumors of the spinal column include a variety of pathologies with variable symptoms, outcomes, and treatment. Knowledge of the lesion's pathology is necessary for proper treatment of any patient presenting with a mass in the bony spinal column. Malignant tumors, such as chordomas, plasmacytomas, osteosarcomas and chondrosarcomas require aggressive surgical resection if the goal is curative intent. Adjuvant chemotherapy and radiation may be needed if the margins of the lesion are compromised, and patients should be followed for several years to monitor for tumor recurrence. In contrast , tumors of benign pathology, such as giant cell tumors and aneurismal bone cysts, may present in younger patients. In all patients, pain is the most common symptom. This chapter will review the symptoms, diagnosis and treatment for primary spinal column tumors, with a focus on the current treatment strategies to optimize patient outcomes.

INTRODUCTION

The axial skeleton is a common site for metastatic disease. However, many primary bony tumors are seen to grow and flourish within the spinal axis. Depending on location, size, and histology, these tumors may produce a variety of neurological symptoms and deficits and may affect patient quality of life and survival. It is well documented that the majority of primary spinal tumors are malignant, adding to the complexity of management. In this chapter we discuss a variety of primary bony tumors of the spine. They each display unique pathophysiological and histologic properties that help determine current diagnostic and treatment modalities. We present these tumors and describe typical presentation, imaging characteristics, diagnostic modalities, histopathological characteristics, and treatment options for each tumor.

DIFFERENTIAL DIAGNOSIS

The differential diagnosis of primary bony tumors of the spine is diverse. It includes pathology such as: multiple myeloma, chordomas, giant cell tumors, hemangiomas, osteosarcomas, chondrosarcomas, aneurysmal bone cysts, hemangiomas, eosinophilic granulomas, osteoid osteomas, and osteoblastomas.

MULTIPLE MYELOMA

Multiple myeloma accounts for over 40 % of primary spinal tumors. Myeloma cells are malignant plasma cells that arise from an overexpansion of a single clone of cells within the bone marrow [1]. Patients are typically in their mid-50s and commonly present with focal pain. Additionally, patients may develop an acute pathological fracture due to the tumor that may cause acute onset pain, as well as radiculopathy if neural foramina are compromised [1]. Patients may have other lesions throughout the body, resulting in focal pain at those sites as well. Finally, patients may present with symptoms related to associated anemia, thrombocytopenia and renal failure from involvement of the bone marrow and kidneys [1]. Infection is common in these patients.

Radiographically, multiple myeloma has a unique appearance. Myeloma tumors demonstrate a classic 'punched-out' lesion on xray without surrounding osteoblastic activity [1]. Computed tomography (CT) scans and magnetic resonance imaging (MRI) scans may demonstrate pathological fracture of the spine with associated foraminal compromise and/or spinal cord compression [1]. Others lesions may be noted throughout the spinal axis, as demonstrated on technetium bone scans showing increased radioactive uptake. Skeletal survey remains a recommended study to identify multiple areas of myeloma involvement throughout the entire skeleton [1].

Diagnostic modalities include bone marrow aspiration, CT-guided biopsy of lesions, serum and urine electrophoresis and a CBC. Bone marrow architecture will yield abnormal plasma cell distribution that often provides the diagnosis immediately [1]. CT guided biopsy of the spinal lesion is rarely indicated, unless diagnosis is still unclear. Hypercalcemia may be noted on the blood work in 40% of patients [1]. Histopathologically, multiple myeloma contains an overabundance of plasma cells, with the quantitative extent of plasma cells determining probability of myeloma. Immunohistochemistry is important to identify lambda and kappa heavy chain and light chain distributions, critical to the specific myeloma diagnosis [1].

Treatment for multiple myeloma is diverse. Patients with stable spinal disease without deformity or spinal cord compromise may be managed non-operatively [1]. Non-operative treatment would consist of radiotherapy for focal disease and chemotherapy for systemic disease [1]. Patients with severe spinal instability, spinal deformity, and spinal cord compromise will require surgical intervention [1]. Surgery would depend on the location, but generally involves affected vertebral body resection through an anterior or posterolateral approach with or without associated posterior decompression and fusion [1]. Despite the above treatment modalities, prognosis remains poor. The 5 year survival remains less than 30% [1].

CHORDOMAS

Chordomas are the most common primary malignant tumors of the spine in adults [2]. They are seen in middle-aged adults and frequently occur in the clivus and sacrum. However, other locations of involvement may include cervical, thoracic, or lumbar spine [3]. Chordomas are derived from notochordal rest cells that undergo transformation. Despite chordomas being classified as benign tumors, they are functionally malignant through their high recurrence rate and propensity to grow indolently into tumors of massive proportions [2, 3]. For example, tumors in the pre-sacral and sacrococcygeal region may reach such significant growth that they may distort surrounding neural structures, causing weakness, perineal numbness, or bowel/bladder dysfunction. Chordomas within the cervical or thoracic spine may present with radiculopathy and/or spinal cord compression causing myelopathy. Lumbar chordomas may present with focal back pain or if larger may present with radicular symptoms and associated weakness/numbness or cauda equina syndrome [2, 3].

Diagnostic modalities include CT and MRI that demonstrate a heterogeneously enhancing and sometimes calcified mass of varying size with possible distortion of surrounding tissues if extensive. Classically, chordomas may remodel the existing bony architecture due to their slow growth, rather than invasion and destruction of bone. Often times, a CT-guided biopsy is needed to make the diagnosis [2].

Histologically, chordomas display their pathognomonic physaliferous cells, which have an unusually vacuolated cytoplasm. Microscopically, chordoma cells react intensely for S-100 and other epithelial markers such as cytokeratins and epithelial membrane [4, 5].

The treatment of spinal chordomas has changed over the last few decades in favor of more aggressive surgical management. Surgical management involves attempted en bloc resection without violation of the tumor capsule. This offers the patient an extended progression free survival of over 60% at 5 years while minimizing local recurrence [6, 7]. Subtotal resection provides a local recurrence rate at 8 months as opposed to over 2 years with en bloc resection [11].

En bloc resection without violation of tumor capsule allows for a decrease two-fold in local recurrence [10]. If en bloc resection is not feasible, pre-operative radiation may be performed to reduce viable tumor at the margins and improve patient outcomes. When performing sacrectomies, recent evidence suggests that salvaging the sacral 2 nerve root is key to restoring a 50% chance of normal bowel and bladder function post-operatively [8, 40]. Sacral 3 root preservation will provide additional guarantee of bowel and bladder function. It has been shown that bilateral sacral 2 nerve root sparing along with unilateral sacral 3 root sparing is associated with normal bowel and bladder function [8, 40].

Cervical chordomas are classified into high cervical, mid cervical and cervicothoracic, with location influencing surgical strategy [7, 8]. Thoracic and lumbar chordomas are managed in multiple staged posterior and anterior instrumentation and fusion procedures with en bloc resection of tumor [6, 7, 8]. Sacro-coccygeal chordomas may be resected with total or partial sacrectomy, through the posterior or combined approach. Preservation of the sacro-iliac joint obviates the need for hardware fixation. Adjunctive treatment for chordomas generally involves post-operative proton beam radiotherapy, as these tumors are classified as radio-resistant [9].

GIANT CELL TUMORS

Giant cell tumors of the spine are benign expansile lesions affecting predominantly female patients between 20-50 years of age [13]. Due to the lytic and locally aggressive qualities of this benign tumor, giant cell tumors functionally act in a malignant manner. Patients may present with focal back pain, or larger lesions may cause pathological fracture with associated radiculopathy or spinal cord compression causing myelopathy [13].

Radiographically, Xrays and CT scans are helpful to define the extent of bony destruction associated with the vertebral body. MRI is useful to identify extent of tumor along the spinal column, along with any foraminal or spinal canal compromise. A radionuclide bone scan may be used and will show decreased uptake in the center of the lytic process and increased uptake along the surrounding [12]. A CT-guided biopsy is often recommended to look for the classic mononuclear stromal cells with giant cells throughout [12]. Based on histology, giant cell tumors are classified under 3 stages with stage 1 most benign and stage 3 highly aggressive [12]. Treatment for giant cell tumor varies based on tumor grade. For localized disease without neurological symptoms, some studies have demonstrated efficacy with radiotherapy [16]. For large lesions with neural compromise, en bloc spondylectomy is recommended, with studies demonstrating more effective local control and lower recurrence [14-16]. However, some studies have demonstrated an unacceptable complication rate post-operatively [14-15]. En bloc resection generally will involve a multiple staged posterior then anterior reconstruction with instrumentation and fusion, depending on site of tumor within the spinal column [15, 41]. The role of post-operative radiotherapy is currently unclear, as malignant transformation of the giant cell tumor has been reported [15, 41]. Local recurrence rates are noted to be at 41%-66.7% within the mobile spine [12-13]. 5%-13% of patients with have pulmonary metastases, which may require surgical resection [12] and whose histology will determine a benign versus malignant diagnosis [12].

HEMANGIOMA

Hemangiomas are very common benign lesions that can be found in the spinal column, typically the vertebral bodies of the thoracic spine. They are often asymptomatic lesions found incidentally on routine imaging [17]. Related symptoms are typically due to the large size or pathological fracture associated with the hemangiomas [17]. Larger lesions may encroach upon the neural foramina and spinal cord causing myelopathy. Focal kyphotic deformity with instability may result from pathological fracture [17]. Radiographically, xrays will show the classic vertical striations of the hemangioma, while CT scans will demonstrate the 'spikes of bone' appearance within the vertebral body. MRI will show an enhancing tumor with hemorrhage and thrombosis on T1 imaging [17]. Histologically, hemangiomas are a collection of thin-walled capillaries with an endothelial lining and surrounding capsule [17]. They may have thrombosed lumens with occasional hemosiderin deposition from vessel rupture [18]. Treatment options will depend on the clinical presentation. Asymptomatic patients only require observation of the lesion and conservative treatment [19]. If the patient has persistent pain associated with the spinal hemangioma, radiation therapy may be offered for symptomatic control with adequate results [19]. For lesions with hypertrophy or ballooning of the posterior cortex of the vertebral body into the spinal canal causing neurologic compromise or intractable pain from deformity, studies have demonstrated acceptable results from either an anterior approach, posterolateral approach, or posterior approach [19] for corpectomy and posterior fusion. Preoperative embolization reduces the risk of intra-operative hemorrhage and should be performed when angiography identifies the arterial blood supply [19].

EOSINOPHILIC GRANULOMA

Eosinophilic granulomas of the spine are benign lesions typically of the thoracic spine that are the localized form of Langerhans Histiocytosis X. Vertebral location is noted to be around 8-25% [20]. Granulomas are typically found incidentally but acute presentations may include pain or deformity from pathological fracture, as well as radiculopathy and myelopathy from spinal cord compression [21]. Radiographically, CT and MRI scans may demonstrate vertebral flattening which precedes eventual vertebral collapse with additional lesions elsewhere within the spinal axis [21]. If patient has not been diagnosed prior with histiocytosis X, then biopsy is indicated to confirm the diagnosis [21]. Histologically, granulomas demonstrate mononuclear histiocytic cells with oval nuclei and Birbeck granules on electron microscopy. Additionally, lipid-laden foam cells and lack of nuclear atypia characterize this tumor [22-23]. Eosinophilic granulomas are usually self-limiting. Chemotherapy is recommended for the systemic form of Langerhans Histiocytosis X. Low dose conventional radiotherapy is recommended for symptomatic lesions without neurological compromise and/or patients who are not operative candidates. If lesions are causing progressively worse intractable pain and instability and/or deformity with neurological compromise, then surgical intervention is warranted [21]. Surgical approach would depend on the level along the spine, with either an anterior corpectomy with fusion or posterior or posterolateral approach for corpectomy with instrumentation [23].

ANEURYSMAL BONE CYST

Aneurysmal bone cysts (ABC) are benign expansile lesions of bone composed of blood filled cavities separated by septa of osteoclastic cells [24]. Typically, patients are in their 20's and most are incidentally discovered. Acute presentations may include severe back pain from pathological fracture and/or radiculopathy or myelopathy from spinal cord compression and kyphotic instability [24]. Radiographicallly, CT and/or MRI are the studies of choice. They will demonstrate a lytic lesion surrounded by a thin shell of cortical bone with areas of cortical disruption causing a blown-out appearance [25]. Lobulated appearance, septations, and fluid-fluid levels are very suggestive. CT scan is helpful to determine the bony anatomy and invasion of bone by tumor in order to decide on required stabilization procedures. MRI is helpful to determine the relationship of the tumor from the adjacent neural structures [25].

On histologic analysis, ABC display cavernous spaces with blood filled centers without endothelial lining separated by fibrous septa composed of fibroblasts and osteoclasts [25].

The literature describes a combination of treatments, ranging from curettage, subtotal excision, en bloc resection, embolization, intralesional injection, and radiation [25]. For lesions that are asymptomatic, conservative treatment with or without bracing is indicated. For larger lesions with neurological compromise, surgical treatment is recommended. Preoperative embolization may play a role in management [26]. Indolent lesions may resolve spontaneously over months [24]. Overall recurrence rate is 28% and they generally occurs within the first 2 years [25].

OSTEOBLASTOMA

Osteoblastomas are rare benign tumors of the spine in young adults that are similar to osteoid osteomas, but are larger than 2 cm in size. In contrast to osteoid osteoma patients, patients with osteoblastomas are less likely to present with severe attacks of night pain, and focal pain is typically not relieved with anti-inflammatory medications such as aspirin [27].

Xrays and CT scans demonstrate the predilection for the posterior elements and show a radiolucent lesion with surrounding reactive bone with or without expansion. Bone scans will show intense isotope uptake at the site of tumor [27]. Biopsy may be performed if diagnosis is unclear. Histologically, osteoblastomas demonstrate significant production of surrounding osteoid and primitive woven bone, with areas of fibrovascular connective tissue nearby. Osteoblasts are seen in great numbers [27].

Treatment will vary depending on symptoms and size of tumor. For tumors that are small, conservative treatment and observation is warranted. For tumors that increase in size, cause mass effect upon nearby neural structures, or cause progressive spinal instability and deformity, surgical treatment is recommended. Some studies advocate intralesional excision while others recommend en bloc resection [29]. For larger lesions and en bloc resections, a staged procedure is performed with both an anterior and posterior approach, along with instrumentation and fusion [28, 29]. For patients with intralesional resection, radiation therapy can be used as an adjunct for local control [29] with good results, though osteoblastomas are not classified as radiosensitive. Malignant transformation has been reported in 12-25% of patients [29].

CHONDROSARCOMA/OSTEOSARCOMA

Osteosarcomas are malignant mesenchymally-derived tumors of the bone seen in adolescents. They rarely affect the spine [30]. Chondrosarcomas are malignant tumors of the cartilage that are seen in patients between ages 30-70 [31]. They are locally aggressive with a high recurrence rate [31]. Both of these tumors are most commonly seen in the thoracic spine [31]. Patients with both tumors may present with focal pain throughout the day [30]. Lesions may grow large enough to cause neurological symptoms such as radicular pain or myelopathy [30]. Radiographically, xrays and CT scans for osteosarcomas demonstrate a destructive lytic lesion with evidence of new bony formation and periosteal reaction, with or without an associated soft tissue mass [30].

Xrays and CT scans for chondrosarcomas demonstrate irregularly mottled calcification with bony destruction and invasion. MRI will demonstrate a heterogeneously enhancing mass with hypointensity on T1 and hyperintensity on T2 imaging. A biopsy may be performed when diagnosis is unclear. Histologically, osteosarcomas have pleomorphic giant and atypical cells with mitotic figures. They produce osteoid with eosinophilic trabecula with occasional areas of calcification. The tumor cells are within the osteoid matrix. Chondrosarcomas demonstrate undifferentiated cartilaginous cells with mitotic figures and atypia [30, 31]. Sarcomas of the spine are quite complex but in cases of neurological compromise from compression and/or instability, surgical treatment is warranted. Recent evidence for chondrosarcomas has emerged showing an increased progression-free survival after en bloc resection without violation of tumor capsule.

This typically involves a multi-stage anterior and posterior reconstruction with instrumentation and fusion [31, 32]. Outcome for chondrosarcomas is based on histology, patient age, and en bloc resection [31, 32]. Metastatic disease is the most important factor for survival in patients with osteosarcoma. With adjunctive therapy such as chemotherapy, osteosarcoma survival is 50% over 5 years. Osteosarcomas are radioresistant and thus surgical resection for appropriate tumors will require aggressive multi-stage approaches [332].

OSTEOID OSTEOMA

Osteoid osteomas are benign tumors typically in males aged 4-30 of the posterior elements of the spine that are less than 2 cm in size. As previously described, osteoblastomas are lesions greater than 2 cm [33]. Patients may present with severe focal night pain that is relieved with aspirin [33]. Radiographically, xrays and CT scans will demonstrate areas of reactive bony formation with a low attenuation nidus and sclerotic border [34]. Technetium bone scans may demonstrate intense uptake at the site of the lesion [33, 34]. MRI demonstrates a T1 nidus with intermediate signal intensity and T2 hypointensity with heterogenous enhancement [34].

Rarely is biopsy needed for the diagnosis. Histologically, osteomas have yellowish to red areas of osteoid and woven bone with interconnected trabeculae, amidst a background of vascularized, fibrous connective tissue [33].

Osteomas are typically self-limiting. Small lesions can be treated conservatively with non-steroidal anti-inflammatory medications such as aspirin. Pain from these lesions typically responds to non-steroidal anti-inflammatory drugs such as aspirin [33, 35]. When pain is intractable or patient's tumor is causing instability or neural compromise, surgery is indicated. Surgical treatment generally involves instrumentation and fusion for tumors that are large and near neural structures [35].

FIBROUS DYSPLASIA

Fibrous dysplasia is a predominantly osteolytic disorder that affects young children and adolescents. It affects males and females equally [36]. Most of the time, patients are asymptomatic [37] but symptomatic patients may present with focal pain or radiculopathy from foraminal compromise.

Radiographically, xrays, CT, and MRI demonstrate a ground-glass appearance with definite sclerotic margins. CT may show an expansile lesion with a blown-out cortical rim. McCune-Albright syndrome is a severe form of polyostotic fibrous dysplasia combined with an endocrinopathy and café-au-lait spots, and should be suspected in patients with severe dysplasia [37]. Histologically, fibrous dysplasia demonstrates curvilinear trabecular woven bone with a background of fibroblasts. Foamy macrophages may also be seen [37].

Patients should undergo metabolic and endocrinological evaluation to treat an underlying vitamin D deficiency, phosphate wasting, and/or hyperparathyroidism. Oral bisphosphonates are effective for relief of pain in fibrous dysplasia [38]. Surgery is indicated in cases of neural compromise and/or instability. Surgical approach would depend on the location along the spinal axis but may require multi-stage corpectomy with instrumentation and fusion [39].

CONCLUSION

The primary bony tumors of the spine are a diverse and heterogenous group of tumors. They each exhibit unique structural and pathophysiological mechanisms that then determine specific diagnosis and treatment modalities. Recent advances such as en bloc resection without violation of tumor capsule in patients with spinal chordomas and chondrosarcomas has significantly advanced progression free survival. Ongoing research continues to establish optimal diagnosis and treatment options for each of these primary spinal tumors.

REFERENCES

[1]   Palumbo A, Anderson K. Multiple myeloma. *New Engl. J. Med.* 2011; 364(11): 1046-1060.
[2]   Healey JH, Lane JM. Chordoma: a critical review of diagnosis and treatment. *Ortho. Clin. North Am.* 1989; 20(3): 417-426.
[3]   Bjornsson J, Wold LE, Ebersold MJ, et al. Chordoma of the mobile spine. A clinicopathologic analysis of 40 patients. *Cancer* 1993; 71:735–40.
[4]   Bergh P, Kindblom LG, Gunterberg B, Remotti F, et. al. Prognostic factors in chordoma of the sacrum and mobile spine: a study of 39 patients. *Cancer.* 2000; 88: 2122–2134.
[5]   Schwab JH, Boland PJ, Agaram NP. Chordoma and chondrosarcoma gene profile: implications for immunotherapy. *Cancer Immunol Immunother.* 2009; 58: 339–349.
[6]   Hsieh P, Gallia G, Sciubba D, et. al. En bloc excisions of chordomas in the cervical spine: review of five consecutive cases with more than 4-year follow-up. *Spine.* 2011; 36 (24): 1581-1587.
[7]   Sciubba D, Gokaslan Z, Black J, et. al. 5-Level spondylectomy for en bloc resection of thoracic chordoma: case report. *Neurosurgery.* 2011; 69: 48-56.
[8]   Samson IR, Springfield DS, Suit HD, et. al. Operative treatment of sacrococcygeal chordoma. A review of twenty-one cases. *J. Bone Joint Surg. Am.* 1993; 73:1476–1484.

[9]   Park L, Delaney TF, Liebsch NJ, et al. Sacral chordomas: impact of high-dose proton/photon-beam radiation therapy combined with or without surgery for primary versus recurrent tumor. *Int. J. Radiat. Oncol. Biol. Phys.* 2006; 65: 1514–1521.

[10]   Kaiser TE, Pritchard DJ, Unni KK. Clinicopathologic study of sacrococcygeal chordoma. *Cancer.* 1984; 53:2574–2578.

[11]   Fuchs B, Dickey ID, Yaszemski MJ, et. al. Operative management of sacral chordoma. *J. Bone Joint Surg. Am.* 2005; 87: 2211–2216.

[12]   Sanjay BK, Sim FH, Unni KK, McLeod RA, et. al. Giant cell tumors of the spine. *J. Joint Bone Surg. Br.* 1993; 75(1):148-154

[13]   Balke M, Henrichs M, Gosheger G, Ahrens H, et. al. Giant cell tumors of the axial skeleton. *Sarcoma.* 2012; epub ahead of print.

[14]   Filder MW. Surgical treatment of giant cell tumors of the thoracic and lumbar spine: report of nine patients. *European Spine Journal.* 2001; 10(1): 69-77.

[15]   Liljenqvist U, Lerner T, Halm H, Buerger H, et. al. En bloc spondylectomy in malignant tumors of the spine. *European Spine Journal.* 2008; 17(4): 600-609.

[16]   Chakravarti A, Spiro IJ, Hug EB, Mankin HJ, et. al. Megavoltage radiation therapy for axial and inoperable giant-cell tumor of bone. *J. Bone Joint Surg. Am.* 1999; 81(11): 1566-73.

[17]   Ng VW, Clifton A, Moore AJ. Preoperative endovascular embolization of a vertebral haemangioma. *J. Bone Joint Surg. Br.* 1997; 79(5): 808-811.

[18]   Kumar V. Robbins and Coltran Pathologic Basis of Disease-8 ed. Philadelphia: *Saunders Elsevier,* 2010; pp 520-521.

[19]   Jankowski R, Nowak S, Zukiel R, Szymas J, et. al. Surgical treatment of symptomatic vertebral haemangiomas. *Neurol. Neurochir. Pol.* 2011; 45(6): 577-582.

[20]   Yeaom JS, Lee CK, Shin HY, et. al. Langerhans' cell histiocytosis of the spine. Analysis of twenty-three cases. *Spine.* 1999; 24: 1740-1749.

[21]   Seimon LP. Eosinophil granuloma of the spine. *J. Pediatr. Orthop.* 1981; 1(4): 371-376.

[22]   Katz RL, Silva EG, deSantos LA, Lukeman JM. Diagnosis of eosinophilic granuloma of bone by cytology, histology, and electron microscopy of transcutaneous bone-aspiration biopsy. *J. Bone Joint Surg. Am.* 1980; 62(8): 1284-90.

[23]   Chen SY, Chao SC, Kao TH, Shen CC, et. al. Surgical treatment using mesh cage and plate fixation in a 9-year-old child with solitary histiocytosis lesion in the cervical spine. *Eur. J. Pediatric. Surg.* 2011; 21: 189-191.

[24]   Papagelopoulos PJ, Choudhury SN, Frassica FJ, Bond JR, ET. AL. Treatment of aneurysmal bone cysts of the pelvis and sacrum. *J. Bone Joint Surg. Am.* 2001; 83 (1): 1674-81.

[25]   Zenonos G, Jamil O, Governale L, Jernigan S, et. al. Surgical treatment for primary spinal aneurysmal bone cysts: experience from Children's Hospital Boston. *J. Neurosurg. Pediatrics.* 2012; 9:305-315.

[26]   Ameli NO, Abbassioun K, Saleh H, Eslamdoost A: Aneurysmal bone cysts of the spine. Report of 17 cases. *J Neurosurg.* 1985; 63: 685-690.

[27]   Boriani S, Capanna R, Donati D, Levine A. Osteoblastoma of the spine. *Clin. Orthop. Relat. Res.* 1992; 278:37-45.

[28] Boriani S, Mendola L, Bandiera S, Simoes CE, et. al. Staging and treatment of osteoblastoma in the mobile spine: a review of 51 cases. *Eur. Spine J.* June 2012; epub ahead of print.

[29] Marsh BW, Bonfiglio M, Brady LP, Enneking WF. Benign osteoblastoma: range of manifestations. *J. Bone Joint Surg. Am.* 1975; 57(1): 1-9

[30] Shives TC, Dahlin DC, Sim FH, Pritchard DJ, et. al. Osteosarcoma of the spine. *J. Bone Joint Surg. Am.* 1986; 68(5): 660-8.

[31] Yang X, Wu Z, Ziao J, Feng D, et. al. Chondrosarcomas of the cervical and cervicothoracic spine. *J. Spinal Disord. Tech.* 2012; 25(1): 1-9.

[32] Hsieh PC, Xu R, Sciubba DM, McGirt MJ, et. al. Long term clinical outcomes following en bloc resections for sacral chordomas and chondrosarcomas: a series of twenty consecutive patients. *Spine.* 2009; 34(20): 2233-9.

[33] Cohen MD, Harrington TM, Ginsburg WW. Osteoid osteomas: 95 cases and a review of the literature. *Semin. Arthritis Rheum.* 1983; 12(3): 265-281.

[34] Ropper A, Cahill K, Hanna J, McCarthy E, et. al. Primary vertebral tumors: a review of epidemiologic, histological, and imaging findings. *Neurosurgery.* 2010; 69(6): 1171-1180.

[35] Lisbona R, Rosenthall L. Role of radionuclide imaging in osteoid osteomas. *Am. J. Roentgenol.* 1979; 132 (1): 77-80.

[36] Harris WH, Dudley HR, Barry RJ. The natural history of fibrous dysplasia: an orthopedic, pathological, and roentgenographic study. *J. Bone Joint Surg. Am.* 1962; 44:207-233.

[37] Kumar V, Robbins SL. *Robbins Basic Pathology.* 8th ed. Philadelphia, PA: Saunders/Elsevier; 2007.

[38] Chapurlat RD. Medical therapy in adults with fibrous dysplasia of bone. *J. Bone Miner Res.* 2006; 21(suppl 2): 114-119.

[39] Medow JE, Agrawal BM, Resnick DK. Polyostotic fibrous dysplasia of the cervical spine: case report and review of the literature. *Spine J.* 2007; 7(6): 712-715.

[40] Wagner TD, Kobayashi W, Dean S, Goldberg SI, et. al. Combination short-course pre-operative irradiation, surgical resection, and reduce-field high-dose postoperative irradiation in the treatment of tumors involving the bone. *Int. J. Radiat. Oncol. Biol. Phys.* 2009; 73(1): 259-266.

[41] Shi W, Indelicato DJ, Reith J, Smith KB, et. al. Radiotherapy in the management of giant cell tumor of the bone. *Am. J. Clin. Oncol.* 2012. Epub ahead of print.

In: Bone Tumors: Symptoms, Diagnosis and Treatment   ISBN: 978-1-62618-190-8
Editor: Moncef Berhouma   © 2013 Nova Science Publishers, Inc.

Chapter 2

CURRENT STRATEGIES IN THE MANAGEMENT OF METASTATIC SPINE DISEASE AND METASTATIC SPINAL CORD COMPRESSION

*Haroon Majeed**

Registrar Trauma and Orthopaedics University Hospitals of North Staffordshire, UK

ABSTRACT

*Introduction.*Management of metastatic spinal disease has changed significantly over the last few years. Cement augmentation techniques like vertebroplasty and kyphoplasty are useful in managing the osteolytic spinal secondary induced pain. Breast, lung and prostate tumours along with myeloma and lymphoma account for majority of spinal metastases. There are approximately 4000 new cases of spinal metastases in England and Wales each year.

*Clinical Presentation and Investigations.*Pain is the most common and disabling symptom. Spinal cord compression can result from pathological fractures and direct invasion of the spinal canal by the tumour. MRI is the most sensitive and specific investigation and should be done in time to allow definitive treatment to be planned.

*Treatment Stretegies.*Goals of treatment are to improve the quality of life, maintain or re-establish spinal stability, improve or preserve neurological function, and improve life expectancy. Pain control is important and is achieved by conventional analgesics and bisphosphonates. Radiotherapy is offered to patients with non-mechanical pain and tumour induced spinal cord compression.

Surgical options include posterior decompression with stabilisation, reinforcement with cement, vertebral body reconstruction with cage or bone graft and en-bloc excision. Research has suggested that patients with lung and renal tumours usually do not do well while the patients with other tumours have better functional outcome after surgical intervention.

Different scoring systems are used in clinical practice for predicting the life expectancy of patients with metastatic spinal disease, however research has suggested that other factors including age, mobility status, primary site and stage of tumour must be taken into account for decision making for surgical intervention.

* E-mail: haroonmajeed@gmail.com.

*Conclusion.*Multiple factors have to be taken in to account in decision making for definitive treatment for patients with metastatic spinal disease along with predicting their life expectancy based on different scoring systems. The available evidence suggests that early surgical intervention is more effective in maintaining or regaining mobility status along with resulting in better functional outcome in patients with metastatic spinal disease and spinal cord compression.

INTRODUCTION

Management of metastatic spinal disease has changed significantly over the last few years. The use of recent advances in spinal instrumentation in conjunction with surgical decompression of the metastatic lesion has resulted in significant improvement in the outcome. Recently evolved minimally invasive vertebral body cement augmentation techniques like vertebroplasty and kyphoplasty are useful in managing osteolytic spinal secondary induced pain and also reduce the need for anterior spinal reconstruction. Computer guided stereotaxic radiation delivery methods have also enhanced our ability to administer high doses of radiation to the target the lesion in the spine with pinpoint accuracy.

Spine is the most common site of skeletal metastasis and represents a continuum of disease process that affects patients with cancer. Management of these patients requires combined efforts from medical oncologists, spinal surgeons and healthcare providers. Breast, lung and prostate tumours account for majority of spinal metastases and tumours from kidney and gastrointestinal tract account for the rest. Lymphoreticular malignancies like lymphoma and myeloma are other common sources of spinal involvement.

Metastatic spinal cord compression (MSCC) is defined as spinal cord or cauda equina compression by direct pressure and or induction of vertebral collapse or instability by metastatic spread or direct extension of malignancy that threatens or causes neurological disability *[NICE, UK, Nov. 2008]*. Evidence from research carried out in Scotland and Canada suggested that the incidence of metastatic spine disease might be up to 80 cases per million people every year [1, 2]. This equates to approximately 4000 cases each year in England and Wales, or more than 100 cases per cancer network each year.

CLINICAL SYMPTOMS AND SIGNS

Metastatic disease of the spine can present with pain or neurological weakness or a combination of both. Pain is the most common symptom and can be severe enough to cause significant disability in performing daily activities including mobilisation [3]. Significant bone destruction can lead to fracture, instability and deformity. Spinal cord compression can result from pathological fractures, direct invasion of the spinal canal by the tumour or osteoblastic bone reaction [4]. Symptoms suggestive of spinal metastases include progressive or unremitting spinal pain, back pain aggravated by straining (during micturition, defecation and cough), localised spinal tenderness and nocturnal pain preventing sleep. Neurological symptoms and signs often begin with radiculopathy and are followed by myelopathy.

INVESTIGATIONS

The urgent work up of a patient with suspected spinal metastasis starts with haematological investigations. These include routinely performed blood tests; including full blood count, renal functions, liver functions, calcium profile along with plasma electrophoresis and tumour markers according to clinically predicted source of primary tumour. Radiological investigations include plain X-rays, which are considered less sensitive as the changes are visible only in the late stages of the disease. Bone scan is more sensitive but less specific. MRI is the most sensitive and specific investigation, unless there is a specific contraindication. Staging CT scan of chest, abdomen and pelvis provides further assistance in the assessment process either with or without bone scan or skeletal survey X-rays. MRI of the whole spine should be done in time to allow definitive treatment to be planned within one week of the suspected diagnosis in the case of spinal pain suggestive of spinal metastases, and within 24 hours in the case of suspected MSCC, and occasionally sooner if there is a pressing clinical need for emergency surgery [NICE, UK, Nov. 2008]. Bone scans rely on an osteoblastic reaction or bone deposition to detect spinal metastases. Therefore patients with rapidly progressive and destructive tumours may not be detected. Bone scan is relatively insensitive for multiple myeloma and tumours confined to the bone marrow. Fractures, degenerative disease, and benign disorders of the spine (haemangioma) all may be positive. Percutaneous biopsy using either image intensifier or CT scan is needed in patients with unknown primary source despite of extensive investigations and is helpful in planning the definitive or palliative surgical intervention. Tissue diagnosis and the amount of visceral and skeletal spread will dictate how aggressive we have to be in treating these patients.

TREATMENT STREGTEGIES

Medical Treatment

Pain control is important in order to improve the quality of life and is usually attempted by using conventional analgesics (NSAIDs, non-opiate and opiate medication). In patients with vertebral involvement from myeloma or breast cancer, bisphosphonates may reduce the pain and the risk of vertebral fracture or collapse. Steroids (Dexamethasone; loading dose 16mg followed by 16mg per day in divided doses) are indicated in patients who present with spinal cord compression till the definitive treatment; thereafter steroid has to be tapered over 5 to 7 days.

Radiotherapy

Radiotherapy is offered to the patients with non-mechanical back pain and tumour induced spinal cord compression. Patients with asymptomatic spinal metastases should not be offered radiotherapy with the intention of preventing MSCC.

Surgical Options

These include posterior decompression with instrumented stabilisation, reinforcement with cement, vertebral body reconstruction with anterior cage or bone graft and en-bloc excision surgery.

Goals of Treatment

Goals of treatment are to improve the quality of life, maintain or re-establish spinal stability, improve or preserve neurological function and improve the overall life expectancy. Definitive treatment options include non-operative and operative methods. Non-operative treatments include radiotherapy and chemotherapy, which are indicated in spinal tumours without significant mechanical pain or neurological deficit. Surgical strategies include various treatments ranging from wide or marginal excision to palliative treatment and care.

Different prognostic scores are used in clinical practice for predicting survival in these patients. One of the commonly used scoring system is Modified Tokuhashi Score (MTS) [5]; according to which, higher the score, better the prognosis and hence more aggressive intervention is indicated. Another commonly used scoring system is Tomita Scoring System [6]; according to which, lesser the score, better the prognosis indicating more aggressive treatment. These scoring systems use parameters including site of the primary cancer, number of systemic and spinal metastasis, spinal cord palsy and general health of the patient, in order to decide whether to perform excision surgery or palliative surgery.

Prior to the 1970s, surgery was considered an overly aggressive treatment for malignant spinal tumours [7]. With improvements in surgical techniques, medical treatment and perioperative care, indications have gradually broadened. Martin and Williamson described their indications for surgery as 'documented progressive neurological deficit, an impending pathological fracture, or obtaining a biopsy sample of a lesion of unknown primary origin' [8].

Recently, aggressive surgery such as total en-bloc spondylectomy has been advocated for solitary spinal metastases from renal or thyroid tumours. For spinal tumours causing instability pain and neurological compromise, the choice of surgical options are mainly between posterior and anterior procedures on the spine and sometimes combination of both in two stages. Posterior decompression of the neural structures with instrumented stabilisation is commonly performed as palliative surgery if the expected survival is less than one year. Vertebral body, after tumour decompression through posterior approach, could be reinforced with cement to avoid the need for another anterior procedure. If the expected survival is longer than one year then vertebral body reconstruction is performed using cages and bone graft in order to provide long-term stability and to achieve better functional outcome. Primary anterior procedures are commonly performed if the tumour is located within the vertebral body and compressing the spinal cord anteriorly. These cases commonly require additional posterior pedicle screw stabilisation as a second procedure.

Cement augmentation of vertebral bodies using vertebroplasty and kyphoplasty techniques is indicated in cases where mechanical pain is resistant to conventional analgesia, particularly in osteolytic spinal secondaries including myeloma. These techniques alone are contraindicated in patients with cord compression and spinal instability but could supplement surgical decompression and stabilisation, reducing the need of additional anterior surgical stabilisation of the spine.

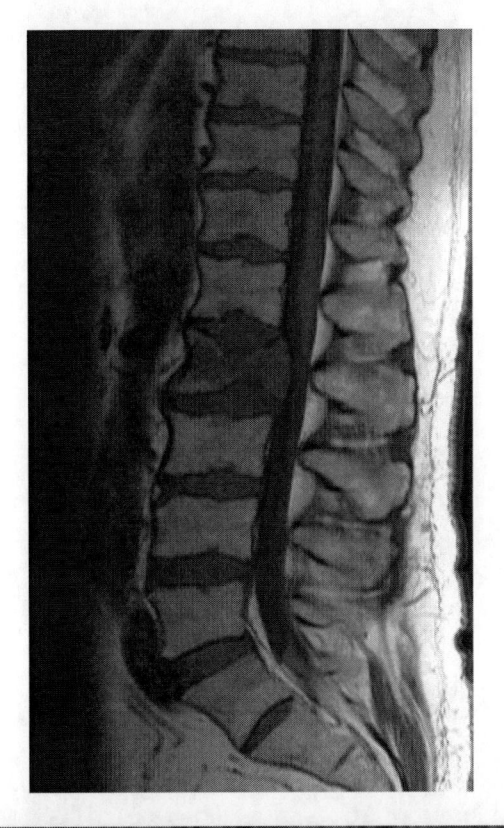

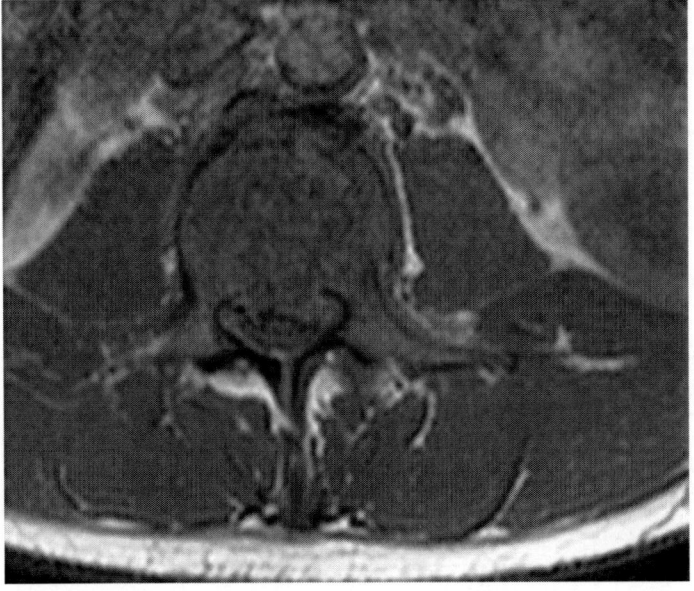

Figure 1. (Continued)

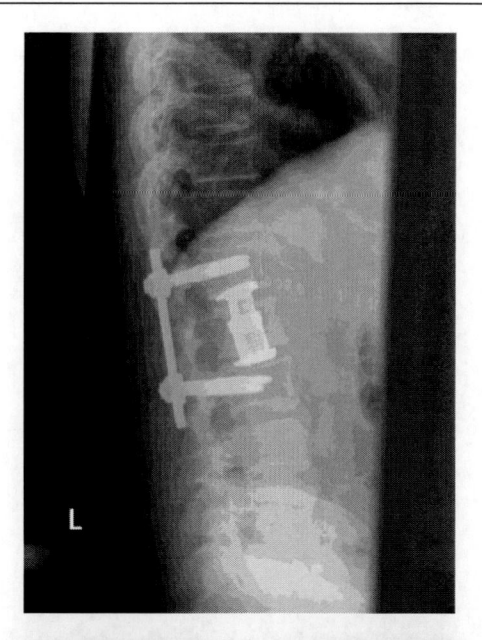

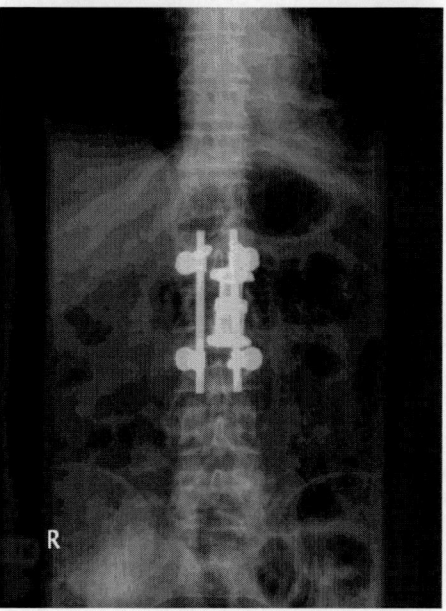

Figure 1.-Myeloma in a 57 years male with severe back pain and unable to mobilise with 2 weeks history, treated with 2-stage (posterior stabilisation + anterior cage fusion, allograft) had good functional outcome and mobility status.

A study done by the author reviewed the patients over 4 years duration (2006-2009) on 55 patients with equal male to female ratio [9]. Average age of patients was 63 years (32-87). Most frequent metastatic lesions were found in thoracic spine followed by lumbar and cervical spine. Twenty-nine patients had posterior instrumented stabilisation, 10 had anterior stabilisation and 16 patients with expected survival of more than one year had both anterior and posterior procedures performed. Twenty-three patients presented with metastatic spinal cord compression. Primary tumours included myeloma (11 patients) [Figure 1], breast CA (9 patients) [Figure 2], lymphoma (8 patients), lung CA (7 patients), renal cell CA (7 patients) [Figure 3], prostate CA (8 patients) and bladder CA (3 patients).

Expected survival based on Modified Tokuhashi Score (MTS) was more than one year in 10 patients, while after surgical stabilisation, 25 patients actually survived for longer than one year. Functional assessment revealed that patients with lung and renal tumours did not do well while the patients with other tumours had better functional outcome.

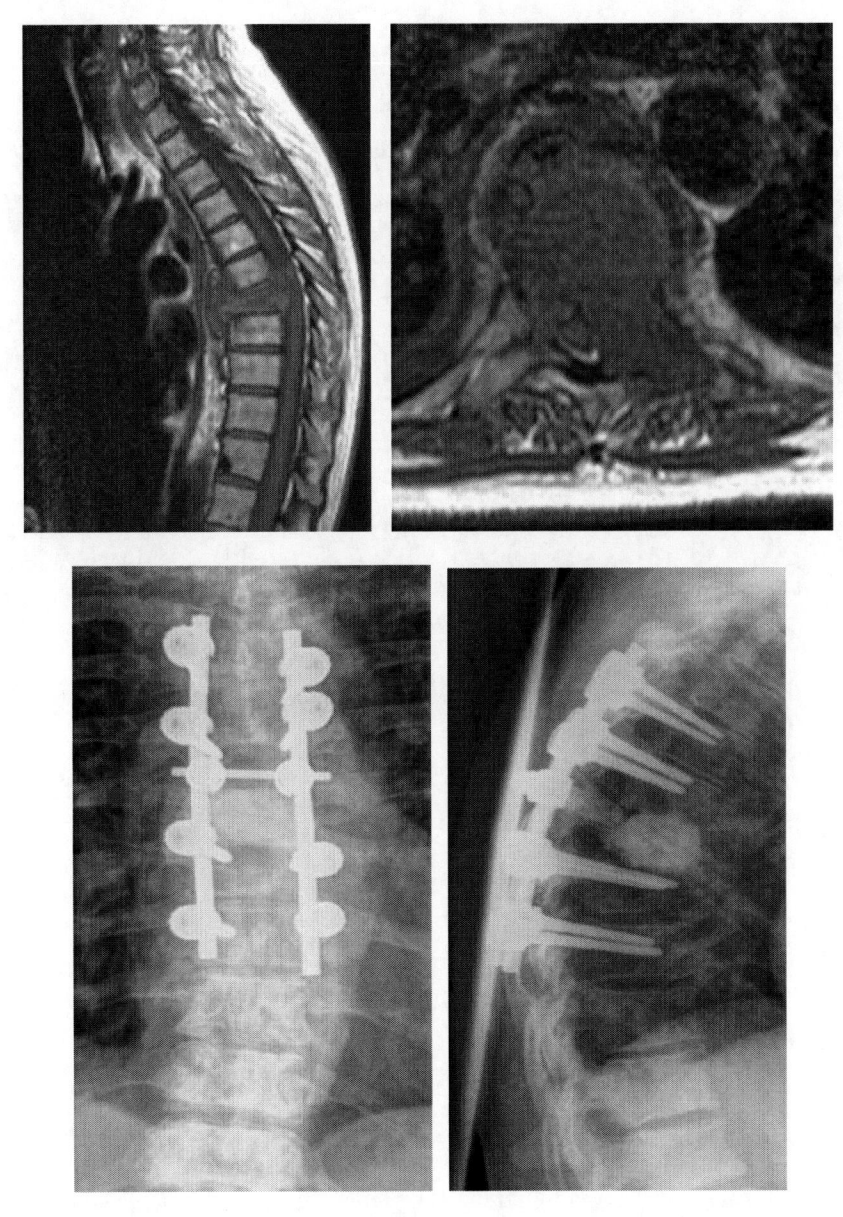

Figure 2. Breast CA, 55 years female with upper thoracic back pain and rapidly progressive parapersis, emergency spinal decompression and stabilisation performed with good outcome.

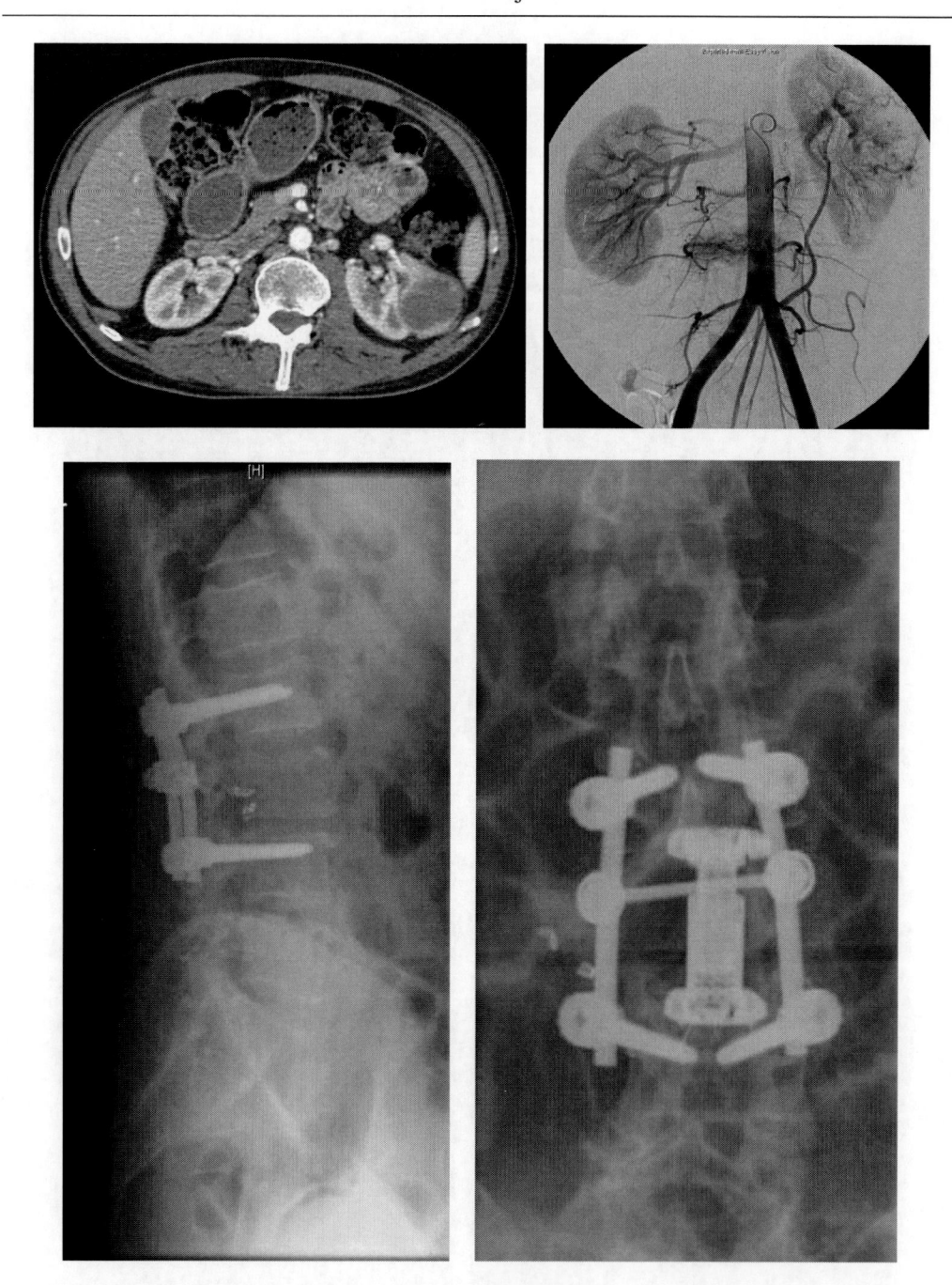

Figure 3. Renal Cell Carcinoma, 57 years male presented with 2 months history of back pain, L3 vertebral body metastasis, had preoperative embolisation followed by decompression and stabilisation with satisfactory outcome.

Based on this research, it was found that the predictive scoring systems are not uniformly effective in all types of primary tumours as some discrepancies were seen in the expected and actual outcome after surgical intervention, especially in cases of lung cancer, lymphoma and renal cell cancer.

Table 1. Karnofsky Performance Score

Able to carry on normal activity and to work; no special care needed.	100	Normal no complaints; no evidence of disease.
	90	Able to carry on normal activity; minor signs or symptoms of disease.
	80	Normal activity with effort; some signs or symptoms of disease.
Unable to work; able to live at home and care for most personal needs; varying amount of assistance needed.	70	Cares for self; unable to carry on normal activity or to do active work.
	60	Requires occasional assistance, but is able to care for most of his personal needs.
	50	Requires considerable assistance and frequent medical care.
Unable to care for self; requires equivalent of institutional or hospital care; disease may be progressing rapidly.	40	Disabled; requires special care and assistance.
	30	Severely disabled; hospital admission is indicated although death not imminent.
	20	Very sick; hospital admission necessary; active supportive treatment necessary.
	10	Moribund; fatal processes progressing rapidly.
	0	Dead

Spinal surgeons frequently face the challenging decisions of how to treat patients with these metastatic spinal lesions. The decision to proceed with operative intervention is not always straightforward. Ability to walk is the single most important factor in decision making process for surgical intervention in patients with spinal cord compression. Findlay et al. [10] have reported 70% of ambulant, 30% of paraperitic, and 5% of paraplegic patients maintained or regained their ambulant status after surgical treatment. Patchell et al. reported 57% with radiotherapy alone and 84% with surgery and radiotherapy maintained the ambulant status after surgery indicating better outcome in surgical group [11].

Thomas et al. showed in their study that the surgical group maintained the ambulant status till they died [12]. Suitable candidates for surgical intervention are those with better life expectancy, who can tolerate surgery and have favourable cancer cell histology and staging. Age of the patient is a poorly validated factor. According to NICE guidelines, surgical intervention should not be denied based on patient's age. However Chi et al. have shown that age is an important variable in predicting preservation of ambulation and survival and there is no difference in the outcome in patients above or below 65 years of age [13]. The main indications for surgical intervention are spinal cord compression causing neurological weakness and instability pain secondary to pathological fracture. The traditional laminectomy operation has shown no better results than radiotherapy alone.

Current evidence indicates that the surgery followed by radiotherapy provides better outcome than radiotherapy alone. Despite of various attempts, so far there are no accurate methods available for predicting life expectancy in these patients [5, 12, 14-16]. Regardless, it is a general consensus that patients in whom expected survival is at least 12 weeks should be considered for palliative surgery. Multiple other factors must be considered including general health, nutrition, mobility status, aggressiveness of the primary tumour and the extent of preoperative neurological deficit [12, 14, 15]. Improvements in oncological management have also increased the survival in patients with skeletal metastases. Typically it is the medical oncologist who makes this life expectancy estimation, on the basis of natural history of the disease itself.

The surgeon, however, must consider the attendant morbidity and negative effects that the surgery itself will have on the patient's survival [4, 12, 15]. It is in the surgeon's best interest to be thoroughly familiar with all the factors involved, in order to achieve favourable outcome for the patient.

Once the decision for surgery has been made, the goals can be more defined. If the neural elements are compressed, the first fundamental step is to undertake decompression surgery, excising either the anterior or posterior elements. Resection of tumour material is also effective for pain relief. With various methods available, reconstruction of the spine, in which cement augmentation, bone graft, and instrumentation can be used, is crucial for achieving fixation [17-21]. There are strong supporters of posterior surgery over anterior surgery, whereas others favour combined approaches [3, 5, 22]. Minimally invasive techniques, such as kyphoplasty, may also play a role for the prophylactic spinal fixation before significant vertebral collapse occurs [23, 24]. At present, relatively few patients with MSCC in the UK receive surgery for this condition. However, research evidence suggests that surgical intervention in early stages may be more effective than radiotherapy. Although not curative, resection and stabilisation can have beneficial effects on neurological status, function, pain, and mobility status [11, 17, 18, 20, 25]. These are important issues, particularly in individuals in whom remaining life expectancy is no more than 1 to 2 years.

Tokuhashi and co-workers have studied the results obtained in 64 patients who underwent surgery for spinal metastases [5]. They included all primary diagnoses and operations performed for a variety of indications including pain and paralysis. They formulated a score based on a number of parameters including general systemic condition, number of extraspinal bone metastases, number of spinal metastases, presence of lesions in other internal organs, location of primary lesion, and the severity of spinal cord injury. Although no single parameter was predictive, scores correlated with survival periods. Scores of 9 or higher were predictive of at least 12 months survival; scores of 8 and lower indicated survival less than 12 months; and scores of 5 or lower predicted survival of 3 months or less. Based on this data, it appears that the Tokuhashi system is a valuable tool in pre-operative discussions and decision making process [Table 2, Figure 4]. However, further research has suggested that other factors must also be taken into account for consideration of surgical intervention [9].

Sioutos and co-workers found that patients who were ambulatory preoperatively and those in whom the disease involved only one vertebra survived statistically longer than patients who were non-ambulatory and those with multilevel disease [15].

Not surprisingly, patients with metastatic renal carcinoma survived the longest, whereas those with breast experienced longer life spans than individuals with lung metastases. Weigel, et al. reported that patients with age 60 years or younger survived statistically longer than those older than 60 years, whereas tumour location was not statistically significant [3].

Table 2. Modified Tokuhashi Score [5]

Variable	Score
General condition (Karnofsky's performance status)	
Poor (PS 10–40%)	0
Moderate (PS 50%–70%)	1
Good (PS 80%–100%)	2
No. of extraspinal bone metastases foci	
≥3	0
1–2	1
0	2
No. of metastases in the vertebral body	
≥3	0
1–2	1
0	2
Metastases to the major internal organs	
Unremovable	0
Removable	1
No metastases	2
Primary site of the cancer	
Lung, stomach	0
Kidney, liver, uterus	1
Other, unidentified	
Thyroid, prostate, breast, rectum	2
Spinal cord palsy	
Complete	0
Incomplete	1
None	2

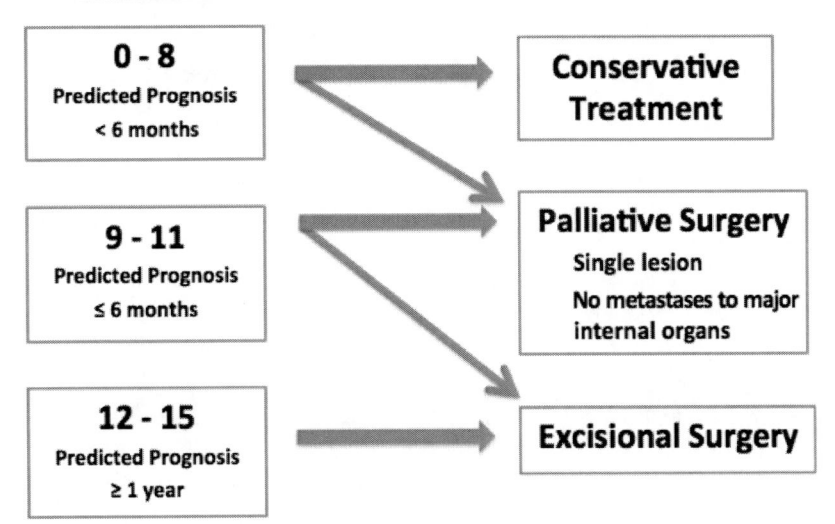

Figure 4. Treatment strategies according to Modified Tokuhashi Scores [5].

In contrast to the findings of Sioutos et al., Weigel, et al. did not find preoperative neurological function to be an important factor in survival.

Patients treated with surgery and radiotherapy together had better overall outcome and mobility status. Patchell, et al. in a study on 101 patients revealed that 84% patients were able to walk following a combined treatment with surgical decompression and radiotherapy compared to 57% with radiotherapy alone [11].

These patients maintained their mobility status for 122 days compared to those with radiotherapy who maintained for only 13 days. In another recent study, Chi et al, found that preservation of mobility status was significantly prolonged in patients younger than 65 years undergoing surgery and radiotherapy compared to radiation alone [13].

This study also showed that as age increases, the beneficial effect of surgery diminishes and becomes equivalent to radiation therapy alone.

CONCLUSION

Multiple factors have to be taken in to account in decision making for definitive treatment for patients with metastatic spinal disease along with predicting their life expectancy based on different scoring systems. The available evidence suggests that early surgical intervention is more effective in maintaining or regaining mobility status along with resulting in better functional outcome in patients with metastatic spinal disease and spinal cord compression.

REFERENCES

[1]   Levack, P., et al., Don't wait for a sensory level--listen to the symptoms: a prospective audit of the delays in diagnosis of malignant cord compression. *Clin. Oncol. (R Coll. Radiol.)*, 2002. 14(6): p. 472-80.

[2]   Durr, H.R., et al., Surgical treatment of osseous metastases in patients with renal cell carcinoma. *Clin. Orthop. Relat. Res.*, 1999(367): p. 283-90.

[3]   Weigel, B., et al., Surgical management of symptomatic spinal metastases. Postoperative outcome and quality of life. *Spine (Phila. Pa. 1976)*, 1999. 24(21): p. 2240-6.

[4]   Enkaoua, E.A., et al., Vertebral metastases: a critical appreciation of the preoperative prognostic tokuhashi score in a series of 71 cases. *Spine (Phila. Pa. 1976)*, 1997. 22(19): p. 2293-8.

[5]   Tokuhashi, Y., et al., Scoring system for the preoperative evaluation of metastatic spine tumor prognosis. *Spine (Phila. Pa. 1976)*, 1990. 15(11): p. 1110-3.

[6]   Tomita, K., et al., Surgical strategy for spinal metastases. *Spine (Phila. Pa. 1976)*, 2001. 26(3): p. 298-306.

[7]   Halnan, K.E. and P.H. Roberts, Paraplegia caused by spinal metastasis from thyroid cancer. *Br. Med. J.*, 1967. 3(5564): p. 534-6.

[8]   Martin, N.S. and J. Williamson, The role of surgery in the treatment of malignant tumours of the spine. *J. Bone Joint Surg. Br.*, 1970. 52(2): p. 227-37.

[9]   Majeed, H., et al., Accuracy of prognostic scores in decision making and predicting outcomes in metastatic spine disease. *Ann. R. Coll. Surg. Engl.,* 2012. 94(1): p. 28-33.

[10]   Findlay, G.F., Adverse effects of the management of malignant spinal cord compression. *J. Neurol. Neurosurg. Psychiatry,* 1984. 47(8): p. 761-8.

[11]   Patchell, R.A., et al., Direct decompressive surgical resection in the treatment of spinal cord compression caused by metastatic cancer: a randomised trial. *Lancet,* 2005. 366(9486): p. 643-8.

[12]   Yamashita, K., et al., Prognostic significance of bone metastases in patients with metastatic prostate cancer. *Cancer,* 1993. 71(4): p. 1297-302.

[13]   Chi, J.H., et al., Selecting treatment for patients with malignant epidural spinal cord compression-does age matter?: results from a randomized clinical trial. *Spine (Phila. Pa. 1976),* 2009. 34(5): p. 431-5.

[14]   Saengnipanthkul, S., et al., Metastatic adenocarcinoma of the spine. *Spine (Phila. Pa. 1976),* 1992. 17(4): p. 427-30.

[15]   Sioutos, P.J., et al., Spinal metastases from solid tumors. Analysis of factors affecting survival. *Cancer,* 1995. 76(8): p. 1453-9.

[16]   Cahill, D.W. and R. Kumar, Palliative subtotal vertebrectomy with anterior and posterior reconstruction via a single posterior approach. *J. Neurosurg.,* 1999. 90(1 Suppl): p. 42-7.

[17]   Nagashima, C., et al., Reconstruction of the atlas and axia with wire and acrylic after metastatic destruction. Case report. *J. Neurosurg.,* 1979. 50(5): p. 668-73.

[18]   Sundaresan, N., et al., An anterior surgical approach to the upper thoracic vertebrae. *J. Neurosurg.,* 1984. 61(4): p. 686-90.

[19]   Rompe, J.D., et al., Decompression/stabilization of the metastatic spine. Cotrel-Dubousset-Instrumentation in 50 patients. *Acta. Orthop. Scand.,* 1993. 64(1): p. 3-8.

[20]   Olerud, C. and B. Jonsson, Surgical palliation of symptomatic spinal metastases. *Acta. Orthop. Scand.,* 1996. 67(5): p. 513-22.

[21]   Hussein, A.A., E. El-Karef, and M. Hafez, Reconstructive surgery in spinal tumours. *Eur. J. Surg. Oncol.,* 2001. 27(2): p. 196-9.

[22]   Barr, J.D., et al., Percutaneous vertebroplasty for pain relief and spinal stabilization. *Spine (Phila. Pa. 1976),* 2000. 25(8): p. 923-8.

[23]   Cortet, B., et al., Percutaneous vertebroplasty in patients with osteolytic metastases or multiple myeloma. *Rev. Rhum. Engl. Ed.,* 1997. 64(3): p. 177-83.

[24]   Deramond, H., et al., Percutaneous vertebroplasty with polymethylmethacrylate. Technique, indications, and results. *Radiol. Clin. North Am.,* 1998. 36(3): p. 533-46.

[25]   King, G.J., et al., Surgical management of metastatic renal carcinoma of the spine. *Spine (Phila. Pa. 1976),* 1991. 16(3): p. 265-71.

In: Bone Tumors: Symptoms, Diagnosis and Treatment
Editor: Moncef Berhouma

ISBN: 978-1-62618-190-8
© 2013 Nova Science Publishers, Inc.

Chapter 3

SURGICAL STRATEGY FOR THE MANAGEMENT OF METASTATIC SPINE TUMORS: INDICATIONS, TECHNIQUES AND OUTCOMES

Cédric Y. Barrey[1], Luis Manera[2], Didier Frappaz[3], Aurélie Fontana[4], Véronique Favrel[5], Jean-Baptiste Pialat[6], Gualter Vaz[7] and Gilles Perrin[1]

[1]Department of Spine Surgery, P Wertheimer Hospital,
Hospices Civils de Lyon and Claude Bernard Lyon 1 University, Lyon, France
[2]Department of Interventional Neuro-radiology, P Wertheimer Hospital,
Hospices Civils de Lyon and Claude Bernard Lyon 1 University, Lyon, France
[3]Department of Oncology, Centre Leon Berard, Lyon, France
[4]Department of Rheumatology and Bone tumors, E Herriot Hospital,
Hospices Civils de Lyon, France
[5]Department of Radiotherapy, Lyon-Sud Hospital, Hospices Civils de Lyon, France
[6]Department of Musculo-skeletal Radiology, E Herriot Hospital,
Hospices Civils de Lyon and Claude Bernard Lyon 1 University, Lyon, France
[7]Department of Orthopaedic Surgery, E Herriot Hospital,
Hospices Civils de Lyon, France

ABSTRACT

Spinal metastases are very frequently observed in cancer patients raising up to 70% and represent the most common tumors of the spine (>90%). Optimal management of spinal metastases is controversial and still under investigation.

With recent progresses in imaging techniques, spinal instrumentation, development of safer surgical approaches, advances in technology and better comprehension of spine biomechanics, surgery appears more efficient than before to manage successfully spinal metastases and is now considered as a primary treatment modality.

The goal of this chapter is to review the existing classifications for metastatic spine tumour, the criteria for surgery, the main surgical techniques and the complications associated with the surgical treatment. A decisional algorithm is proposed at the end of the chapter to help the spine surgeon to choose the right strategy and therefore optimally manage spine metastatic patients.

INTRODUCTION

Spinal metastases are very frequent considering that 70% of metastatic bone tumors are located in the spine. In fact spinal metastases account for more than 90% of all spine tumors [1,5,9]. Optimal management of metastatic lesions is essential for cancer patients since these lesions may lead to spinal cord compression in approximately 20% of cases [1,3]. Otherwise, improvement of life expectancy of cancer patients is associated with an increased incidence of metastatic spinal disease, making this pathology more frequent than before for the spine surgeon.

GENERAL CONSIDERATIONS

The origin of spinal metastases (arising most commonly from adenocarcinomas) is summarized in table 1. Breast represents the most common primary cancer in women, whereas it is lung and prostate for men. The average patient age is around 50 years-old with a slight male predominance.

Table 1. Origin of primary cancer for spinal metastases

ORIGIN	FREQUENCY
Unknown	10-20%
Breast	20-25%
Lung	15%
Prostate	7.5%
Gastro-Intestinal	5%
Kidney	5%
Thyroid	2.5%

The most common pathway for spread of spinal metastasis consists of systemic embolism via the epidural venous plexuses (Batson's plexus). The highly vascularised bone marrow of the vertebral body thus represents a natural barrier for these tumor emboli, especially at the site of the basi-vertebral veins. This explains why metastatic spinal lesions are most frequently located within the vertebra, at the posterior part of the vertebral body, and why breast and lung cancers typically metastasize to the thoracic spine whereas prostate cancers most frequently metastasize to the lumbar spine and pelvis.

In descending order of frequency, metastatic spine tumors are observed in the lumbar spine, thoracic spine and in the cervical spine.

Axial pain is a very frequent symptom involving more than 80% of patients with metastatic spinal tumors. Pain secondary to a spinal tumor is typically localized, progressive and worse during night [9].Neurologic deficit may be due to different mechanisms: direct spinal cord compression by epidural extension, spinal instability secondary to vertebral fracture or vascular phenomenon with spinal cord ischemia.

The cause of the neurologic deterioration is very important to consider for the surgical strategy. Neurological status is generally appreciated by using Frankel functional classification from grade E to A, table 2.

Table 2. Frankel functional classification [4]

GRADE	DESCRIPTION
A	No motor or sensory function
B	Preserved sensation only, no motor function
C	Non ambulatory, wheelchair bound, some motor function
D	Ambulatory but with neurological symptoms D1 with walker D2 with cane D3 independently
E	Normal neurological functions

Prognostic factors associated with spinal metastatic tumors are summarized in table 3.

Table 3. Prognostic factors for spinal metastases

FACTOR RELATED TO	PROGNOSTIC FACTOR	INCLUDED in TOKUHASHI SCALE
Cancer	Histology	+
	Visceral extension	+
Metastasis	Location (cerv./thor./lum.)	-
	Number	+
	Volume	-
	Epidural extension	-
Patient	Age	-
	General status	+

Pre-operative evaluation for spinal metastatic patients includes:

- Assessment of general status: patient age, Karnofsky index, co-morbidity
- Clinical data: pain pattern, neurologic deficit
- Origin of spinal metastases (site of the primary tumor?)
- Disease extension: spine, bone, visceral metastatic tumors

Full spine MRI is a mandatory examination prior to manage a metastatic spine tumor permitting to fully evaluate spinal extent of the disease. MRI allows excellent assessment of the neurological structures and soft tissue tumor involvement. Metastasis generally demonstrates hypo-signal on T1, enhanced signal on T1-gado and hyper-signal on T2. In addition MRI is highly sensitive to detect the bone marrow replacement by tumor tissue at other spinal levels. MRI can be usefully completed by a CT-scan to fully investigate the bony vertebral destruction, figure 1.

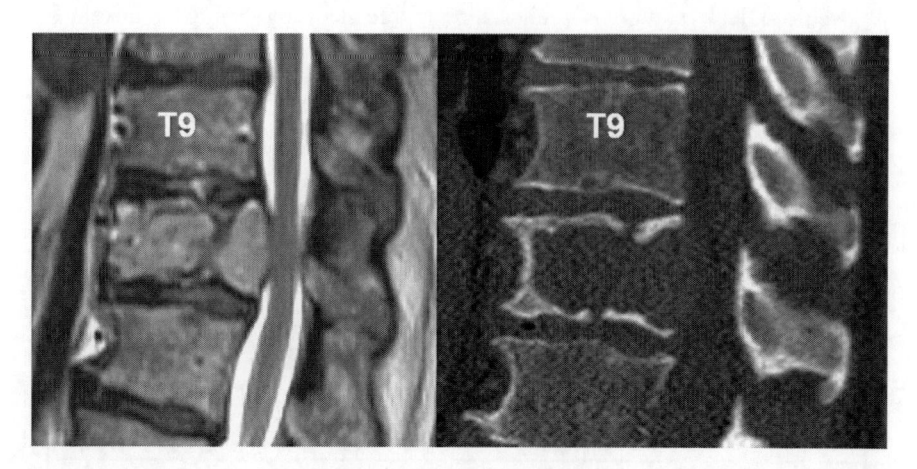

Figure 1. CT-scan allows for a better assessment of bony vertebral destruction, compared to MRI, as demonstrated in this case of T10 spinal metastatic tumor (myeloma).

CT-scan thus allows for better assessment of the risk of mechanical failure and vertebral collapse. Bone scan is a highly sensitive procedure to detect osteoblastic lesions; however one must care that some metastatic lesions (especially osteolytic tumors like multiple myeloma or hypernephroma) may not be detectable on bone scan. In such cases, PET-scan should be preferred, figure 2. Angiography is an effective tool in evaluating the vascularisation of spinal tumors.

Angiography with embolization is strongly recommended prior to operate thyroid or renal metastases.

In addition angiography permits to localize the Adamkiewicz spinal cord artery. When initial manifestation is spinal metastasis, investigation in order to localize the primary tumor should include: chest radiograph, chest-abdomino-pelvic CT-scan, serum analysis (full blood count, electrolytes, creatinin ± tumoral markers), mammography for women and whole body bone scan. Prior to treat a spinal metastatic tumor, knowledge of the type of primary tumor cancer is very important for the overall management. The primary cancer influences the overall surgical strategy considering that the histology of primary tumor is highly correlated with patient survival prognosis and also determines radio/chemo-sensitivity of the spinal metastasis.

CLASSIFICATIONS

Staging

Staging of spinal metastatic tumors allows for providing a common language and more precise analysis of treatments and outcomes.

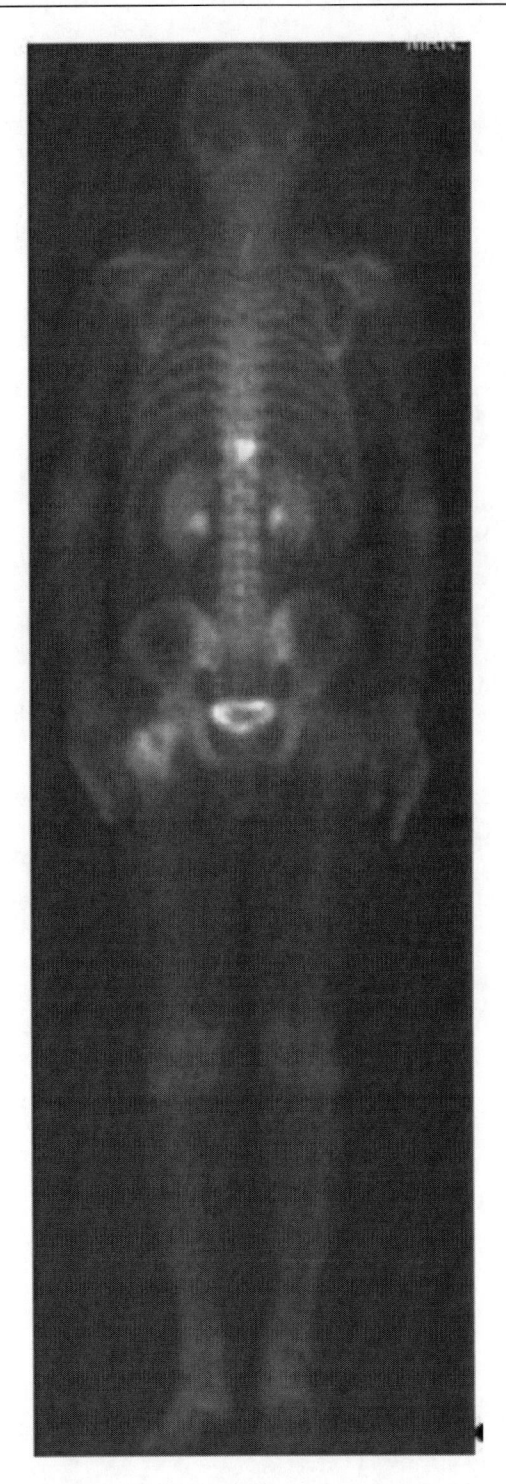

Figure 2. PET-scan are very efficient to detect tumoral lesions, especially for spinal metastases with a higher specificity than bone-scans. This is the case of a cancer patient with solitary T11 metastasis involving the right part of the vertebra.

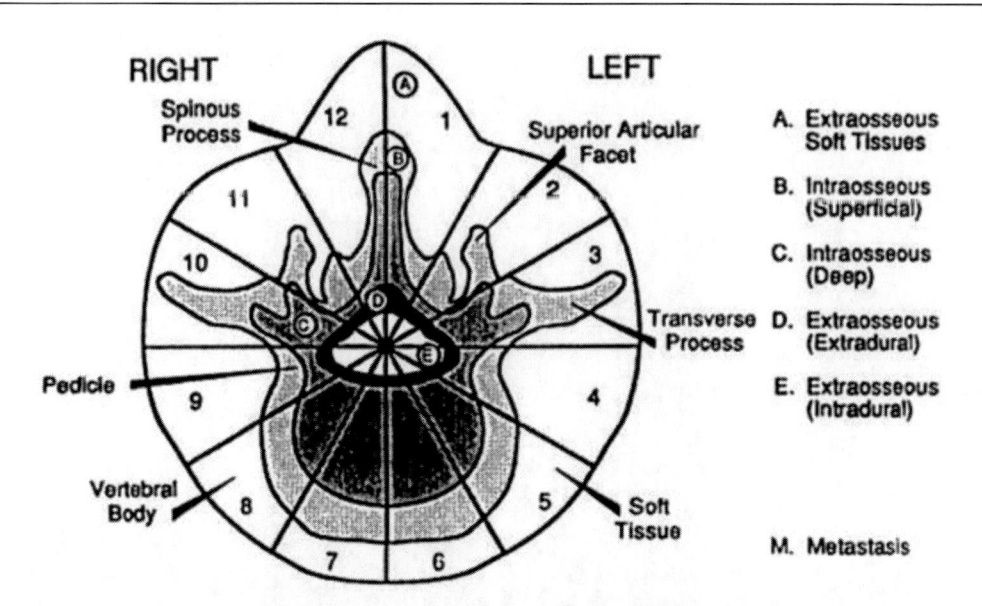

Figure 3. WBB (Weinstein, Boriani, Biagnini) Surgical Staging System. The transverse extension of the vertebral tumor is described with reference to 12 radiating zones (numbered 1 to 12 in a clockwise order) and to five concentric layers (A to E, from the paravertebral extraosseous compartments to the dural involvement). The longitudinal extent of the tumor is recorded according to the levels involved [10].

The Weinstein-Boriani-Biagini (WBB) system has been developed to describe spinal tumors (initially for primary spinal tumors), figure 3. This system provides a 3D evaluation of tumor extent by referring to anatomical zones, concentric layers and vertebral level. In 2001, Tomita et al proposed a classification based into 3 groups and 7 types, figure 4.

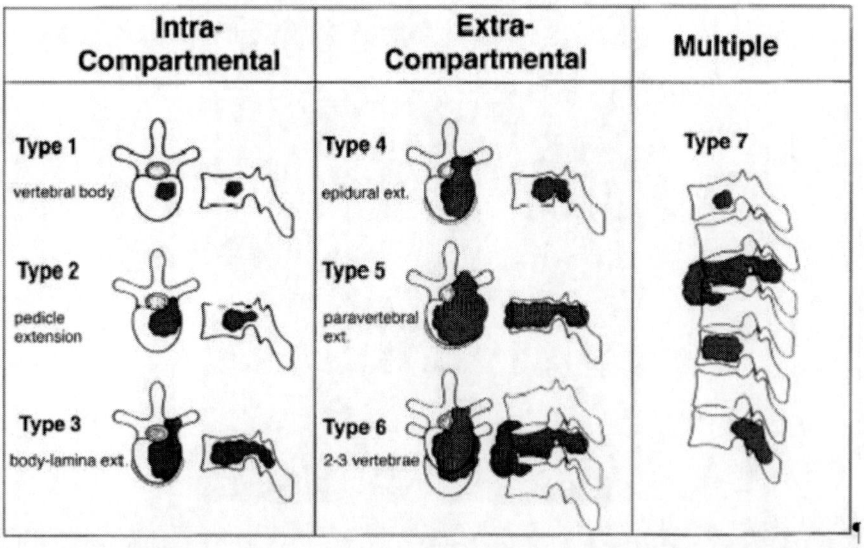

Intra-Compartmental	Extra-Compartmental	Multiple
Type 1 vertebral body	Type 4 epidural ext.	Type 7
Type 2 pedicle extension	Type 5 paravertebral ext.	
Type 3 body-lamina ext.	Type 6 2-3 vertebrae	

Figure 4. Tomita classification of spinal tumors [8]. Palliative surgery is recommended for type 7, partial vertebrectomy for types 4 to 6 and total vertebrectomy for types 1 to 3.

Prognosis

Overall prognosis of cancer patients with metastatic spine tumors can be evaluated by the Tokuhashi scale (table 4). This scale is highly correlated with the patient's survival. Therefore, surgery is recommended for a score superior to 9 whereas it is unlikely to be beneficial for a score less than 6.

Table 4. Modified Tokuhashi score [7]

CRITERIA			POINTS
1	General status	Poor	0
		Mild	1
		good	2
2	Neurologic deficit	Complete (Frankel A, B)	0
		Incomplete (Frankel C, D)	1
		none	2
3	Primary cancer	Lung, stomach, GI, ENT, pancreas, sarcoma	0
			1
		bladder	2
		other, unknown	3
		Kidney, uterus	4
		Rectum	5
		Thyroid, breast, prostate, carcinoïd tumor	
4	Number of vertebra involved	≥ 3	0
		2	1
		1	2
5	Extra-spinal bone metastases	≥ 3	0
		1-2	1
		0	2
6	Visceral metastases	Unresectable	0
		resectable	1
		none	2
n=6	TOTAL		/15

One limitation of this scale is that some of the data required to measure the score are most often unavailable in an emergency context.

Expected life expectancy:

— Less than 6 months for a score ≤ 8
— From 6 to 12 months for a score from 9 to 11
— More than 1 year for a score ≥ 12

Radiation therapy is an efficient treatment for metastatic spinal lesions by stopping metastasis growth, promoting reossification of the vertebral body and reducing tumor volume.

Table 5. Radio-sensitivity/resistance of tumors

RADIOSENSITIVE	RADIORESISTANT +	RADIORESISTANT +++
Lymphoma	Breast	Renal cell carcinoma
Leukemia	Lung	Melanoma
	Prostate	
	Thyroid	
	GI adeno-carcinoma	
	Myeloma	

Radio-sensitivity/resistance according to the tumor type is presented in table 5.

SURGICAL TREATMENT

Treatment options for metastatic spinal lesions includes conservative treatment with external bracing and steroids, radiotherapy, chemotherapy, hormonal therapy, surgery and most commonly a combination of these different options. In general, systemic disease requires chemotherapy.

Except in few cases, most of the surgical procedures for metastatic spine are palliative. The two main objectives of the surgery are to prevent neurologic deterioration and reduce pain.

Pain control and postponing spinal cord compression with preservation of ambulation and continence remain worthwhile therapeutical goals. Contrary to primary bone tumors for which the goal is to excise the tumor, the objective of surgery for metastatic spinal tumors is to improve the quality of life.

Indications

Indications for surgical procedure for metastatic spinal tumors include:

- Need for a histological diagnosis
- Deterioration of neurologic status due to spinal cord compression
- Spinal instability (pathologic fracture or kyphotic deformity)
- Intractable pain resistant to conservative treatment
- Radio-resistant tumors
- Isolated spinal metastatic spinal lesion

Contra-Indications

Patients who present with one (or more) of the following criteria should be excluded from a surgical planning:

- Expected lifespan less than 3 months
- Numerous spinal metastatic lesions involving the cervical, thoracic and lumbar regions
- Widespread visceral or brain metastases
- Severe immune-suppression
- Poor general status (Karnofsky ≤ 40)

Principles of Surgical Treatment

Principles of spinal metastases surgery are:

- Decompression of neurological structures (nerve roots and spinal cord)
- Stabilization of the spine and correction of deformity
- Most complete reduction of volume tumor (most commonly performed intra-lesionally)

After successful surgical management, radiotherapy is classically recommended to treat the residual tumoral disease, included after gross total removal.

Outcomes

Overall outcomes for spinal metastasis are related to several prognosis factors such as type of primary cancer, general conditions, neurological status and number of spinal and extra-spinal metastases.

Surgery is associated with approximately 20% complications rates (40% for sacral localizations), [11]. The most frequent complication is wound infection requiring most often re-operation for cleaning and debridement.

Post-operative complications include (in decreasing frequency order):

- Wound infections
- Urinary tract infections
- Hardware failure
- -Thrombo-embolic complications
- Local recurrence
- Death
- Disseminated Intra-Vascular Coagulation (DIVC)
- Deterioration of neurological status

In 1999, Wise et al reported 25% of complications in a series of 80 spinal metastatic patients [11]. They found that the occurrence of complications was related to the presence of pre-operative neurological deficit and pre-operative radiotherapy.

Through the literature, neurological status and general conditions seem to be the two most significant predictive factors for post-operative complications.

SURGICAL TECHNIQUES

Surgical Approaches

Different surgical approaches are described to achieve these goals depending on the characteristics of the tumor: posterior approach, postero-lateral approach, anterior approach and combined approach in 1 or 2 stages.

In general, for compression coming from anteriorly, anterior or combined approach is preferred. On the contrary, for posteriorly predominant compression, posterior approach is suitable. Factors that influence the choice for surgical approach are presented in table 6.

Laminectomy

Laminectomy alone is rarely a relevant procedure to treat a metastatic spinal lesion. In cancer patients with spinal metastatic tumors, most spinal cord compressions arise from the anterior epidural space (> 70%). In fact, neurologic compression from posterior epidural space is observed in only 10% of patients.

Table 6. Factors that influence the choice for surgical approach

1	Location of the tumor (cervical/thoracic/lumbar)
2	Presence and type of spinal cord compression
3	Number of vertebra involved
4	Spinal instability
5	General status/ co-morbidities

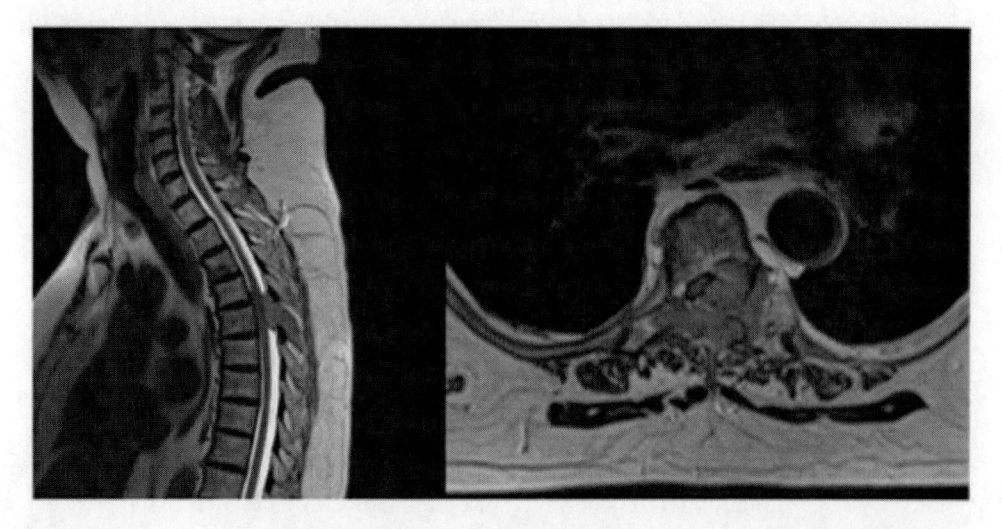

Figure 5. Spinal cord compression due to posterior epidural extent of a T6 metastatic tumor (lung origin) with no or minimal involvement of the vertebral body. The patient underwent an isolated laminectomy procedure without need for stabilization.

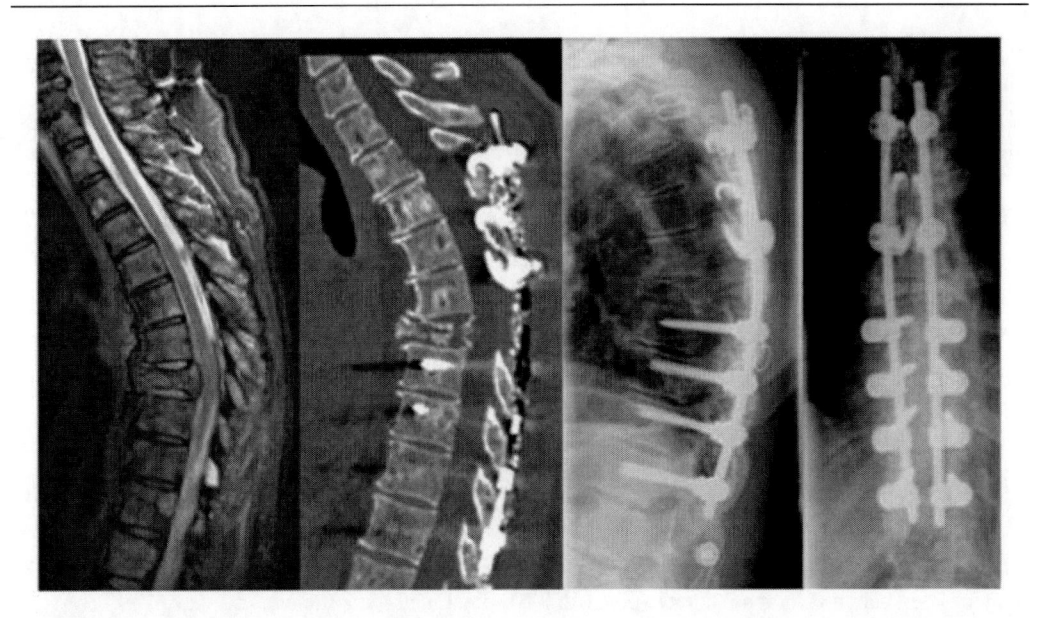

Figure 6. As in this example (metastasis from breast cancer), posterior stabilization most commonly requires long construct with segmental posterior instrumentation by pedicles screws and/or laminar hooks.

Therefore, it is unlikely to achieve an adequate decompression of the spinal cord via a pure laminectomy.

In addition, potential destabilization effect of laminectomy may result in increase of kyphotic deformity and thus induce neurological deterioration. Weinstein et al [10] reported that a better outcome was observed for patients with spinal cord compression treated anteriorly (80% of improvement) in comparison with those treated posteriorly (only 37% of improvement).

We consider that the only pertinent indication for laminectomy as a stand-alone procedure is represented by a posterior epidural compression with no or minimal anterior spinal column involvement by metastasis, figure 5. In most cases additional posterior stabilization is necessary after laminectomy.

Posterior Stabilization

In the presence of spinal instability and/or kyphotic deformity posterior segmental spinal instrumentation is generally required, figure 6. For metallic devices, titanium is preferred to minimize MRI artefacts.

Postero-lateral Approach

In the thoraco-lumbar spine, postero-lateral approach allows for an adequate decompression of neurological structures and anterior reconstruction of the anterior column (with PMMA for example).

Postero-lateral approach is generally conducted bilaterally with costo-transversectomy in the thoracic spine and pediculo-transversectomy in the lumbar spine, figures 7 and 8.

Due to difficult access anteriorly, postero-lateral approach represents an attractive option for T3-T4 spinal metastatic tumors.

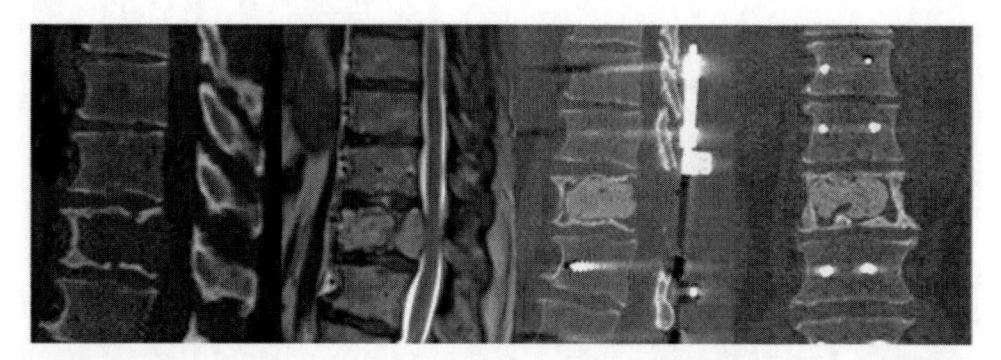

Figure 7. Example of anterior reconstruction performed with PMMA inserted through a bilateral postero-lateral approach in the thoracic pine (for T10 spinal metastatic tumor).

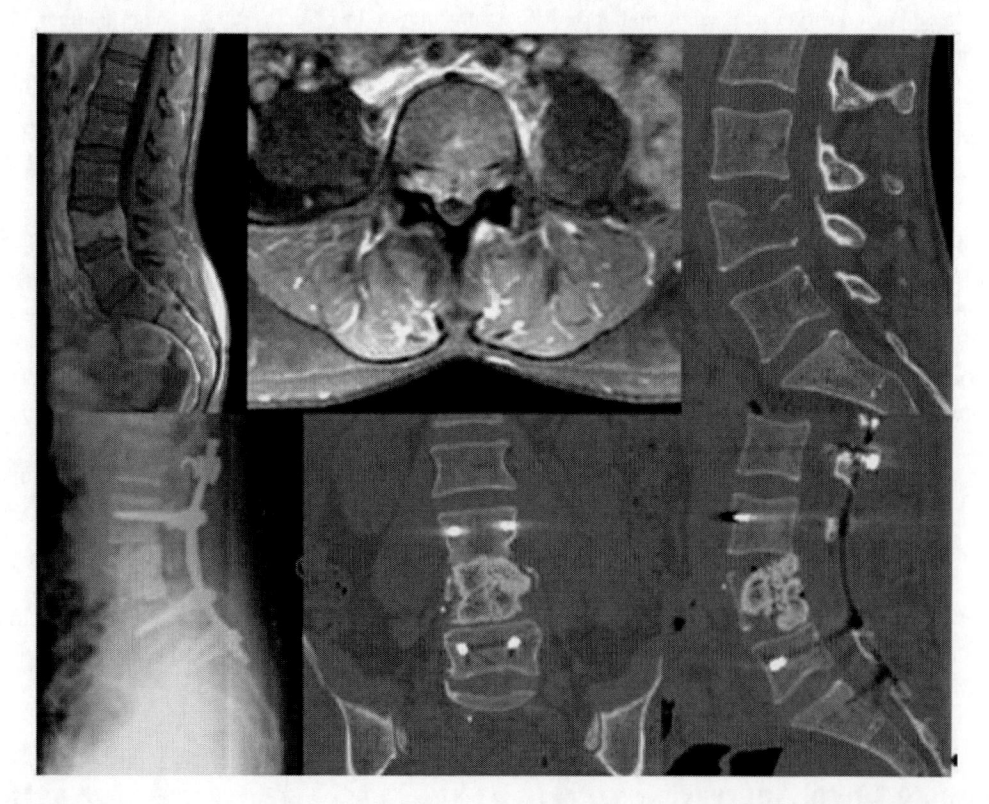

Figure 8. This is the case of decompression, stabilization and anterior reconstruction realized through a postero-lateral approach in the lumbar spine (for L4 spinal metastatic tumor from GI cancer). Reconstruction of anterior column was achieved with PMMA inserted bilaterally after sub-total corpectomy.

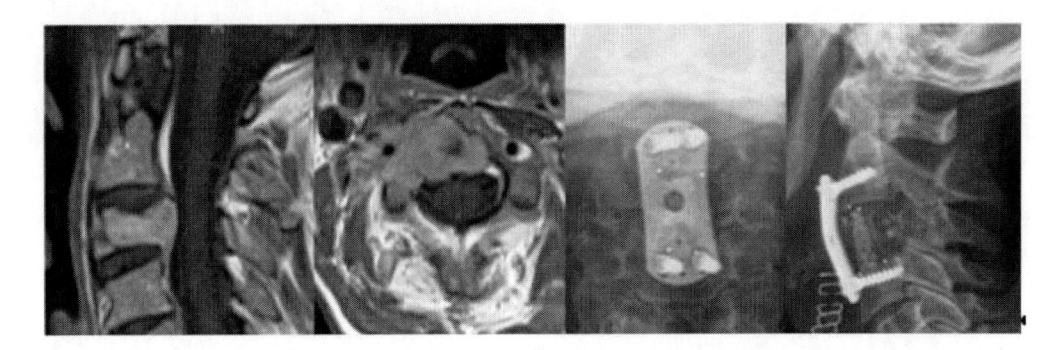

Figure 9. Anterior approach is most commonly performed in the cervical spine to address spinal instability and/or spinal cord compression secondary to spinal metastatic tumors. In the present case (kidney cancer), the anterior approach at C3 allowed for satisfying spinal cord decompression and adequate segmental stabilization with PEEK cage and anterior plating.

Table 7. Anterior approach according to spinal level involved

SPINAL LEVEL	ANTERIOR APPROACH
C0-C2	Trans-oral
C3-T2	Antero-lateral pre-SCM
T3-T4	Manubrial window
T5-T11	Thoracotomy
T12-L1	Thoraco-phrenotomy
L2-L4	Lateral retroperitoneal
L5-S1	Anterior retroperitoneal

Anterior Approach

Anterior approach offers the advantage of direct access to the involved vertebral body which is the predominant site of metastatic tumor growing. Therefore, anterior approach is highly efficient to remove the involved vertebral body, perform decompression of neurological structures and reconstruct the anterior spinal column with the spinal dura under direct vision.

In general, stabilization is achieved by using intervertebral spacer like titanium or PEEK cage and most rarely PMMA. The use of autologous bone like allograft strut is less and less recommended. Additional plating is most frequently required, especially in the case of significant instability.

Anterior approach is the rule in the cervical spine, contrary to thoraco-lumbar spine, figure 9. Type of anterior approach recommended according to spinal level is presented in table 7.

Although anterior procedures may be sufficient in some degenerative or traumatic conditions, spinal metastatic tumor generally require a 360° stabilization due to the severity of the destructive process in the spine.

Therefore, stand-alone anterior approach is rarely sufficient in the context of malignant diseases.

Combined Approach

The antero-posterior approach combines the advantages of each surgical approach: i.e. the quality of the stabilization provided by pedicle-screw fixation systems during the posterior approach and the quality of tumor resection and dural sac decompression achieved during the anterior approach, figure 10. It is now well-accepted that anterior approach alone provides only limited stabilization in case of metastatic spinal tumors and that complementary posterior stabilization is generally required, figures 11 and 12.

Vertebrectomy

Total vertebrectomy is rarely indicated for spinal metastatic tumors. It can be proposed for some solitary kidney or thyroid metastasis.

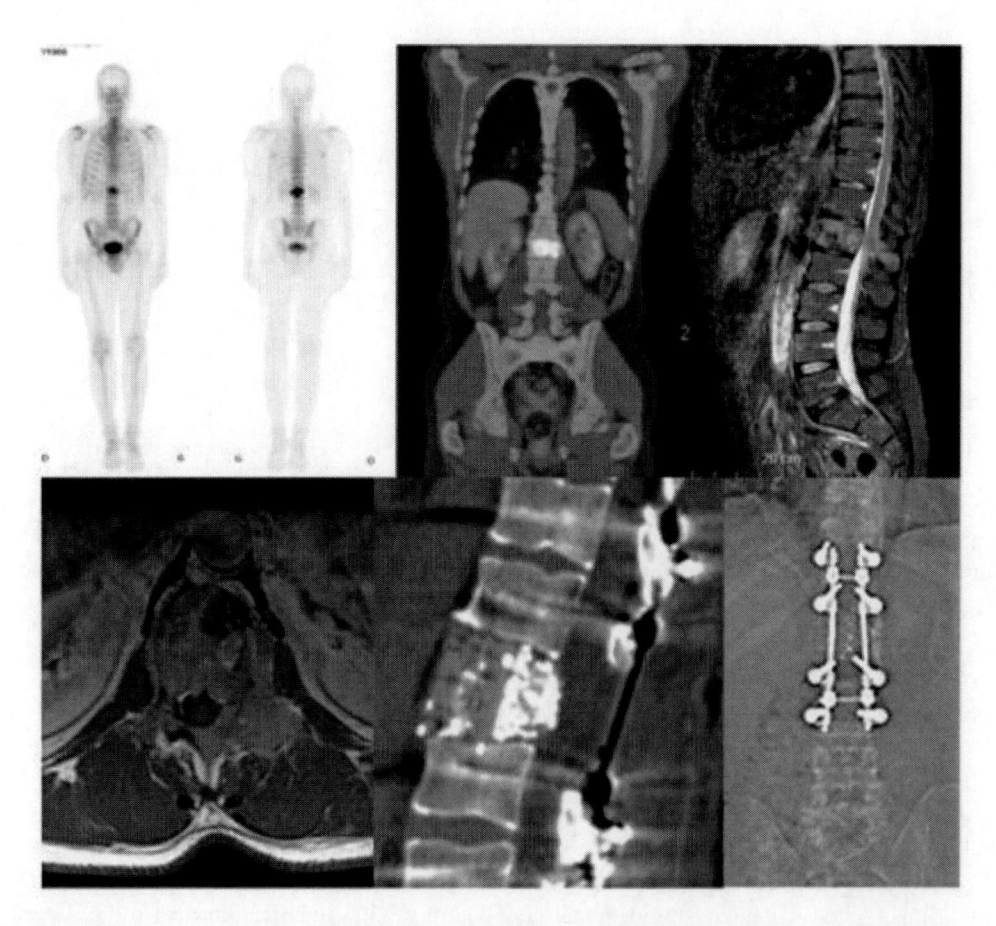

Figure 10. Solitary spinal metastasis in L1 from an unknown primary tumor. Large resection by a combined posterior then anterior approach was conducted. After posterior stabilization (2 levels above and 2 levels below) and posterior arch removal, the vertebral body was resected in a piece-meal fashion and then replaced by a PEEK cage filled with bone substitutes. Histological findings confirmed adenocarcinoma of unknown origin.

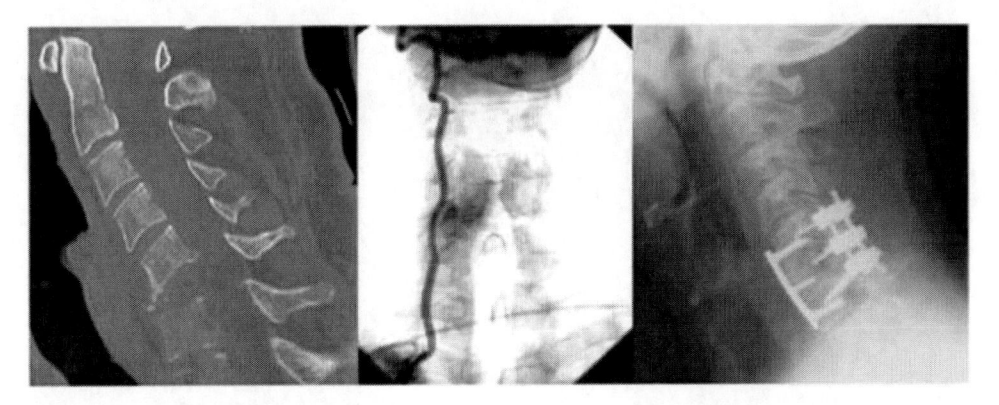

Figure 11. Severe spinal instability in the cervical spine due to C6 involvement by metastasis (from kidney cancer). Stabilization of the spine was restored by a combined approach with iliac crest graft. Instrumentation consisted of anterior plating and C5/C6 lateral mass screws and C7 pedicle screws posteriorly.

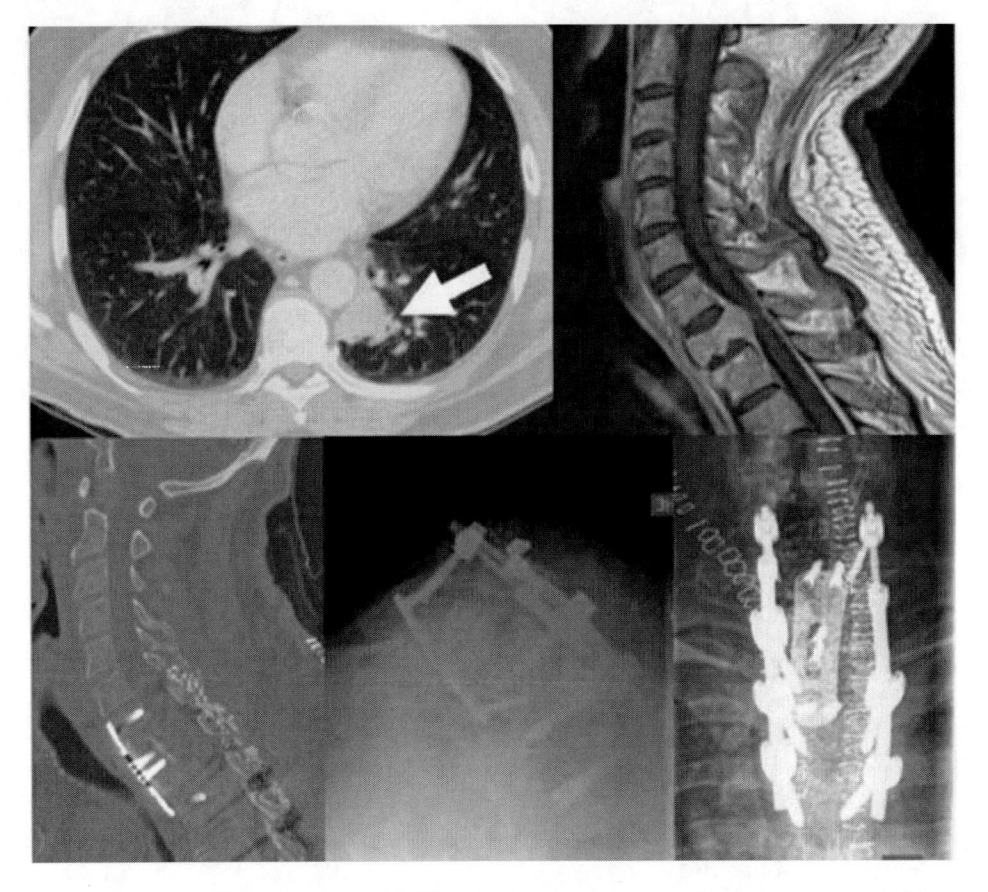

Figure 12. 52 years-old male patient with T1 spinal metastatic tumor from lung cancer (white arrow). T1 vertebra was sub-completely resected via a combined approach, anterior then posterior. After the anterior step of spinal cord decompression, posterior stabilization with pedicles screws in C7, T2, T3 and T4 provided a strong fixation of the cervico-thoracic spine.

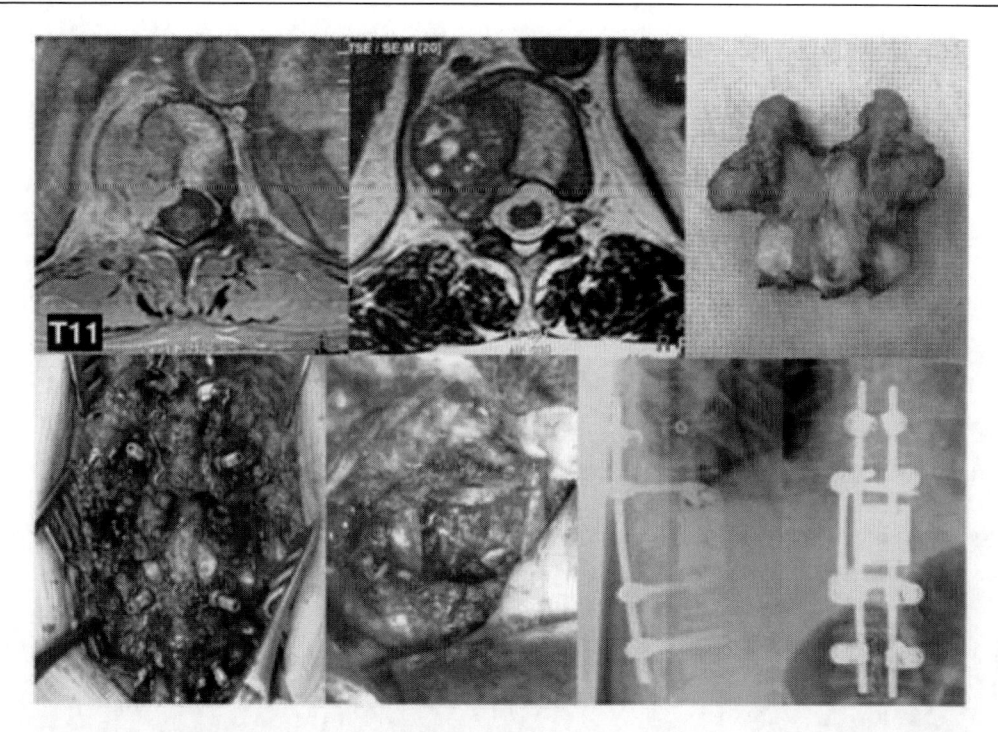

Figure 13. 54 years-old male patient with solitary spinal metastatic tumor (kidney) who underwent total resection with T11 vertebrectomy by combined approach. Spinal stabilization was achieved by segmental posterior instrumentation with pedicle screws and laminar hooks combined with anterior column reconstruction by titanium expandable cage and lateral plating.

In such cases, and contrary to primary malignant spinal tumors, "En bloc" removal is not really justified and piece-meal total vertebrectomy is preferred (gross total resection method), figure 13.

Pre-Operative Embolization

Preoperative embolization may be useful in case of hyper-vascular spinal metastasis (especially from renal cell carcinoma, thyroid carcinoma, and hepato-carcinoma) resulting in reduction of operative blood loss. It is recommended to perform pre-operative embolization 3 days maximum prior to the surgery because of the risk of repermeabilization or collateral compensation. Selective catheterisation is not really necessary and proximal plugging of segmental feeding arteries should be preferred (at the index level, at the level above and at the level below), figure 14.

Anterior Reconstruction

Different strategies can be used to achieve anterior column reconstruction: cages (synthetic or metallic devices), bone autograft (or allograft) or PMMA (figures 15, 16 and 17).

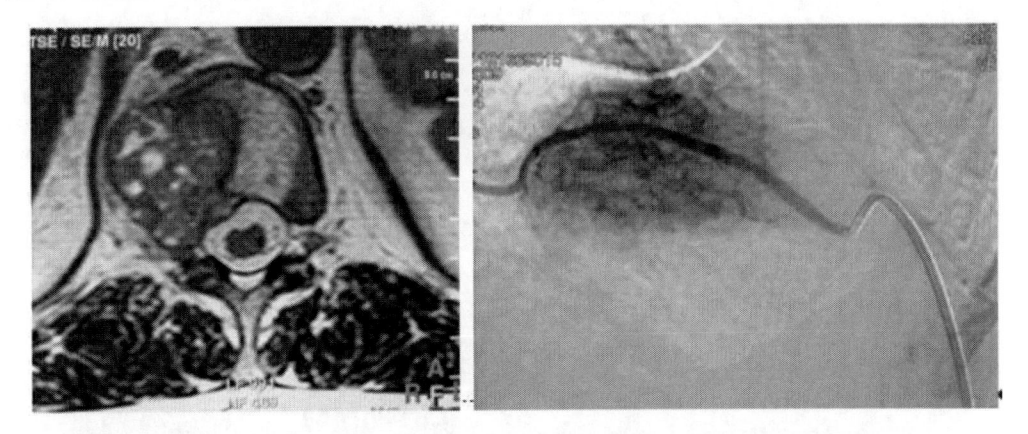

Figure 14. Pre-operative angiography of a T11 metastatic tumor (from kidney cancer) demonstrating hypervascularization arising from the right T11 segmental artery. Embolization of feeding arteries with micro-particles and glue was performed prior to surgical procedure.

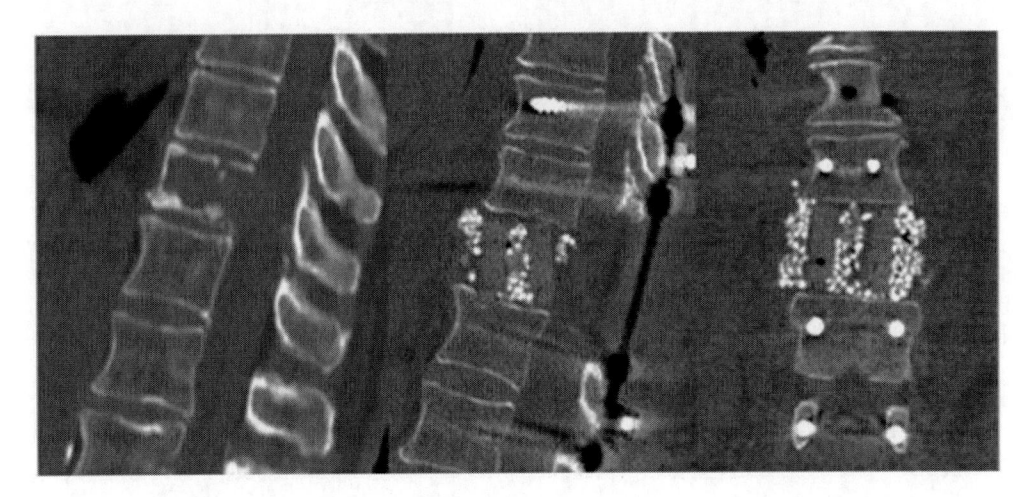

Figure 15. Reconstruction of the anterior column in the thoraco-lumbar spine (L1) by using PEEK cage filled with phospho-calcic bone substitutes.

Although autograft or allograft allow for intervertebral fusion in some cases, there is a high risk for non-union due to post-operative radiotherapy and potential local recurrence.

Otherwise, primary stability provide is satisfying with PMMA, methyl methacrylate may be associated with mechanical complications at mid-term and should not be used for patients with more than 1 year of life expectancy.

SURGICAL STRATEGY

Factors to take into account when choosing the right surgical strategy for patients with a metastatic spine tumor are summarized in table 8.

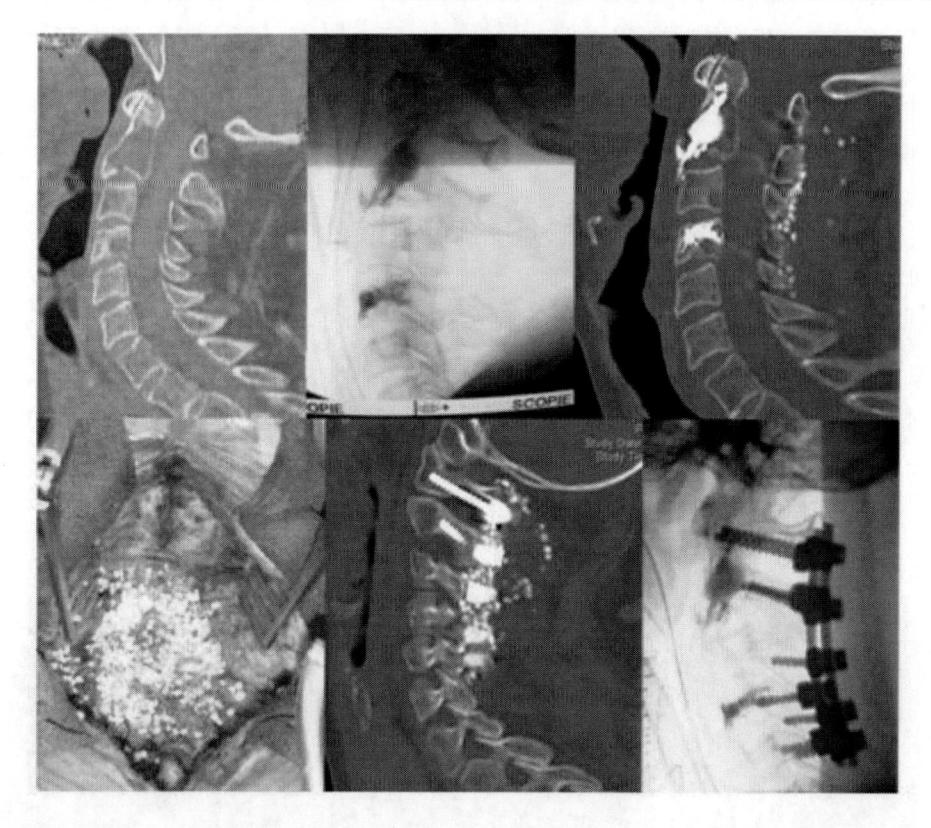

Figure 16. This is the case of anterior column reconstruction achieved with PMMA in the cervical spine (C2 and C4). Additional segmental posterior instrumentation was performed from C1 to C5 under the same general anaesthesia.

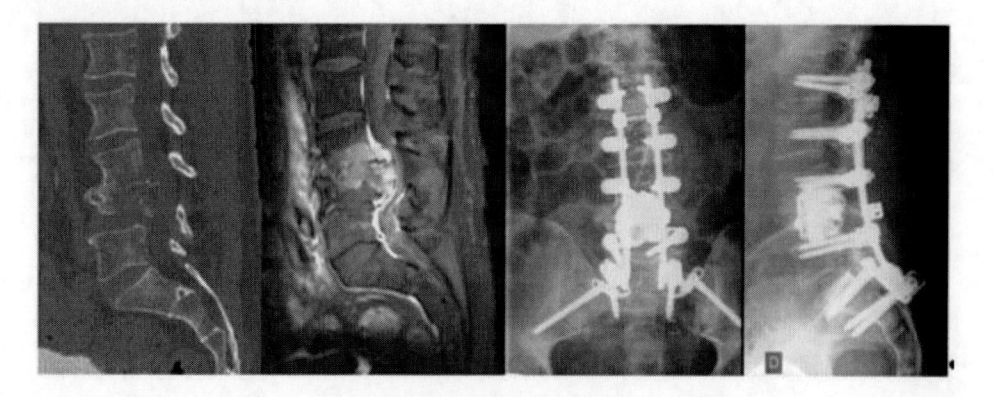

Figure 17. Spinal instability and dural sac compression in the lumbar spine secondary to osteolytic spinal metastatic tumors at L3 and L4 (GI primary cancer). Anterior reconstruction was achieved by insertion of PMMA through bilateral postero-lateral approach. Long construct from L1 to S1 and strong pelvic fixation with ilio-sacral plating were realized.

Finally, we propose a decisional algorithm based on the most significant prognostic factors:

Table 8. Factors that influence the overall surgical strategy

1	Life expectancy
2	Type of cancer
3	Location of the tumor
4	Number of metastases
5	Neurologic status
6	Extent of spinal involvement
7	General status and co-morbidity
8	Patient preference

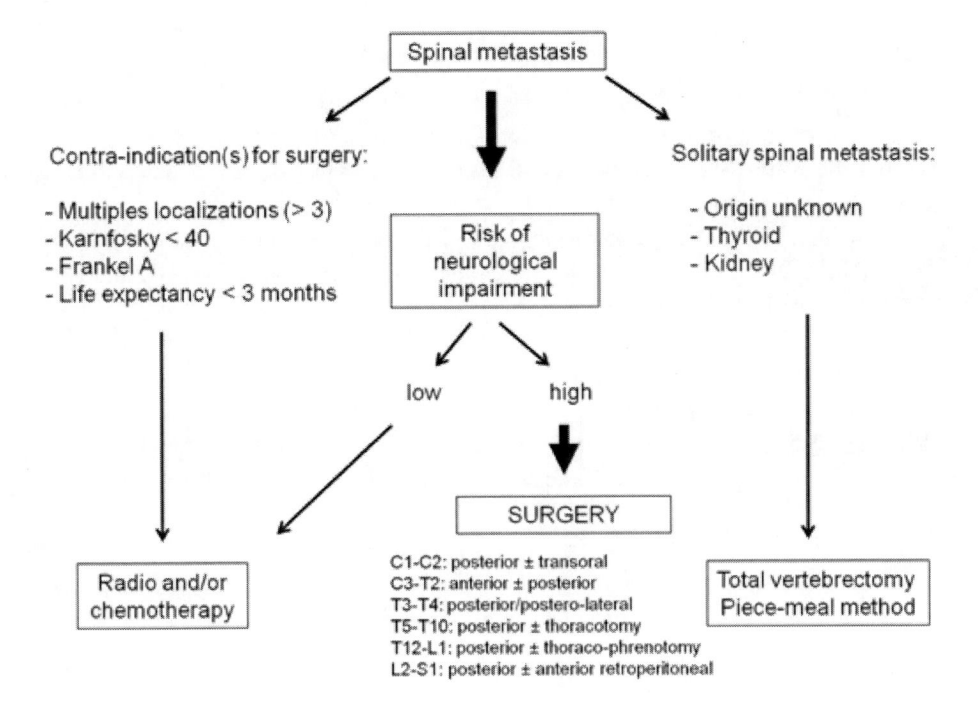

Figure 18. Decisional algorithm for the management of spinal metastatic tumors.

ABBREVIATIONS

PMMA   Poly-methyl-methacrylate
PEEK   Poly-ether-ether-ketone

REFERENCES

[1]   Anderson G, Vaccaro AR. Decision making in spinal care. Book chapter: metastatic spinal tumors by Puschak TJ and Sasso RC. In Thieme, New York, (2006).

[2]   Boriani S, Weinstein JN, Biagini R. Primary bone tumors of the spine. Terminology and surgical staging. *Spine.* 22(9):1036-44, (1997).

[3]   Delvin VJ. Spine secrets. Book chapter: Metastatic spine tumors by Davies MR and Wang JC. Hanley and Belfus, Inc., Philadelphia, (2003).

[4]   Frankel HL, Hancock DO, Hyslop G. The value of postural reduction in the initial management of closed injuries of the spine with paraplegia and tetraplegia. *Paraplegia.* 7:179-92, (1969).

[5]   Kaye AH, Black PM. Operative neurosurgery, volume 2. Book chapter: management of spinal metastases by Comey CH and Haid RW. In Churchill Livingstone, China, (2000).

[6]   Kim DH, Chang UK, Kim SH, Bilsky MH. Tumors of the spine. Book chapter: metastatic evaluation by Cheng ML and S Jaikumar. In Saunders Elsevier, China, (2008).

[7]   Tokuhashi Y, Oda H, Oshima M, Ryu J. A revised scoring system for preoperative evaluation of metastatic spine tumor prognosis. *Spine.* 30:2186-91, (2005).

[8]   Tomita K, Kawahara N, Kobayashi T. Surgical strategy for spinal metastases. *Spine.* 26(3):298-306, (2001).

[9]   Vaccaro AR. Spine, core knowledge in orthopaedics. Book chapter: primary and metastatic spinal tumors by Austin LS, Grauer JN, Beiner JM, Kwon BK and Hilibrand AS. Elsevier Mosby, Philadelphia, (2005).

[10]   Weinstein JN. The adult Spine – Principles and practices. Book chapter: differential diagnosis and treatment of primary benign and malignant neoplasms. Frymoyer eds, Raven Press, New York, (1991).

[11]   Wise JJ, Fishgrund JS, Herkowitz HN. Complications, survival rates and risk factors of surgery for metastatic disease of the spine. *Spine.* 24(18):193-51, (1999).

In: Bone Tumors: Symptoms, Diagnosis and Treatment
Editor: Moncef Berhouma

ISBN: 978-1-62618-190-8

Chapter 4

SPINAL CHORDOMAS

Paul E. Kaloostian, Patricia Zadnik, Ziya L. Gokaslan and Daniel M. Sciubba

The Johns Hopkins Hospital, Baltimore, MD, US

ABSTRACT

Spinal chordomas are a rare group of primary bony tumors of the axial skeleton. Though histologically they are classified as benign tumors, their indolent growth pattern allowing for sizable tumors at presentation and a high rate of recurrence place them into the category of functionally malignant spinal tumors.

Histologically, they have unique cellular architecture that are often pathognomonic for their diagnosis. Management and surgical treatments have advanced significantly over the last few years allowing for an increase in progression free survival.

Despite all that is known about spinal chordomas, there is much more that needs to be studied and learned. But it remains true that treating a patient with a spinal chordoma requires a multidisciplinary team approach, with neurosurgeons, neurologists, oncologists, radiation therapists and nurses working together. In this chapter, we discuss each of these topics in more detail.

INTRODUCTION

Chordomas are rare benign tumors of the axial skeleton that are the most common primary malignant tumors of the spine in adults, typically occurring in middle-age adults [1]. They are most commonly seen along the clival skull base and sacrum, but may occur along the cervical, thoracic, or lumbar spine as well [2]. They present a unique challenge to neurosurgeons due to their growth within the spine and spinal canal, and their propensity to grow to immense sizes in the pelvis prior to clinical detection.

Chordomas are derived from undifferentiated notochord remnants that are found within the developing axial skeleton. [3]. Molecular studies have confirmed that these particular cells are the neoplastic cells that undergo transformation and uncontrolled division in chordoma tumors [4].

PRESENTATION AND NATURAL HISTORY

Spinal chordomas are indolent tumors of the spine and skull base [5]. Due to their slow growth pattern, surrounding tissues are able to accommodate to the presence of this growing tumor [6]. This leads to the presentation of these tumors as extensive lesions with significant distortion of neighboring bone, tissue, and neural elements [6].

Thus, though these tumors are classically benign on histopathology, through their indolent growth pattern and high recurrent nature they functionally act as malignant oncologic lesions [6].

Sacral chordomas comprise 30% of spinal chordomas [1]. Spinal chordomas of the cervical, thoracic and lumbar spine are rare, with the lumbar spine being the more commonly encountered of the three [1]. Of known primary tumors of the sacral elements, chordomas account for over 50% of these tumors [7]. Chordomas are not classically seen in the pediatric population [1]. They are most commonly seen in males around 50-60 years of age [1].

The Surveillance, Epidemiology, and End Results (SEER) database detailed a median survival of 6.29 years with 5 year, 10 year, and 20 year survival decreasing abruptly to 68%, 40%, and 13%, respectively [1]. Factors that have been noted to affect survival include incomplete margins at the time of resection, large tumor burden initially, and degree of expansion of chordoma into nearby vital structures [8].

The clinical presentation of chordomas varies depending on the location. For example, patients with sacral chordomas most commonly present with localized low back pain with or without radicular symptoms [9]. Depending on the extent of tumor burden, patients may or may not present with bowel or bladder dysfunction.

Patients with cervical or thoracic chordomas may present with early myelopathy due to spinal cord compression [10]. Lumbar chordomas may present with focal back pain and/or radiculopathy from nerve root involvement of tumor [10]. Compared to cervical spine chordomas, sacral chordomas are less likely to present with neurological compromise [10].

IMAGING

Chordomas may present in a variety of ways on imaging modalities. X-rays of the lumbosacral spine may demonstrate spotty areas of calcification, usually in tumors that are quite large.

The sacral spine may demonstrate remodeling on x-ray due to local growth. However x-rays typically do not capture the distal sacrum and so may miss tumors in this area [10]. Computerized tomography (CT) of the lumbosacral spine may also demonstrate areas of bony remodeling much more clearly than x-ray.

Further, chordomas presenting along the foramina may cause widening of the sacral foramina, visible on CT or x-ray. Chordomas along the posterior border of the vertebral bodies may demonstrate thinning and remodeling of the body locally. Magnetic resonance imaging of the lumbosacral spine will more clearly demonstrate an enhancing mass with associated soft tissue involvement around the spinal elements as well as nearby neural structure compression.

Additionally, chordomas typically invade the disc space in the spine, distinguishing them from other tumors [10]. PET CT may be used to detect any metastatic disease elsewhere upon presentation [10].

DIFFERENTIAL DIAGNOSES

Spinal chordomas can mimic many other tumors of the spine. The differential diagnosis for these tumors include chondromas, chondrosarcomas, giant cell tumors the spine, multiple myeloma, and metastatic disease.

MANAGEMENT

The histology of tumors is critical forproviding an accurate clinical diagnosis which will guide appropriate and focused treatments. For example, differentiating between a metastatic tumor, chordoma and chondrosarcoma is paramount in determining treatment and prognosis [10]. Therefore, it is often recommended to perform a fine needle CT-guided biopsy to obtain tissue diagnosis prior to any surgical or adjunctive therapy.

PATHOLOGY

Chordomas classically are described as lobulated and rubbery tumors with a grayish-white color on gross pathology [11]. They are noted to have multiple fibrotic septae isolating various compartments of the tumor. They typically are not locally invasive or malignant. However, theirindolent growth processallows for remodeling of the neighboring bony structures of the spine as well as slow compression and distortion of nearby neural elements without the classical erosion seen in other bony tumors [11].

Histopathologically, chordoma cells have round nuclei with vacuolated cytoplasm. This abundant cytoplasm is what distinguishes this group of tumors from all others. The term given to chordoma cells due to their microscopic appearance is physaliferous, denoting presence of bubbles or vacuoles. Microscopically, chordoma cells react intensely for S-100 and other epithelial markers such as cytokeratins and epithelial membrane [12, 13].

There are various histopathologic varieties of chondromas. They may manifest as classical, chondroid or de-differentiated [14]. Chondroid chondromas classically show features of both chordoma and chondrosarcoma, a malignant cartilaginous tumor [14]. Brachyury, a notochordal developmental transcription factor, has recently emerged as a factor in the diagnosis of chordomas [15]. Identifying brachyury as a biomarker, along with cytokeratin staining, enhances the specifity and sensitivity of chondroma diagnosis to 100% and 98%, respectively [15]. These markers have proved helpful in distinguishing chondromas from other tumors of chondroid origin.

Significant research has been performed studying the various genetic properties of chordomas. It has been shown that certain receptors are overexpressed in these tumor cell lines, such as platelet-derived growth factors A/B and KIT receptors [16]. Studies demonstrating reactivity of imatinib and sunitinib, a tyrosine-kinase inhibitor acting at the platelet-derived growth factor receptor level, have shown decreased tumor volume in patients with chordomas [17]. Other tumor markers include epidermal growth factor [EGF] receptor overexpression with EGF receptor inhibition studies done showing decreased tumor volume [18].

CONSERVATIVE/ADJUNCTIVE TREATMENT STRATEGIES

Medical management in the treatment of spinal chordomas is typically done in anticipation of future surgical curative procedures. Pre-operative chemotherapy with alkylating agents and cisplatin have shown a better response rate in the de-differentiated subytpes [19]. The typical chemotherapeutic agents have been shown in multiple reviews to be a minimal clinical significance in the treatment of spinal chordomas [20].

Radiotherapy alone has been proven to be ineffective for the treatment of chordomas and has given them the classification of radioresistant tumors [10]. Doses of 40-60 Gy provide a 5-year local control of 10-40 % [10]. Proton beam therapy has gained momentum as an adjunctive treatment for chordomas with decreasing tissue injury and local control of tumor volume with 5-year local control rate of 50-60% [21].

Other radiation treatments currently under investigation include the use of carbon ion radiotherapy, along with helium and neon radiotherapy. Generally, the current recommendations are en bloc surgical resection along with post-operative proton beam radiotherapy, especially in patients with primary chordomas as opposed to recurrent tumors [22]. Recurrence may be managed with both re-operation or continued chemotherapy and radiation treatments, depending on the particular case [22].

SURGICAL TECHNIQUE

Recent evidence in the literature confirms that en bloc resection of sacral chordomas with wide margins provides a significantly increased progression free survival. This strategy was first described in 1970 by Gunterberg et. al. in an attempt to cure these tumors [23].

Surgical technique depends on the location of the tumor. For example, surgical treatment for cervical chordomas is quite complex. Cervical chordomas are classified into three different types based on location in the cervical spine: C1-C3 are high cervical tumors, C5-C6 are mid cervical tumors, and C7-T1 are cervicothoracic tumors. En bloc resection is almost impossible for all types of cervical chordomas often due to the inability to sacrifice surrounding structures such as nerve roots and the vertebral artery, without causing significant neurological compromise [24].

Thus cervical chordomas are often treated with intralesional resection. The general approach for cervical chordomas is to perform release osteotomies and posterior tumor dissection with placement of instrumentation and posterolateral arthrodesis in the first stage. During the first stage, any sacrifice of nerve roots or the vertebral artery is performed. The second stage, typically 2-5 days after stage 1, involves anterior tumor dissection, en bloc excision of tumor, and anterior vertebral reconstruction [25].

High cervical chordomas generally require sacrifice of C1-4 nerve roots without risk of significant neurological deficits. However, vertebral artery sacrifice here can lead to severe neurological impairment. A cerebral angiogram with temporary balloon occlusion test is recommended pre-operatively. To achieve an en bloc resection for high cervical chordomas, a submandibular or transmandibular approach is needed. A high rate of posterior occipito-cervical fusion constructs is seen with this fusion and reconstruction procedure [25].

Mid cervical chordomas do not allow for sacrifice of the nerve roots or the vertebral artery. Pre-operative cerebral angiogram is once again recommended. An anterior approach using a modified Smith-Robinson approach with radical dissection of the soft tissues of the spine is performed with standard anterior and posterior column reconstruction [25].

Cervicothoracic chordoma resection does not allow nerve root sacrifice due to neurological impairment that may result. Vertebral arteries may be dissected free and preserved in this area. Anterior transcervical approach or median sternotomy may be performed for en bloc resection. Anterior and posterior reconstructions are then performed in standard fashion [25].

Thoracic chordomas may be approached in multiple stages as well. Typically stage 1 involves the posterior approach for long segment cervicothoracic instrumentation with vertebral release at the levels of interest.

Thoracic nerve roots may be sacrificed and the plane between the segmental arteries needs to be dissected to access anterior to the spinal canal. Tomita saws are then tunneled anterior to the spinal cord in preparation for the next stage. The ribs at the appropriate levels are subtotally resected as well. In stage 2, a lateral thoracotomy is performed to separate the soft tissue attachments to the vertebral bodies and tumor, and to reposition the Tomita saws. In stage 3, the vertebrectomy is completed via a left thoracotomy and appropriate reconstruction is performed [26].

Lumbar and sacrococcygeal chordomas are surgically managed in the standard 2 stage approach, with an initial posterior multilevel instrumentation and fusion with posterior element release, followed by an anterior en bloc resection with or without vertebral reconstruction, depending on extent of sacrectomy and preservation of sacroiliac joints [27]. Additionally, excision of the tumor must also include the removal of the biopsy tract and may involve the removal of a large region of skin. Multidisciplinary approaches with plastic surgery involvement should be considered for closure of large, complex skin defects.

An important factor to consider when performing sacrectomies is attempting to salvage the S2 nerve root. This is associated with a 50% chance of normal bowel and bladder function post-operatively, with sacral 3 root preservation increasing that percentage even higher. It has been shown that bilateral sacral 2 nerve root sparing along with unilateral sacral 3 root sparing is associated with normal bowel and bladder function [27]. If en bloc resection dictates resection of the sacral nerve roots, unilateral resection can result in acceptable clinical outcomes.

Unilateral preservation of S2-S5 results in satisfactory bowel control and minimal bladder and sexual dysfunction.

For ambulation, bilateral L5 and above must be spared for satisfactory gait, however bilateral S2 and above must be spared to walk normally (23-25).

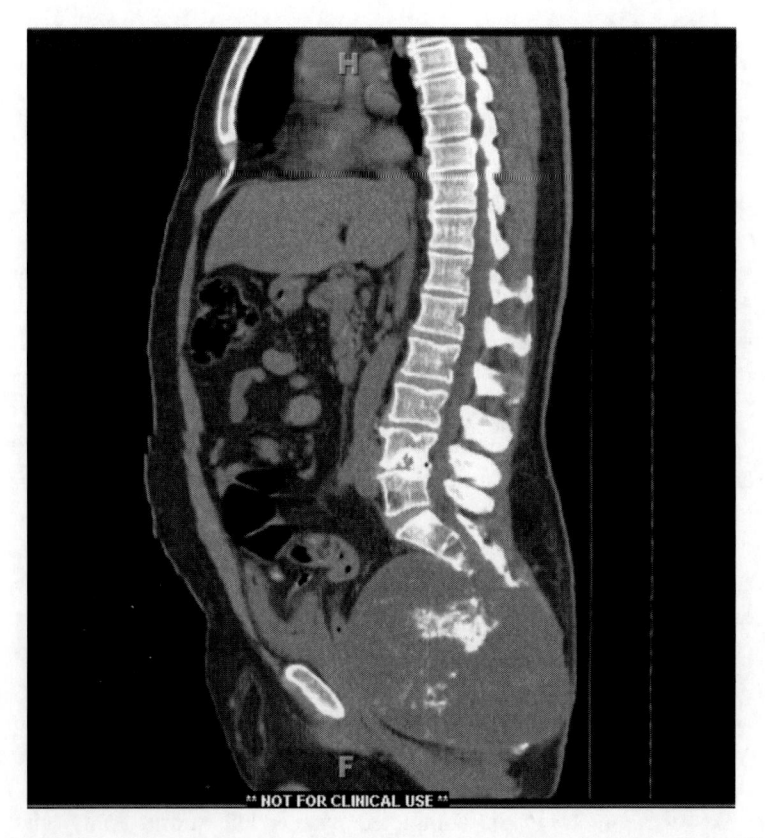

Figure 1. Pre-operative CT of sacrum showing large expansile tumor of the sacrum (The Johns Hopkins Hospital).

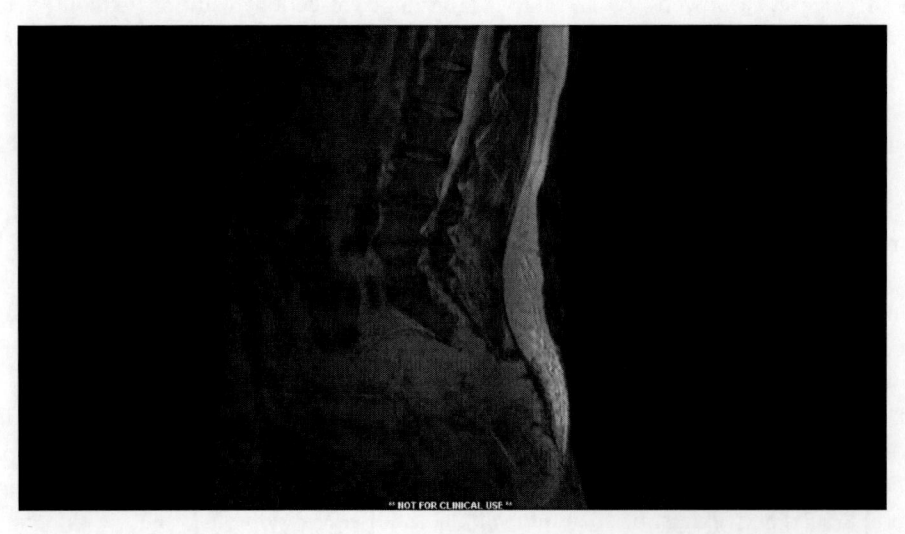

Figure 2. Pre-operative MRI of the sacrum showing a large expansile tumor of the sacrum with significant distortion of the surrounding tissues (The Johns Hopkins Hospital).

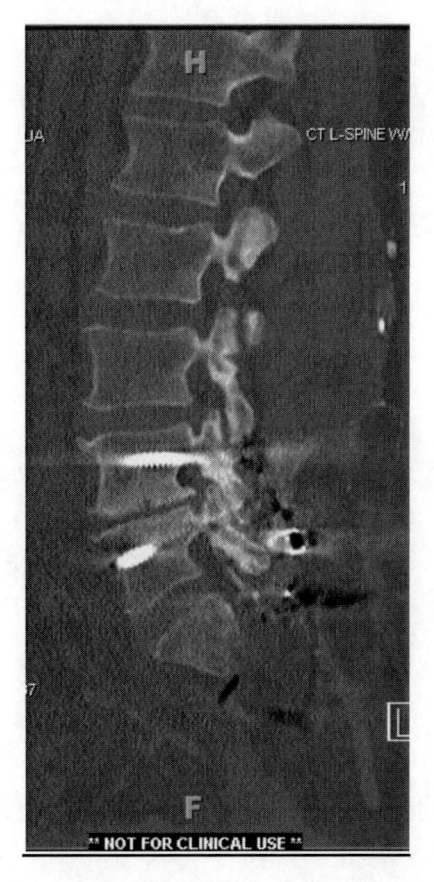

Figure 3. Post-operative CT scan of the lumbosacral spine showing a long segment lumbo-iliac posterior fixation and fusion and complete sacrectomy (The Johns Hopkins Hospital).

OUTCOMES

En bloc resection of sacral chordoma affords the best prognosis for patients. [28] A two fold higher rate of local recurrence has been reported if the tumor capsule is violated during en bloc resection [29]. Subtotal resection recurrence rates have been reported to be around 8 months compared to the over 2 years recurrence rate with en bloc resection [28].

Metastatic disease for chordomas is quite rare but 5% of patients may present with lesions in the bone, lungs, and brain [28, 29]. Typically, however, local disease is considered the main problem affecting survival rather than metastatic disease [30].

RECENT GENETIC AND MOLECULAR ADVANCES

The recent advent of using brachyury, a notochordal developmental transcription factor, along with cytokeratin staining has increased the diagnostic accuracy of chordomas dramatically. This gene is commonly seen in patients with the familial and sporadic chordomas [31].

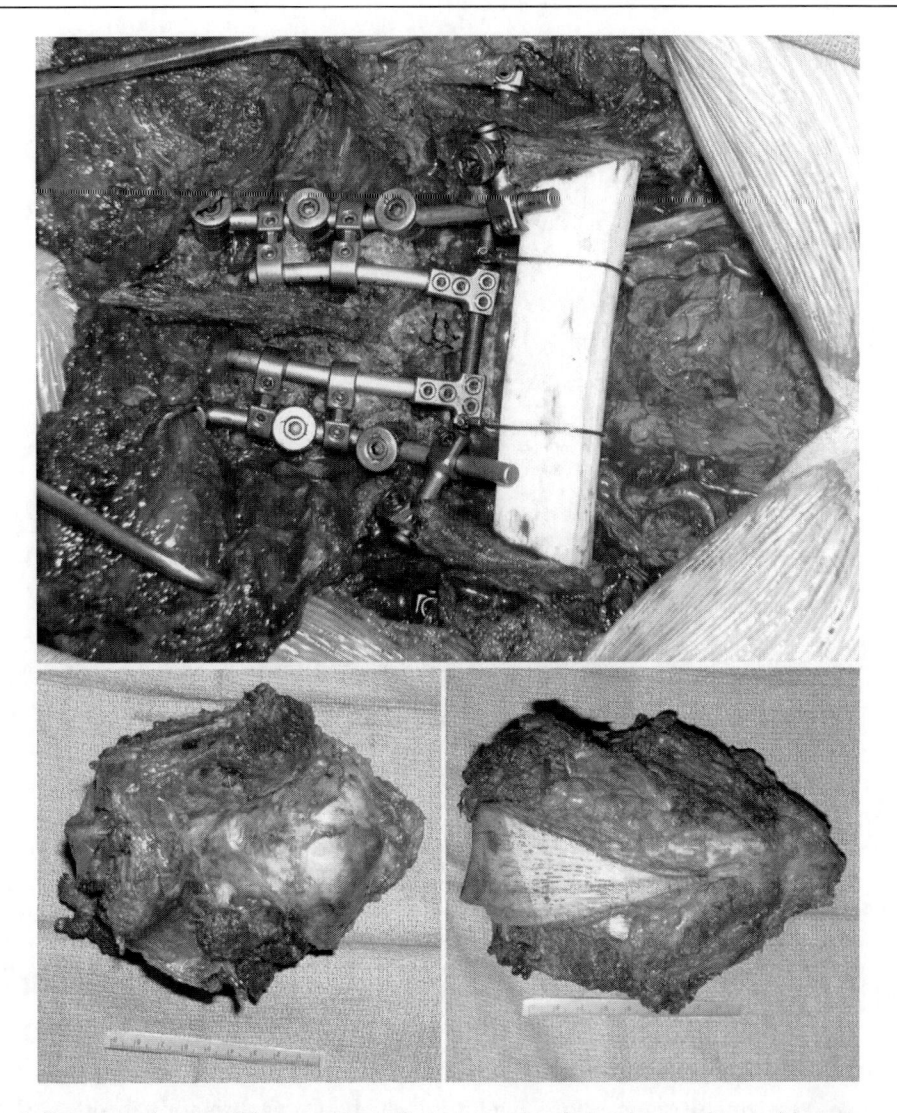

Figure 4. Gross specimen en bloc resection of sacrococcygeal chordomas along with post-operative posterior instrumentation (The Johns Hopkins Hospital).

Additionally, the discovery of tyrosine kinases and epidermal growth factor receptors, in addition to the platelet-derived growth factor receptors have led to ongoing clinical projects looking for possible inhibitory effects on chordoma tumor volume [32].

SUMMARY

1) There are a wide variety of tumors along the sacral spine that may mimic chordomas requiring accurate diagnostic strategies prior to any surgical procedure.
2) En bloc resection of chordomas without violation of tumor capsule have demonstrated increased survival compared to en bloc resection with violation of tumor capsule.

3) Surgical treatment depends on location of tumor along spinal axis but generally involves multiple stages.
4) Adjunctive proton-beam radiotherapy is recommended after surgical resection.
5) Note that despite the more aggressive surgical approach toward patients with sacral chordomas, the ultimate goal is preservation of a patient's neurological function and quality of life, ahead of the desire for gross total resection.

CONCLUSION

Spinal chordomas are rare benign tumors that may act aggressively through growth and expansion of surrounding neural and bony tissues. Patients may present with or without neurological disturbance depending on the level of the chordoma. Diagnosis involves magnetic resonance imaging of the spine demonstrating this tumor. Diagnosis often involves needle biopsy with pathology demonstrating the classic physaliferous cells of the chordoma. Surgical treatment includes multiple stages with an initial posterior segmental instrumentation followed by anterior en bloc resection of the pathologic sacrum and tumor with wide margins as appropriate. Chemotherapy and/or radiation may be used as pre-operative or post-operative adjunctive treatments. Finally, optimal care for the patient with sacral chordoma requires a true team approach, including members of neurosurgery, plastic surgery, nursing, oncology, and radiation therapy.

REFERENCES

[1] McMaster ML, Goldstein AM, Bromley CM, et al. Chordoma: incidence and survival patterns in the United States, 1973–1995. *Cancer Causes Control.* 2001; 12:1–11.
[2] Bjornsson J, Wold LE, Ebersold MJ, et al. Chordoma of the mobile spine. A clinicopathologic analysis of 40 patients. *Cancer.* 1993; 71:735–40.
[3] Horten BC, Montague SR. In vitro characteristics of a sacrococcygeal chordoma maintained in tissue and organ culture systems. *Acta Neuropathol.* 1976; 35: 13-25.
[4] Vujovic S, Henderon S, Presneau N, et al. Brachyury, a crucial regulator of notochordal development, is a novel biomarker for chordomas. *J. Pathol.* 2006; 209: 157–165.
[5] Bergh P, Kindblom LG, Gunterberg B, Remotti F, et al. Prognostic factors in chordoma of the sacrum and mobile spine: a study of 39 patients. *Cancer.* 2000; 88: 2122–2134.
[6] Schwab JH, Boland PJ, Agaram NP. Chordoma and chondrosarcoma gene profile: implications for immunotherapy. *Cancer Immunol. Immunother.* 2009; 58: 339–349
[7] Cheng EY, Ozerdemoglu RA, Transfeldt EE, Thompson RC. Lumbosacral chordoma: prognostic factors and treatment. *Spine.* 1999; 24: 1639–1645.
[8] Wold LE, Laws ER. Cranial chordomas in children and young adults. *J. Neurosurg.* 1983; 59: 1043–1047.
[9] Fourney DR, Gokaslan ZL. Current management of sacral chordoma. *Neurosurg. Focus.* 2003; 15: 9.
[10] Boriani S, Chevalley F, Weinstein JN, et al. Chordoma of the spine above the sacrum. Treatment and outcome in 21 cases. *Spine.* 1996; 21: 1569–1577.

[11] Healy JH, Lane JM. Chordoma: a critical review of diagnosis and treatment. *Orthop. Clin. North Am.* 1989; 20: 417–426.

[12] Crapanzano JP, Ali SZ,Ginsberg MS, Zakowski MF. Chordoma: a cytologic study with histologic and radiologic correlation. *Cancer.* 2001; 93:40–51.

[13] Mitchell A, Scheithauer BW, Unni KK, et al. Chordoma and chondroid neoplasms of the spheno-occiput. An immunohistochemical study of 41 cases with prognostic and nosologic implications. *Cancer.* 1993; 72: 2943–2949.

[14] Chugh R, Tawbi H, Lucas DR, et.al. Chordoma: the nonsarcoma primary bone tumor. *Oncologist.* 2007; 12: 1344–1350.

[15] Oakley GJ, Fuhrer K, Seethala RR. Brachyury, SOX-9, and podoplanin, new markers in the skull base chordoma vs chondrosarcoma differential: a tissue microarray-based comparative analysis. *Mod. Pathol.* 2008; 21:1461–1469.

[16] Negri T, Casieri P, Miselli F, et al. Evidence for PDGFRA, PDGFRB and KIT deregulation in an NSCLC patient. *Br. J. Cancer.* 2007; 96: 180–181.

[17] George S, Merriam P, Maki RG, et al. Multicenter phase II trial of sunitinib in the treatment of nongastrointestinal stromal tumor sarcomas. *J. Clin. Oncol.* 2009; 27:3154–3160.

[18] Weinberger PM, Yu Z, Kowalski D, et al. Differential expression of epidermal growth factor receptor, c-Met, and HER2/neu in chordoma compared with 17 other malignancies. *Arch. Otolaryngol. Head Neck Surg.* 2005; 131:707–711.

[19] Yang C, Hornicek FJ, Wood KB, et al. Characterization and analysis of human chordoma cell lines. *Spine.* 2010; 35:1257–1264.

[20] Azzarelli A, Quagliuolo V, Cerasoli S, et al. Chordoma: natural history and treatment results in 33 cases. *J. Surg. Oncol.* 1988; 37:185–191.

[21] Suit HD, Goitein M, Munzenrider J, et al. Definitive radiation therapy for chordoma and chondrosarcoma of base of skull and cervical spine. *J. Neurosurg.* 1982; 56: 377–385.

[22] Park L, Delaney TF, Liebsch NJ, et al. Sacral chordomas: impact of high-dose proton/photon-beam radiation therapy combined with or without surgery for primary versus recurrent tumor. *Int. J. Radiat. Oncol. Biol. Phys.* 2006; 65: 1514–1521.

[23] Stener B, Gunterberg B. High amputation of the sacrum for extirpation of tumors. Principles and technique. *Spine.* 1978; 3:351–366.

[24] Barrenechea IJ, Perin NI, Triana A, et al. Surgical management of chordomas of the cervical spine. J Neurosurg Spine. 2007; 6:398–406.

[25] Hsieh P, Gallia G, Sciubba D, et al. En bloc excisions of chordomas in the cervical spine: review of five consecutive cases with more than 4-year follow-up. *Spine.* 2011; 36 (24): 1581-1587.

[26] Sciubba D, Gokaslan Z, Black J, et al. 5-Level spondylectomy for en bloc resection of thoracic chordoma: case report. *Neurosurgery.* 2011; 69: 48-56.

[27] Samson IR, Springfield DS, Suit HD, et al. Operative treatment of sacrococcygeal chordoma. A review of twenty-one cases. *J. Bone Joint Surg. Am.* 1993; 73:1476–1484.

[28] Fuchs B, Dickey ID, Yaszemski MJ, et al. Operative management of sacral chordoma. *J. Bone Joint Surg. Am.* 2005; 87: 2211–2216.

[29] Kaiser TE, Pritchard DJ, Unni KK. Clinicopathologic study of sacrococcygeal chordoma. *Cancer.* 1984; 53:2574–2578.

[30] Chambers PW, Schwinn CP. Chordoma: a clinicopathologic study of metastasis. *Am. J. Clin. Pathol.* 1979; 72:765–776.

[31] Yang XR, Ng D, Alcorta DA, et al. T (brachyury) gene duplication confers major susceptibility to familial chordoma. *Nat. Genet.* 2009; 41:1176–1178.

[32] Nikoghosyan AV, Karapanagiotou-Schenkel I, Münter MW, et al. Randomized trial of proton vs carbon ion radiation therapy in patients with chordoma of the skull base, clinical phase III study HIT-1-Study. *BMC Cancer.* 2010; 10: 607.

Chapter 5

IMAGING OF NOTOCHORDAL TUMORS

Prabhakar Rajiah[1,], Hakan Ilaslan[1] and Murali Sundaram[1]*

[1]Musculoskeletal Imaging Section, Imaging Institute, Cleveland Clinic, OH, US

ABSTRACT

Notochord is a midline axial structure that is a major structural organizer in the development of the spine. Tumors originating from notochordal remnants are rare and are typically seen in the midline of the body, commonly in the sacrococcygeal and spheno-occipital regions. Classic chordoma is a malignant notochordal tumor that is pathologically characterized by strands of atypical chordoid cells and myxoid matrix. Radiologically, chordoma presents as an osteolytic mass, with a large calcified soft tissue mass that shows contrast enhancement. Chordomas are locally aggressive and are treated with radical resection and adjuvant radiation therapy. Chondroid chordoma and extra-axial chordoma are variants of chordoma that are associated with a better prognosis than that of classic chordoma. Dedifferentiated chordoma is a histogenetically distinct high-grade tumor arising in a pre-existing chordoma; prognosis in these cases depends on the dedifferentiated element, which is usually a high-grade spindle cell tumor. Benign notochordal cell tumors (BNCT) are intra-osseous benign lesions of notochordal cell origin, with clinical and histopathological features distinct from those of chordoma and notochordal rests. Pathologically, there is no myxoid matrix with BNCT as there is with chordoma. Radiographs and scintigraphy results are usually normal with BNCT, whereas computed tomography shows subtle sclerosis with no evidence of osteolysis and magnetic resonance imaging shows homogeneous low T1 and high T2 signal without contrast enhancement or soft tissue mass. With long-term follow-up, these benign tumors do not show progression to chordoma. Incipient chordoma has histological features between those of BNCT and chordoma. For all tumors of notochordal origin, pathological features should be correlated with imaging findings to ensure accurate diagnosis and appropriate management.

---

[*] E-mail: radprabhakar@gmail.com.

INTRODUCTION

Notochord is a midline axial structure that is a major structural organizer in the development of the spine, acting as an inducer of chondrogenesis and segmentation of mesenchymal elements of the spine. Although notochord is not present in an adult, several tumors can originate from the notochordal remnants within bones.

These tumors are typically seen in the midline of the body, more commonly in the sacrococcygeal and spheno-occipital regions. Notochordal tumors are characterized by the presence of physaliferous cells, in which multiple cytoplasmic vacuoles are seen indenting the nucleus. On immunochemistry, these tumors express epithelial cells that are positive for cytokeratins (AE/1, AE/3, CK18), epithelial membrane antigen (EMA), S-100 protein, vimentin, and the antigenic phenotype of cartilage [1].

This chapter discusses the common and uncommon tumors of notochordal origin, including classic chordoma, chondroid chordoma, extra-axial chordoma, dedifferentiated chordoma, benign notochordal cell tumor (BNCT), and incipient chordoma.

CLASSIC CHORDOMA

Classic chordoma is a rare low- to intermediate-grade malignant notochordal tumor. Classic chordoma accounts for 2% to 4% of all primary bone malignancies, with an overall incidence of 0.08 per 100,000 people [2]. This type of tumor is more common in men, particularly in the fifth and sixth decades of life. Classic chordoma occurs in the axial skeleton, usually in the extremes of the spine, with 50% of cases occurring in the sacrococcygeal region and 35% occurring in the spheno-occipital region; 15% of cases occur in the mobile vertebra, more commonly in the cervical spine than in the lumbar or thoracic spine [3]. Chordoma constitutes 50% of all primary malignant sacral tumors, and is commonly seen below the level of S3 [4]. Lesions in the skull base occur in younger patients than those in the sacrococcygeal region, and lesions occur in equal male and female distributions in the mobile vertebra. The tumor is usually solitary and originates from the midline of the bone of origin [4].

Pathologically, classic chordoma is seen as a multilobulated soft white mass with a fibrous pseudocapsule. Fluid and mucoid matrix, hemorrhage, calcification, and bone fragments are typically also seen. Microscopically, strands of atypical chordoid cells (physaliferous cells, which are large epithelioid cells with prominent vacuoles and clear to eosinophilic cytoplasm) and a frothy myxoid matrix can be observed. Infiltration and destruction of the underlying bone are also seen, along with chronic inflammation at the interface between the involved and uninvolved bone. Expression of cytokeratins (AE/1, AE/3, CK18), S-100 protein, EMA, and vimentin and demonstration of brachyury distinguish chordoma from chondrosarcoma and other similar neoplasms. The presence of chondroid tissue alone is not enough to allow for a diagnosis of chordoma, since this could also be indicative of BNCT (see below).

On radiographs, chordoma is seen as an osteolytic lesion in the involved bone with an associated soft tissue mass. Sclerosis, although uncommon, may be seen in a spinal chordoma [5]. Detecting a lesion may be difficult in the sacral region. Scintigraphy results will be negative because of the absence of reactive bone formation. On computed tomography (CT), a destructive lesion with an associated large lobulated extra-osseous soft tissue mass can be seen; sclerosis may also be seen in the periphery of the destructive lesion. In the sacral region, the soft tissue mass is more likely to occur in the anterior than the posterior aspect, and in the spheno-occipital region, this mass can be seen in the retropharyngeal region. In the soft tissue mass, calcification and bone fragments may be seen, as well as low attenuation because of the gelatinous matrix [6].

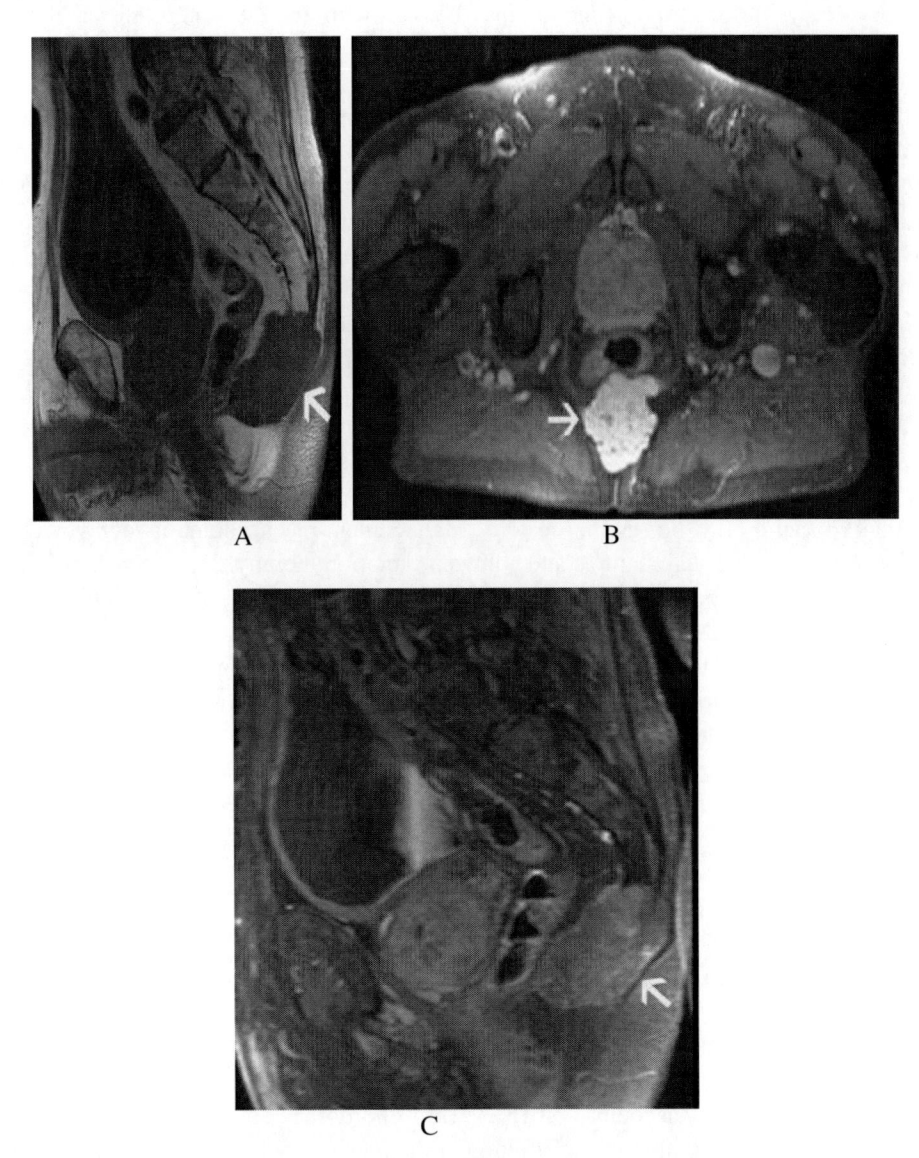

Figure 1. Chordoma in a 43-year-old man. (A) Sagittal T1-weighted magnetic resonance (MR) image shows a lesion with low signal intensity originating from the **S5** vertebra, with large soft tissue component (arrow). (B) In the short T1 inversion recovery (STIR) image, the lesion has high signal intensity (arrow). (C) The lesion shows heterogeneous enhancement (arrow) after administration of gadolinium-based contrast agent.

On magnetic resonance imaging (MRI), chordoma displays low T1 (Figure 1a) and high T2 signal (Figure 1b). Alternatively, high T1 signal may be as a result of hemorrhage. Contrast enhancement is variable and heterogeneous (Figure 1c), with less enhancement in the myxoid areas and moderate enhancement in the vascular fibrous septa, which may appear as a crisscross pattern [7]. In cases of chordoma, MRI is useful in assessing involvement of nerve roots, pelvic organs, bones, joints, and muscles. Coronal and 3-dimensional reconstructions are particularly useful in evaluating nerve root involvement; this is important, as rectal, urinary, and sexual dysfunction may be seen with involvement of all sacral roots or may be preserved if the upper 3 sacral nerves on 1 side and at least 2 on the other side are spared. MRI of the entire spine should be performed to assess for associated lesions and to exclude metastasis. Differential diagnosis for chordoma includes chondrosarcoma, metastasis, and tuberculosis.

In the vertebra, chordoma originates from the center of the body and has associated anterior, lateral, and posterior soft tissue masses (Figure 2). Cranio-caudal spread with involvement of multiple vertebra may be seen, with sparing of the intervertebral disc space until late in the disease. On MRI, extension to the epidural space produces a curtain sign, and invasion of the epidural space produces the epidural tail sign of contrast enhancement. Cranio-caudal spread, including satellite lesions, can be seen once the epidural space has been breached.

Classic chordoma is locally aggressive, but clinical presentation is often delayed because of the low grade and slow growth of these tumors. Distal metastases are seen in 37% of patients, often very late in the presentation [8]. Metastasis is more common in vertebral (30%-40%) than in sacral (10%) or cranial lesions. Management of chordoma involves wide local resection with wide surgical margins and adjuvant radiation therapy. The mean survival is 5.7 years [9]. Prognosis depends on patient age (better prognosis if the patient is <40 years old), site of involvement (better prognosis if the tumor is in the sacrococcygeal region), and tumor size (better prognosis if the tumor is small). Dedifferentiation to a higher-grade tumor may be seen in up to 5% of patients [10] (see below). Recurrence is seen in up to 20% of patients [11], primarily due to the deep location of the tumor in the pelvis and close relationship with vital organs, as a result of which complete resection with wide surgical margins is often not possible. Recurrence, which can be seen as multiple tumor nodules at the resection site, is more effectively detected with MRI than with CT [12]. Radiation is used to reduce the recurrence rate.

Chondroid Chordoma

Chondroid chordoma is a chordoma variant that is characterized by the presence of hyaline cartilaginous elements along with the typical chordoma [13].

Chondroid chordoma accounts for 15% of all chordomas and is more common in the spheno-occipital region. Pathological differential diagnosis for chondroid chordoma includes chondrosarcoma. Both chondroid chordoma and chondrosarcoma express S-100 protein, but chondroid chordoma also expresses EMA, carcinoembryonic antigen (CEA) and cytokeratin and demonstrates brachyury [14]. The imaging features of chondroid chordoma are similar to those of classic chordoma, but chondroid chordoma is associated with lower T1 and higher T2 MRI signal as a result of higher water content [12].

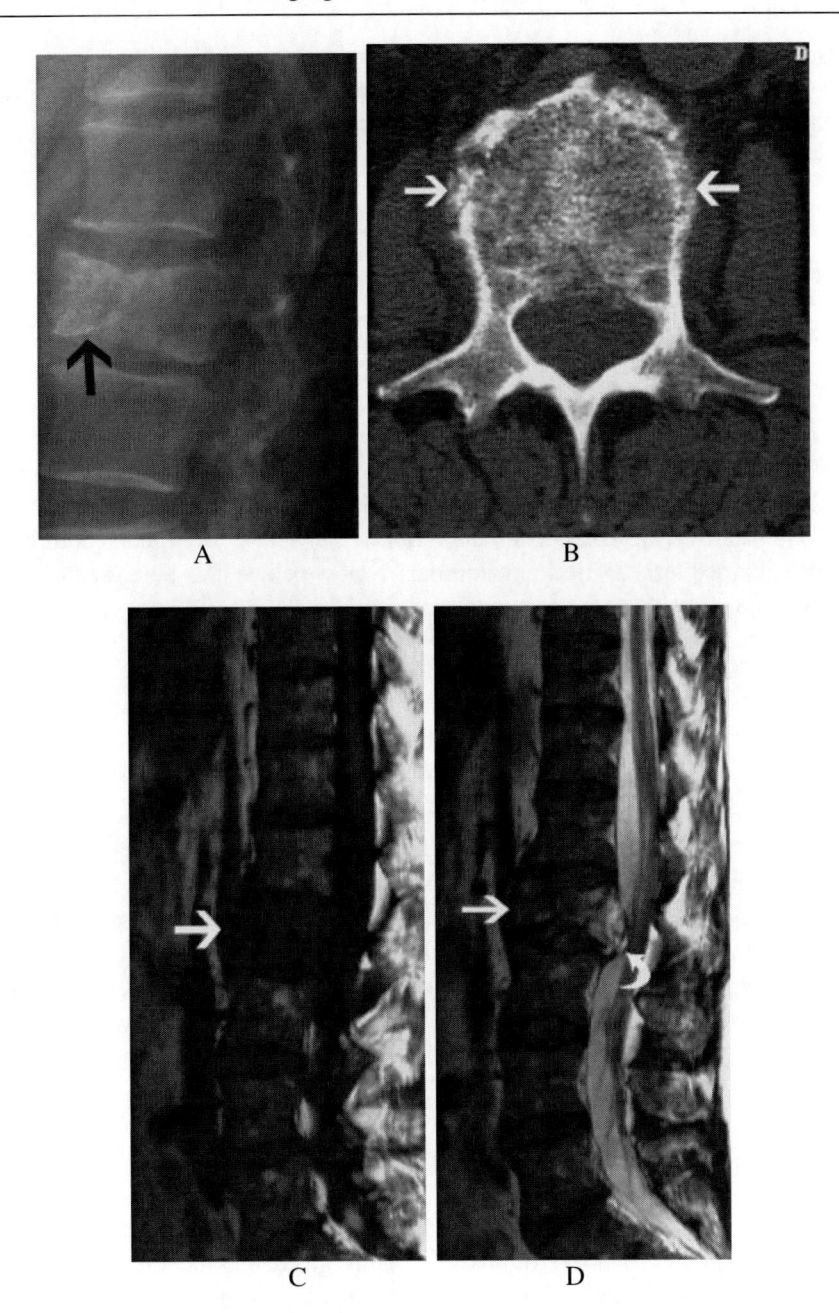

Figure 2. Chordoma in a 73-year-old man. (A) Lateral radiograph shows mixed sclerotic lytic lesion in the L2 vertebra (arrow) with decreased height of the vertebral body (arrow). (B) Axial computed tomography (CT) scan shows mixed lytic-sclerotic lesion in the L2 vertebral body (arrow). (C) Sagittal T1-weighted magnetic resonance (MR) image shows a low signal intensity lesion (arrow) in the L2 vertebral body with a soft tissue component extending posteriorly in the spinal canal. (D) T2-weighted image shows a lesion with heterogeneous high signal (straight arrow) and soft tissue component extending into the spinal canal and indenting on the cauda equine (curved arrow).

Contrast enhancement in chondroid chordoma is heterogeneous, with no lobular and only mildly septal enhancement, compared with lobular, rings and arcs, nodular, or diffuse enhancement in chondrosarcoma. The behavior of the tumor is similar to that of classic chordoma.

Extra-Axial Chordoma

Extra-axial chordoma (also known as chordoma periphericum) is the occurrence of chordoma in the appendicular skeleton. The origin of this tumor is uncertain but may potentially be caused by the presence of ectopic notochordal tissue. The pathology, imaging findings, and behavior of extra-axial chordoma are similar to those of classic chordoma. However, the prognosis with this type of tumor is better than that of classic chordoma, as extra-axial chordoma has an earlier presentation and can be completely resected, as no vital structures are nearby [2]. Extra-axial chordoma is different from parachordoma, which typically does not express CK19. Parachordoma is now believed to be a tumor belonging to the mixed tumor/myoepithelioma group of tumors [2].

Dedifferentiated Chordoma

Dedifferentiated chordoma is characterized by the development of a higher-grade, histogenetically distinct tumor in a pre-existing chordoma. The most common type of dedifferentiated chordoma is high-grade spindle cell/pleomorphic sarcoma.

Dedifferentiation is seen in up to 5% of patients with chordoma [10]. Although this type of tumor can be seen in primary chordoma, dedifferentiation is more commonly seen in recurrences [15] and after radiotherapy. Development of new symptoms and a rapid increase in tumor size should raise suspicion for dedifferentiation. Prognosis depends on the higher-grade element and is usually poor because of the tumor's faster growth rate and distal metastasis.

Benign Notochordal Cell Tumor

BNCT is an intra-osseous benign lesion of notochordal cell origin with clinical and histopathological features distinct from those of chordoma and notochordal rests [16]. BNCT is believed to originate from pre-existing notochordal remnant in the vertebra or from displacement of diskal notochordal remnants through Schmorl's nodes into the vertebral bone marrow, where they proliferate. This type of tumor is more common in men. The mean age of affected patients is 63 years. In an autopsy series, BNCT was more commonly seen in the sacrococcygeal region, followed by the clival, cervical, lumbar, and thoracic regions [16]; in a clinical series, BNCT was more common in the lumbar region than in the cervical, sacral, thoracic, or coccygeal vertebra [17].

Pathologically, BNCT demonstrates intraosseous sheets of chordoid cells with vacuolated cytoplasm and bland nuclei but no mitotic activity. Differential diagnosis for this condition includes fatty marrow and chordoma. Expression of cytokeratins (AE/1, AE/3, CK18), S-100 protein, EMA, and vimentin distinguishes BNCT from fatty marrow but not from chordoma. However, unlike a chordoma, BNCT shows no cortical destruction, trabecular distortion, soft tissue extension, lobulation, or myxoid matrix. There is a sharp transition with normal marrow, with no chronic inflammation at the interface with the uninvolved bone.

BNCT is usually asymptomatic and is often an incidental imaging finding. The lesion presents with variable size. Radiograph (Figure 3a) and scintigraphy (Figure 3b) results are usually normal. Variable degrees of sclerosis may be seen. CT shows subtle sclerosis (Figures 3c, 3d) with no evidence of osteolysis and a sharp zone of transition. No soft tissue mass is seen [18-20].

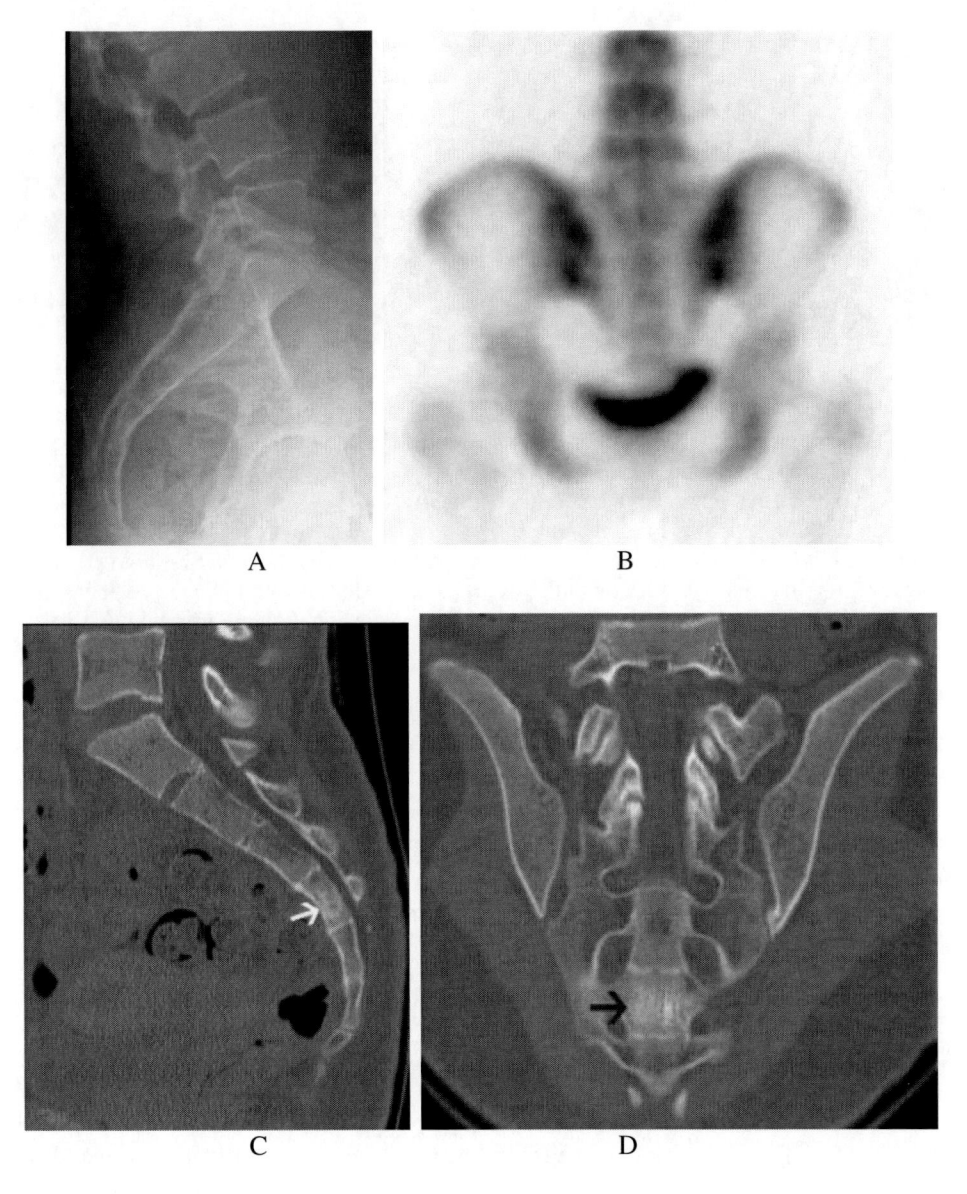

A B

C D

Figure 3. (Continued).

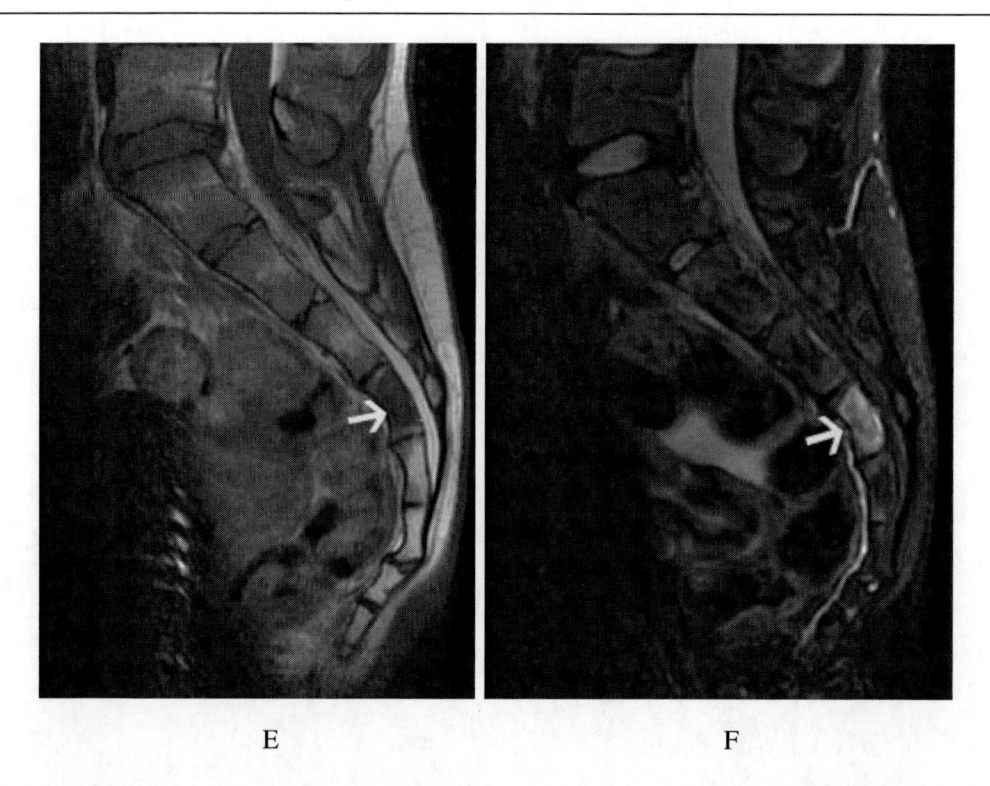

E   F

Figure 3. Benign notochordal cell tumor in a 17-year-old female patient. (A) Lateral radiograph shows a normal-appearing lumbosacral vertebra. (B) 99Tc-methylene diphosphonate (MDP) bone scan shows no abnormal uptake in the pelvis. (C) Sagittal and (D) coronal reconstructed computed tomography (CT) images of the sacral spine show a focal area of sclerosis (arrows) in the S3 vertebra. There is no bone destruction or associated soft tissue. (E) Sagittal T1-weighted magnetic resonance (MR) image shows a lesion with low signal intensity (arrow) in the S3 vertebra. (F) Sagittal short T1 inversion recovery (STIR) image shows a lesion with high signal intensity (arrow) in the S3 vertebra.

MRI shows a sharply demarcated lesion with homogeneous low T1 and high T2 signal (Figures 3e, 3f) without contrast enhancement or soft tissue mass. Pathological features should be correlated with imaging findings to distinguish BNCT from chordoma and to avoid unwarranted surgery, which is inevitably extensive and almost always results in impotence and loss of bladder and rectal functions. On long-term follow-up, these benign tumors do not show progression to chordoma. BNCT does coexist with chordoma in 7.3% of cases [21]. The general consensus is that these lesions should have long-term follow-up with imaging and should be managed expectantly.

Incipient Chordoma

Incipient chordoma has histological features between those of BNCT and chordoma [22]. Pathologically, infiltrative sheets of cells are seen with vacuolated cytoplasm, bland nuclei, and a cord of cells with scanty matrix and delicate fibrous septae. The lesion has no specific clinical or imaging features [22].

CONCLUSION

Rare tumors from notochordal remnants can be seen in the midline of the body in the axial skeleton. Classic chordoma, a low- to intermediate-grade malignancy, is the most common notochordal tumor. The presence of notochordal tissue in a biopsy sample does not necessarily indicate chordoma but could represent BNCT. Correlation of biopsy with imaging features is necessary to accurately diagnose and appropriately manage these tumors.

ACKNOWLEDGMENT

The authors wish to thank Ms. Megan Griffiths, Scientific Writer, Imaging Institute, Cleveland Clinic, for her help in the preparation of this chapter.

REFERENCES

[1]   Crapanzano JP, Ali SZ, Ginsberg MS, Zakowski MF. Chordoma: cytologic study with histologic and radiologic correlation. *Cancer.* 2001;93(1):40-51.

[2]   Tirabosco R, Mangham DC, Rosenberg AE, Vujovic S, Bousdras K, Pizzolitto S, et al. Brachyury expression in extra-axial skeletal and soft tissue chordomas: a marker that distinguishes chordoma from mixed tumor/myoepithelioma/parachordoma in soft tissue. *Am. J. Surg. Pathol.* 2008;32(4):572-80.

[3]   McMaster ML, Goldstein AM, Bromley CM, Ishibe N, Parry DM. Chordoma: incidence and survival patterns in the United States, 1973-1995. *Cancer Causes Control.* 2001;12(1):1-11.

[4]   York JE, Kaczaraj A, Abi-Said D, Fuller GN, Skibber JM, Janjan NA, et al. Sacral chordoma: 40-year experience at a major cancer center. *Neurosurgery.* 1999;44(1): 74-9.

[5]   DeBruine FT, Kroon HM. Spinal chordoma: radiological features in 14 cases. *AJR. Am. J. Roentgenol.* 1988;150(4):861-3.

[6]   Meyer JE, Lepke RA, Lindfors KK, Pagani JJ, Hirschy JC, Hayman LA, et al. Chordomas: their CT appearance in the cervical, thoracic and lumbar spine. *Radiology.* 1984;153(3):693-6.

[7]   Sung MS, Lee GK, Kang HS, Kwon ST, Park JG, Suh JS, et al. Sacrococcygeal chordoma: MR imaging in 30 patients. *Skeletal Radiol.* 2005;34(2):87-94.

[8]   McPherson CM, Suki D, McCutcheon IE, Gokaslan ZL, Rhines LD, Mendel E. Metastatic disease from spinal chordoma: a 10-year experience. *J. Neurosurg. Spine.* 2006;5(4):277-80.

[9]   Cheng EY, Ozerdemoglu RA, Transfeldt EE, Thompson RC Jr. Lumbosacral chordoma: prognostic factors and treatment. *Spine* (Phila Pa 1976). 1999;24(16): 1639-45.

[10]   Al-Adnani M, Cannon SR, Flanagan AM. Chordomas do not express CD10 or renal cell carcinoma (RCC) antigen: an immunohistochemical study. *Histopathology.* 2005;47(5):535-7.

[11] Fuchs B, Dickey ID, Yaszemski MJ, Inwards CY, Sims FH. Operative management of sacral chordoma. *J. Bone Joint Surg. Am.* 2005;87(10):2211-6.

[12] Rosenthal DI, Scott JA, Mankin HJ, Wismer GL, Brady TJ. Sacrococcygeal chordoma: magnetic resonance imaging and computed tomography. *AJR. Am. J. Roentgenol.* 1985;145(1):143-7.

[13] Heffelfinger MJ, Dahlin DC, MacCarty CS, Beabout JW. Chordomas and cartilaginous tumors at the skull base. *Cancer.* 1973;32(2):410-20.

[14] Vujovic S, Henderson S, Presneau N, Odell E, Jacques TS, Tirabosco R, et al. Brachyury, a crucial regulator of notochordal development, is a novel biomarker for chordomas. *J. Pathol.* 2006;209(2):157-65.

[15] Meis JM, Raymond AK, Evans HL, Charles RE, Giraldo AA. "Dedifferentiated" chordoma: a clinicopathologic and immunohistochemical study of three cases. *Am. J. Surg. Pathol.* 1987:11(7):516-25.

[16] Yamaguchi T, Suzuki S, Ishiiwa H, Shimizu K, Ueda Y. Benign notochordal cell tumors: a comparative histological study of benign notochordal cell tumors, classic chordomas, and notochordal vestiges of fetal intervertebral discs. *Am. J. Surg. Pathol.* 2004;28(6):756-61.

[17] Yamaguchi T, Iwata J, Sugihara S, Sugihara S, McCarthy EF Jr, Karita M, et al. Distinguishing benign notochordal cell tumors from vertebral chordoma. *Skeletal Radiol.* 2008;37(4):291-9.

[18] Darby AJ, Cassar-Pullicino VN, McCall IW, Jaffray DC. Vertebral intra-osseous chordoma or giant notochordal rest? *Skeletal Radiol.* 1999;28(6):342-6.

[19] Mirra JM, Brien EW. Giant notochordal hamartoma of intraosseous origin: a newly reported benign entity to be distinguished from chordoma. Report of two cases. *Skeletal Radiol.* 2001;30(12):698-709.

[20] Kyriakos M, Totty WG, Lenke LG. Giant vertebral notochordal rest: a lesion distinct from chordoma: discussion of an evolving concept. *Am. J. Surg. Pathol.* 2003;27(3):396-406.

[21] Deshpande V, Nielsen GP, Rosenthal DI, Rosenberg AE. Intraosseous benign notochord cell tumors (BNCT): further evidence supporting a relationship to chordoma. *Am. J. Surg. Pathol.* 2007;31(10):1573-7.

[22] Yamaguchi T, Wannabe-Ishiiwa H, Suzuki S, Igarashi Y, Ueda Y. Incipient chordoma: a report of two cases of early-stage chordoma arising from benign notochordal cell tumors. *Mod. Pathol.* 2005;18(7):1005-10.

In: Bone Tumors: Symptoms, Diagnosis and Treatment
Editor: Moncef Berhouma
ISBN: 978-1-62618-190-8
© 2013 Nova Science Publishers, Inc.

Chapter 6

AMINOBISPHOSPHONATES AND NANO TECHNOLOGICALLY-MODIFIED AMINOBISPHOSPHONATES: A NEW DAWN IN THE TREATMENT OF BONE AND EXTRA-BONE TUMORS?

Michele Caraglia[1], Gabriella Misso[1] and Daniele Santini[2]
[1]Department of Biochemistry, Biophysics and General Pathology,
Second University of Naples, Naples, Italy
[2]Campus Biomedico University of Rome, Section of Oncology, Rome, Italy

ABSTRACT

Therapy with aminobisphosphonates (ABP) and specifically with zoledronic acid (ZOL) is a standard for patients with malignant bone disease. The present chapter will describe the main results achieved with ABP and ZOL in the treatment of bone metastases from solid tumours including prostate, breast, lung and renal cancer. The possible direct anti-cancer effects of ABP and particularly of ZOL will be also discussed with the description of the effects of ZOL in preventing the occurrence of metastases in breast cancer patients. Although the direct anti-cancer effects of ZOL are widely demonstrated in preclinical setting, the clear evidence of a clinical activity of ZOL is still far from being achieved. ZOL blocks protein isoprenylation, a pleiotropic and basic biochemical processes within the cells regulating the activity of several proteins involved in survival and proliferating pathways. The challenge in demonstrating the clinical activity of ZOL is mainly based on its pharmacokinetic properties that limit its distribution in tumour tissues and prevalently allow its accumulation in bone tissue in osteolytic areas and consequently in osteoclasts. Emerging data suggest that the encapsulation of ABP in nanodevices could allow their delivery in tumour tissues and could increase the accumulation of the drug also in the "tumour niche" in bone tissue compromised by cancer metastases. In conclusion, ABP and ZOL have still underestimated anti-cancer properties that could be completely exploited though their pharmacological modification and encapsulation in appropriate nanodevices.

INTRODUCTION

Bisphosphonates (BPs) are synthetic analogues of naturally occurring pyrophosphate compounds that inhibit calcification. They represent the treatment of choice for different diseases affecting bone,such as metabolic bone disease, osteoporosis, Paget's disease and bone metastases. Calcium phosphate, in the form of calcium hydroxyapatite, is the main constituent of the skeletal system.Inorganic pyrophosphate (PPi) can inhibit the precipitation of calciumcarbonate, thus inhibiting the transformation of amorphous calcium phosphate into its crystalline form [1]. It had been known since the 1930s that trace amounts of pyrophosphate were capable of acting as water softeners by inhibiting the crystallization of calcium salts, such as calcium carbonate [2]. In the 1960s Fleisch et al. showed that inorganic pyrophosphate, a naturally occurring polyphosphate and a known product of many biosynthetic reactions in the body, was present in serum and urine and could prevent calcification by binding to newly forming crystals of hydroxyapatite [3]. It was proposed that inorganic pyrophosphate might be the body's own natural "water softener" that normally prevents calcification of soft tissues and regulates bone mineralization [3]. It subsequently became clear that calcification disorders might be linked to disturbances in PPi metabolism. The first example was an inherited disorder, hypophosphatasia, in which lack of alkaline phosphatase is associated with mineralization defects of the skeleton and elevated PPi levels, indicating that alkaline phosphatase might be the key extracellular enzyme responsible for hydrolyzing pyrophosphate [3]. Alkaline phosphatase present in bone destroy pyrophosphate locally, thereby allowing a morphous phase calcium phosphate to crystallize and inducing mineralisation of bone [3].Orally administered pyrophosphate was inactive because of its hydrolysis in the gastrointestinal tract. During the search for more stable analogues of pyrophosphate that might also have the antimineralization properties of pyrophosphate but would be resistant to hydrolysis, several different chemical classes were studied. The bisphosphonates (at that time called diphosphonates), characterized by P-C-P motifs, were among these classes [1]. The fundamental property of BPs, which has been exploited by industry and medicine, is their ability to form bonds with crystal surfaces and to form complexes with cations in solution or at a solid–liquid interface.Since BPsare synthetic analogues of pyrophosphates, they have the same chemical activity, but greater stability [1]. Like pyrophosphate, BPs had high affinity for bone mineral and they were found to prevent calcification both *in vitro* and *in vivo* but, unlike pyrophosphate, they were also able to prevent experimentally induced pathologic calcification when given orally to rats *in vivo*. This property of being active by mouth was key to their subsequent use in humans. Perhaps the most important step toward the successive use of BPs occurred when it was attributed them the new property, already shown for PPi, of being able to inhibit the dissolution of hydroxyapatite crystals. This finding led to following studies designed to determine if they might also inhibit bone resorption [2].

Once evidenced this new property, BPs remained the most widely used and effective antiresorptive agents for the treatment of diseases in which there was an increase in the number or activity of osteoclasts, including tumor-associated osteolysis and hypercalcemia [4].After more than three decades of research, first-, second- and third-generation bisphosphonates have been developed. Changes in chemical structure have resulted in increased potency, without demineralisation of bone [1].

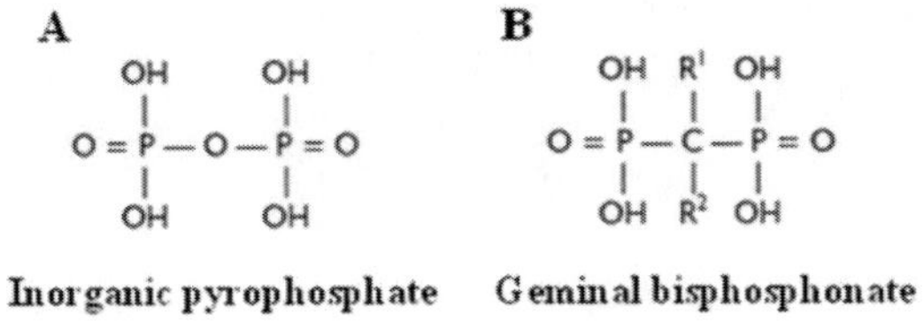

Figure 1. Structures (**A**) and (**B**) show the basic structures of inorganic pyrophosphate and germinal bisphosphonate, respectively, where R1 and R2 represent different side-chains for each bisphosphonate.

There is now a growing body of evidence regarding the efficacy of these drugs in clinical settings.All BPs that act significantly on the skeleton are characterized, as stated above,by P–C–P bond (Figure 1A), in contrast to pyrophosphate,which has a P–O–P bond (Figure 1B).

This peculiarity confers stability both to heat and to most chemical reagents and is one of the most important properties of these compounds. Extensive chemical research programmes have produced a wide range of molecules with various substituents attached to the carbon atom. Variations in potency andin the ability of the compounds to bind to crystals in bone is determined by the chemical and three-dimensional structure of the two side chains, R_1 andR_2, attached to the central, geminal carbon atom [1].

The addition of a hydroxyl (OH)or primary amino (NH_2) group increases the affinity for calcium ions, resulting in preferential localisation of these drugs to sites of bone remodelling. Increasing the number of carbonatoms in the side-chain (i.e. the length) initially increase and then decrease the magnitude of the effect on bone resorption [1]. The early compounds, clodronate (CLO) and etidronate (ETI), contained simple substituents (H, OH, Cl, CH3) and lacked a nitrogen atom (Figure 2).

Subsequently, more complex and potent compounds were produced by the insertion of a primary, secondary or tertiary nitrogen function in the R_2 side chain, for example, pamidronate (PAM), alendronate (ALN), ibandronate (IBA) and incadronate (INC), which have an alkyl R_2 sidechain, or risedronate (RIS), zoledronate(ZOL) and minodronate (MIN), which have heterocyclic rings in the R_2 side chain (Figure 2). Variation of the substituents modulates the pharmacologic properties and gives each molecule its unique profile [5].The most active compound in this class, ZOL, which is up to 10,000-fold more potent than both CLO and ETI in some experimental systems (Figure 3), contains animidazole ring. Extensive structure/activity studies have resulted in several very useful drugs that combine potent inhibition of osteoclastic bone resorption with good clinical tolerability [2]. The pronounced selectivity of BPs for bone rather than other tissues is the basis for their value in clinical practice. Their preferential uptake by and adsorption to mineral surfaces in bone bring them into close contact with osteoclasts. During bone resorption, BPs are probably internalized by endocytosis along with other products of resorption. Many studies have shown that BPs can affect osteoclast-mediated bone resorption in a variety of ways, including effects on osteoclast recruitment, differentiation, and resorptive activity, and may induce apoptosis.

Because mature, multinucleated osteoclasts are formed by the fusion of mononuclear precursors of hematopoietic origin, BPs could also inhibit bone resorption by preventing osteoclast formation, in addition to affecting mature osteoclasts. *In vitro*, BPs can inhibit dose-dependently the formation of osteoclast-like cells in long-term cultures of human bone marrow. In organ culture, also, some BPs can inhibit the generation of mature osteoclasts, possibly by preventing the fusion of osteoclast precursors [2].

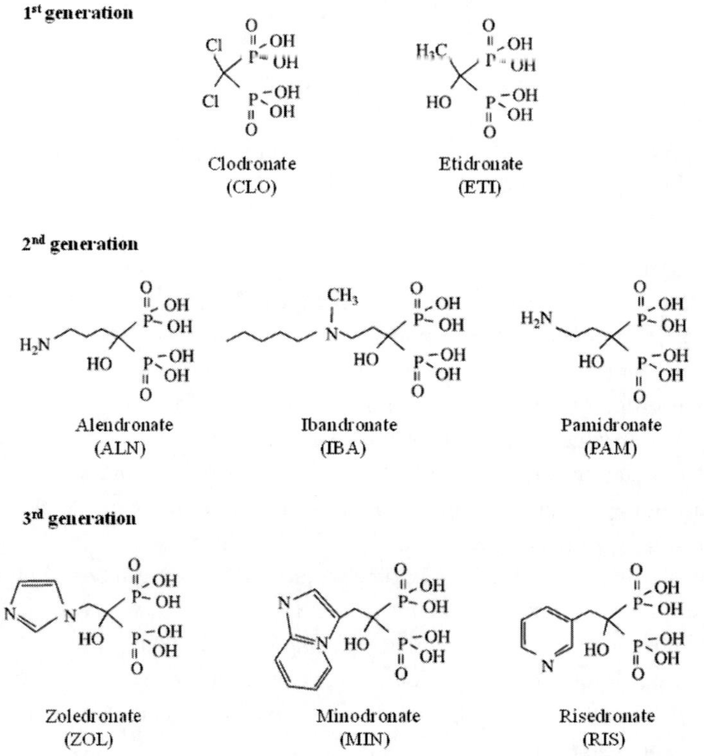

Figure 2. Structures of simple bisphosphonates (1st generation), N-BPs with primary, secondary or tertiary nitrogen function in the R_2alkyl side chain (2nd generation) and N-BPs with heterocyclic rings in the R_2 side chain (3rd generation).

In contrast to their ability to induce apoptosis in osteoclasts, which contributes to the inhibition of resorptive activity, some experimental studies suggest that BPs may protect osteocytes and osteoblasts from apoptosis induced by glucocorticoids [6].

The antiresorptive effect cannot be accounted simply by adsorption of BPs to bone mineral and prevention of hydroxyapatite dissolution. It became clear that BPs must inhibit bone resorption by cellular effects on osteoclasts rather than simply by physicochemical mechanisms [2].

Since the early 1990s there has been a systematic effort to elucidate the molecular mechanisms of action of BPs and, not surprisingly, it has been found that they could be divided into 2 structural subgroups [7;8].

The first group comprises the non–nitrogen-containing bisphosphonates that perhaps most closely resemble pyrophosphate, such as CLO and ETI, and these can be metabolically incorporated into nonhydrolyzable analogues of adenosine triphosphate (ATP) -methylene-containing (AppCp) nucleotides - by reversing the reactions of aminoacyl–transfer RNA synthetases [9]. The resulting metabolites contain the P-C-P moiety in place of the β,γ-phosphate groups of ATP[10]. Intracellular accumulation of these metabolites within osteoclasts inhibits their function and may cause osteoclast cell death, most likely by inhibiting ATP-dependent enzymes, such as the adenine nucleotide translocase, a component of the mitochondrial permeability transition pore [11].

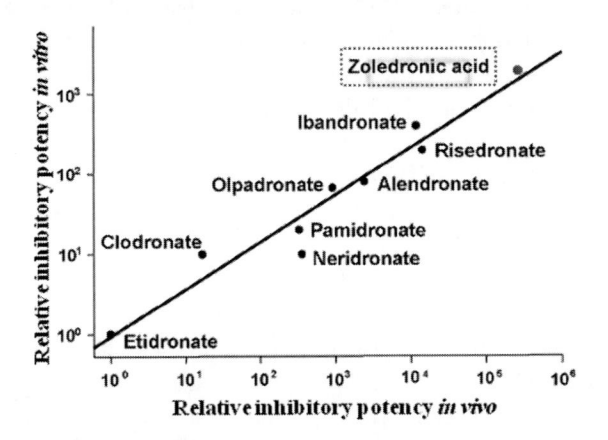

Figure 3. *In vivo* potency of bisphosphonates correlates with *in vitro* potency. Differences in structure of the bisphosphonates have strong influence on the potency.

Induction of osteoclast apoptosis seems to be the primary mechanism by which the simple BPs inhibit bone resorption, since the ability of CLO and ETI to inhibit resorption *in vitro* can be overcome when osteoclast apoptosis is prevented using a caspase inhibitor [12].

In contrast the second group, comprising the nitrogen-containing bisphosphonates (N-BPs), which are several orders of magnitude more potent at inhibiting bone resorption *in vivo* than the simple bisphosphonates, is not metabolized to toxic analogues of ATP [13]. N-BPs act by inhibiting farnesyl diphosphate (FPP) synthase, a key enzyme of the mevalonate pathway (Figure 4). This enzyme is inhibited by nanomolar concentrations of N-BPs. ZOL and the structurally similar MIN are extremely potent inhibitors of FPP synthase [4] and inhibit the enzyme even at picomolar concentrations. Importantly, studies with recombinant human FPP synthase revealed that minor modifications to the structure and conformation of the R_2 side chain that are known to affect antiresorptive potency also affect the ability to inhibit FPP synthase.

These studies strongly suggest that FPP synthase is the major pharmacologic target of N-BPs in osteoclasts *in vivo* and help to explain the relationship between bisphosphonate structure and antiresorptive potency [4].Clinical and experimental evidence indicates that N-BPs suppress the progression of bone metastases, and recent observations suggest that this effect may be independent of the inhibition of bone resorption [14]. Tumour progression and metastasis formation are critically dependent on tumour angiogenesis [15]. Anti-angiogenic treatments suppress tumour progression in animal models, and many anti-angiogenic substances are currently being tested in clinical trials for their therapeutic efficacy against human cancer [16].Recent research indicates that ZOL possesses anti-angiogenic activities [17].

The exact mechanism by which N-BPs inhibit FPP synthase is only just becoming clear. The recent generation of X-ray crystal structures of the human FPP synthase enzyme, cocrystallized with RIS or ZOL [18], revealed that N-BPs bind the geranyl diphosphate (GPP) binding site of the enzyme, with stabilizing interactions occurring between the nitrogen moiety of the N-BP and a conserved threonine and lysine residue in the enzyme. Enzyme kinetic analysis with human FPP synthase indicates that the interaction with N-BPs is highly complexand characteristic of "slow tight binding" inhibition [18].By inhibiting FPP synthase, N-BPs prevent the synthesis of FPP and its downstream metabolite geranylgeranyl diphosphate. These isoprenoid lipids are the building blocks for the production of a variety of metabolites, such as dolichol and ubiquinone, but are also required for post-translational modification (prenylation) of proteins, including small GTPases.

The loss of synthesis of FPP and geranylgeranyl diphosphate therefore prevents the prenylation, at a cysteine residue in characteristic C-terminal motifs, of small GTPases, such as Ras, Rab, Rho, and Rac (Figure 4). Small GTPases are important signaling proteins that regulate a variety of cell processes important for osteoclast function, including cell morphology, cytoskeletal arrangement, membrane ruffling, trafficking of vesicles, and apoptosis. Prenylation is required for the correct function of these proteins because the lipid prenyl group serves to anchor the proteins in cell membranes and may also participate in protein-protein interactions [2;17].

Recent evidence suggests that ZOL is a potent inducers of apoptosis in several cancer cell types [19].It has recently been demonstrated in vitro that N-BPs, PAM and ZOL, induce apoptosis and growth inhibition in human epidermoid cancer cells, together with depression of Ras-dependent Erk and Akt survival pathways. These effects occurred together with poly (ADP ribose) polymerase (PARP) fragmentation and the activation of caspase 3 [20]. Moreover, the latter seems to be essential for apoptosis induced by N-BPs in this experimental model. Furthermore, it was reported that ZOL induced growth inhibition on both androgen-dependent LnCaP and androgen-independent PC3 prostate cancer cell lines with G1 accumulation.

Recent studies showed that the effects of ZOL were caspase-dependent. In human breast cancer cell lines ZOL induced a modulating expression of Bcl-2 and subsequent caspase-3 activation. These events might be precipitated by inhibition of Ras activation, which requires protein farnesylation [21]. In human colon carcinoma HCT-116 cells ZOL strongly inhibited the proliferation paralleled by a G1 cell cycle accumulation and induction of apoptosis via a caspase-dependent mechanism [22]. Recent studies by Fujita et al. demonstrated the involvement of the mevalonate pathway in the antiproliferative and pro-apoptotic effects of ZOL on ACHN renal cell carcinoma cells [23]. Several in vitro studies have shown that, by inhibiting protein prenylation and Ras signalling, ZOL inhibits adhesion of tumour cells to extracellular matrix proteins, thereby impairing the process of tumour-cell invasion and metastasis [24]. ZOL has also been shown to have anti-angiogenic properties both in vitro and in vivo [25].

Differences in structure of the bisphosphonates have strong influence on their potency (Figure 3) and induce substantial biological and clinical implications. Presently, ZOL is considered the most potent N-BP, and is clinically available in the treatment of skeletal complications secondary to bone metastases derived from different solid tumours including hormone-refractory prostate cancer (HRPC), breast cancer (BC), lung cancer (LC) and renal cell carcinoma (RCC).

CLINICAL RESULTS OF ABPS AND ZOL IN PREVENTING SKELETAL RELATED EVENTS

The skeleton is the most common organ to be affected by metastases arising from breast, prostate, thyroid, lung, and kidney cancer.

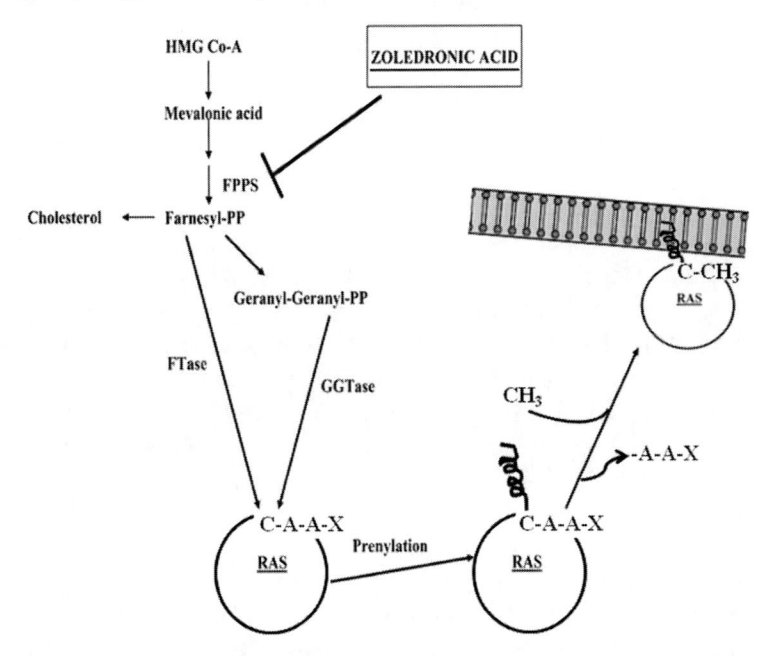

Figure 4. Isoprenoids are synthesized from the mevalonate pathway that starts from reaction catalyzed by the 3-hydroxy-3-methylglutaryl CoA(HMGCoA) reductase (the rate-limiting reaction in cholesterol biosynthesis) that catalyzes the conversion of HMGCoA to mevalonic acid.The pathway triggered by this reaction can lead to the synthesis of a key isoprenoid molecule, the farnesyl-pyrophosphate (Farnesyl-PP) whose formation is catalyzed by the farnesyl-pyrophosphate synthase (FPPS). Farnesyl-PP can be either converted by a series of reactions incholesterol or can be transferred on target cellular proteins as Farnesyl-PP itself (reaction catalyzed by farnesyltransferase, FTase) or firstlyconverted in geranyl-geranyl-pyrophosphate (Geranyl-Geranyl-PP) and then transferred on cellular proteins by type I or type II geranylgeranyl-transferases (GGTase).FTase and GGTase-I catalyze the prenylation of substrates with a carboxy-terminal tetrapeptide sequence called a CAAX box; where C refers to cysteine, A refers to an aliphatic residue and X typically refers tomethionine, serine, alanine or glutamine for FTase or to leucine for GGTase-I. Following prenylation of physiological substrates,the terminal three residues (AAX) are subsequently removed by a CAAX endoprotease and the carboxyl group of the terminal cysteine is methyl esterified by a methyl transferase. Thereafter,prenyl substrates, such as Ras, are ready to be located on the inner side of the biological membranes to receive signals mediated by external factors. ZOL specifically inhibits the FPPS activity required for the synthesis of farnesyl and geranylgeranyllipidic residues blocking prenylation of Ras that regulate the proliferation, invasive properties and pro-angiogenic activity of human tumour cells.

About 75% of patients affected by breast and prostate cancer with advanced metastatic disease present bone metastases. These patients have a relatively long median survival - of 2-3 years -after diagnosis of bone metastases, compared with patients with other cancers (e.g., lung and renal cancer), resulting in a high prevalence of bone metastases [26]. Anyhow, patients with disease that remains confined to the skeleton have a better prognosis than those with subsequent visceral involvement [27]. Metastatic bone disease causes substantial morbidity among cancer patients. In these patients, the decline in quality of life (QoL) and eventual death is due almost entirely to skeletal complications and their subsequent treatment. Complications from bone metastases include pathological fracture, hypercalcaemia, nerve root compression, spinal cord compression, bone marrow infiltration, pain, and reduced mobility [28]. Breast carcinoma, the most prevalent malignancy, causes the greatest morbidity, however pathologic fractures are relatively late complications of bone involvement. For patients with breast carcinoma, good prognostic factors for survival after the development of bone metastases are good histologic grade, positive estrogen receptor status, bone disease at initial presentation, a long disease free interval, and increasing age. For patients with prostate carcinoma, adverse prognostic features include poor performance status, involvement of the appendicular skeleton and visceral involvement, whereas for patients with multiple myeloma, the levels of serum β2-microglobulin and lactate dehydrogenase and the immunologic phenotype are the most important factors. Hypercalcemia occurs in 5-10% of all patients with advanced cancer but is most common in patients with breast carcinoma, multiple myeloma, and squamous carcinomas of the lung and other primary sites. Recent evidence suggests that pain caused by bone metastasis may also be related to the rate of bone resorption [27]. Patients with metastatic bone disease continue to represent a major therapeutic challenge for the clinician. Although there are many therapeutic options for the treatment of such complications, none is completely satisfactory, even when used in combination [28]. Of great clinical importance is the observation that metastatic bone disease may remain confined to the skeleton [27].

Several scientific evidence attesting the role of N-BPs in reducing both bone resorption and bone formation, has led to the development of N-BPs therapies, thereby reducing the risk of skeletal complications in patients with bone metastases. Consequently, N-BPs have become the standard treatment for tumor-induced bone disease. In clinical trials, therapy with N-BPs is associated mainly with mild to moderate adverse events, while severe adverse events are rare. In fact, ZOL induces a clinical benefit and improves the QoL of patients with bone metastases. Moreover, the occurrence of bone clinical response is often related to a reduced risk of skeletal related events (SRE) [29;30].

A recent study, which is part of an overall ZOL clinical trial program culminating in larger phase III trials in cancer patients with metastatic bone disease, evaluate the dose–response relation for 2.0–4.0 mg ZOL given as a 5 minute infusion, comparing it to a 2 hours 90 mg PAM infusion in patients with malignant osteolytic disease [31]. Both ZOL and PAM, at the previously indicated doses, significantly reduced the need for radiation therapy to bone (p = 0.05). SREs of any kind, pathologic fractures, and hypercalcemia also occurred less frequently in patients treated with a single infusion of 4.0 mg ZOL than a single 90 mg PAM infusion Increases in lumbar spine bone mineral density (6.2–9.6%) and decreases in the bone resorption marker N-telopeptide (range, 237.1 to 260.8%) were observed for all treatment groups. Both ZOL and PAM were well tolerated [31].

A phase I trial in patients with bone metastases demonstrated that a single short infusion of ZOL was safe and well tolerated at doses up to 16 mg [32]. Another phase I study studied the effects of ZOL in 58 patients with malignant osteolysis evaluated doses of 0.1 to 8.0 mg given every 4 weeks for 3 dosages. Doses of 2.0–8.0 mg effectively suppressed urinary bone markers in a dose-dependent manner within the first 4 weeks after treatment, with sustained inhibition at 12 weeks [33]. The consistent results obtained with ZOL in these trials indicated that longer term use of ZOL would be effective in minimizing bone loss and reducing skeletal complications in patients with metastatic bone disease.

For lung cancer in particular, ZOL is the only BP that has been extensively studied and that has gained regulatory approval based on the results of large pivotal trials. The efficacy of ZOL for the treatment of bone metastases in patients with lung cancer was demonstrated in a large, randomized, placebo-controlled trial in which a total of 773 patients received ZOL (4 mg or 8 mg) or placebo via a 15 min infusion every 3 weeks for 21 months. Fewer patients treated with ZOL developed at least 1 SRE compared with patients treated with placebo (39% of those treated at the 4-mg dose and 36% of those treated at the 8 mg dose, compared with 46% of those treated with placebo). Furthermore, 4 mg of ZOL significantly delayed the median time to first SRE (236 days with 4 mg vs. 155 days with placebo) and significantly reduced the annual incidence of SREs (1.74 per year with the 4-mg dose vs. 2.71 per year with placebo). Moreover, the 4 mg dose of ZOL was found to reduce the risk of developing a skeletal event by 31% (hazard ratio of 0.693). ZOL was also well tolerated in long-term use [34].

Recent trials demonstrate the need for early diagnosis and treatment with BPs for preventing skeletal morbidity in lung cancer patients with bone metastases. In patients with non-small cell lung cancer (NSCLC) and other solid tumors (n=773), ZOL (4 mg via 15 min infusion every 3 weeks) delayed the median time to first SRE by >80 days compared with placebo (p=0.009). Moreover, ZOL significantly reduced the ongoing risk of SREs by 32% versus placebo (p=0.016). Early therapies with ZOL resulted essential for delay the onset of potentially debilitating SREs and preserve patients' QoL [35].

The use of ZOL as a valid weapon in the treatment of skeletal localization of tumour disease was also demonstrated by Facchini et al.Patients with bone metastases from breast and lung cancer were enrolled in order to evaluate the impact of the addition of BP therapy to standard treatments in terms of pain control, QoL and toxicity and to evaluate any relations between clinical activity and the occurrence of SREs [30]. A total of 60 patients were included in the study. Median age was 76 years (range 40-83). The majority of patients were treated with chemotherapy or hormonal therapy. All patients received ZOL (4 mg) every 3-4 weeks for at least 3 cycles. No significant improvement in Performance Status of patients after 12 cycles of ZOL (p = 0.1672) was recorded. A statistically significant early and long-lasting amelioration of both pain, narcotic scores and QoL was found. Twenty-one patients (48%) experienced at least one SRE during the study. The most common SRE was radiation to bone (30% of patients). An inverse correlation between bone tumour response and SREs was also found (p = 0.019) [30].

Based on data from a Phase III, randomized trial, Rosen et al. compared a treatment with a dose of 4 mg or 8 mg of ZOL with 90 mg of PAM in 1,130 breast carcinoma patients who had all types of bone metastases (osteolytic, mixed, or osteoblastic by radiology). Among all patients with breast carcinoma, the proportion of those who had a SRE was comparable between treatment groups (43% of patients who received 4 mg of ZOL vs. 45% of patients who received PAM). Among patients who had breast carcinoma with at least 1 osteolytic lesion (528 patients), the proportion with SRE during the 13 months of the trial was similar between treatment groups (43% in the 4-mg ZOL group, 45% in the 8 mg ZOL group, and 45% in the PAM group), but this did not reach statistical significance (p = 0.058). Among patients with lytic lesions, ZOL demonstrated a statistically significant clinical benefit compared with PAM in several protocol-specified secondary efficacy analyses; treatment with 4 mg of ZOL significantly prolonged the time to first SRE compared with PAM (median, 310 vs. 174 days; p = 0.013)and was comparable to PAM in the nonlytic subgroup. Moreover, multiple-event analysis demonstrated significant further reductions in the risk of developing SREs over the reduction achieved with PAM (30% in the osteolytic subset [p = 0.010] and 20% for all patients with breast carcinoma [p = 0.037]) [36].

One of the best clinical trials studied 600 patients with bone metastasis resulting from advanced prostate cancer [37]. Patients treated with ZOL had a significant reduction in the number of SRE (pathological fractures: vertebral or nonvertebral) and an alleviation in bone pain. All these were achieved with a minimum of toxicity compared with placebo. The patients received doses of 4 mg iv every 4 weeks [38]. In a placebo-controlled randomized clinical trial, Saad et al evaluated also the long-term role of ZOL in the prevention of skeletal events in metastatic prostate cancer patients [37]. ZOL (4 mg via a 15 minute infusion every 3 weeks for 15 months) reduced the incidence of SREs in men with hormone-refractory metastatic prostate cancer. Among 122 patients who completed a total of 24 months on study, fewer patients in the 4 mg ZOL group than in the placebo group had at least one SRE (38% versus 49%, difference = -11.0%, 95% confidence interval [CI] = -20.2% to -1.3%; p = 0.028), and the annual incidence of SREs was 0.77 for the 4 mg ZOL group versus 1.47 for the placebo group (p = 0.005). The median time to the first SRE was 488 days for the 4 mg ZOL group versus 321 days for the placebo group (p = 0.009). Compared with placebo, 4 mg of ZOL reduced the ongoing risk of SREs by 36% (risk ratio = 0.64, 95% CI = 0.485 to 0.845; p = 0.002). Therefore it was concluded that long-term treatment with 4 mg of ZOL was safe and provided sustained clinical benefits for men with metastatic hormone-refractory prostate cancer [37].

Confirming and complementing the study of Saad et al., a multi-centered observational study evaluated the efficacy of ZOL for improving pain and mobility, and preventing SRE (fracture, spinal compression, pain-relieving radiotherapy), in patients with prostate cancer and bone metastases [39].Males (n = 218) with prostate cancer and bone metastases undergoing oncologic therapy received ZOL (4 mg iv/month) for 6 months.There was a measurable statistically significant reduction in pain at rest and on movement as well as an improvement in the quality of life compared with baseline. Best results were obtained with early treatment. Overall incidence of bone events was 11.2%. Of the 212 patients (97.2%) evaluable for safety, 16% suffered adverse events and 66% expressed satisfaction with the treatment. ZOL was then effective for reducing pain, improving mobility, and increasing the QoL in patients with prostate cancer with bone metastasis [39]. Its easy administration and good tolerability made ZOL one of the principal therapeutic tools in the management of patients with pain associated with bone metastasis from prostate cancer.As has been cited by various authors [40;41;42;37], the use of BPs in patients with bone metastases from prostate cancer has two main objectives: to reduce pain and to help avoid bone fractures and adverse skeletal events. Skeletal lesions appear more frequently with the hormonal treatment employed in these patients because of the resultant loss in bone mass which, in addition to the metastasis, makes fractures more likely [43]. The low frequency of adverse effects (fever, arthralgia, constipation) and good tolerability observed with ZOL appeared not too different from that observed with other BPs, particularly that of PAM, and with less severe side-effectsat the pharmacologically efficacious dose of 4 mg iv a month [39].

Skeletal metastases occur also in around one third of patients with advanced or metastatic renal cell carcinoma (RCC), however, compared with bone metastases in breast and prostate cancer, there is a paucity of data relating to the demographics of bone metastases in RCC and their *sequelae* in terms of SREs and survival. A retrospective analysis of patients with RCC enrolled in a multicenter, randomized, placebo-controlled study of ZOL demonstrated its significant clinical benefit in patients with bone metastases [44]. Patients (n=74) received ZOL (4 or 8 mg as a 15-minute infusion) or placebo with concomitant antineoplastic therapy every 3 weeks for 9 months. ZOL was found to significantly reduce the proportion of patients with an SRE (37% vs. 74% for placebo; p = 0.015). Similarly, ZOL significantly reduced the mean skeletal morbidity rate (2.68 vs. 3.38 for placebo; p = 0.014) and extended the time to the first event (median not reached vs. 72 days for placebo; p = 0.006). A multiple event analysis demonstrated that the risk of developing an SRE was reduced by 61% compared with placebo (hazard ratio of 0.394; p = 0.008). The median time to progression of bone lesions was significantly longer for patients who were treated with ZOL (p = 0.014 vs. placebo). ZOL appeared also to be well tolerated [44].

One goal of N-BPs therapy in metastatic cancer is to keep patients functional and mobile for as long as possible, thus preserving their QoL and delaying its deterioration. Reduction and postponement of SRE is essential for this purpose.Controlled clinical studies have shown N-BPs therapy, apart from its benefits in terms of skeletal morbidity, to reduce bone pain including opioid-resistant pain, and over the course of progressive disease to maintain it at lower levels compared with controls [45].

PRELIMINARY EVIDENCE OF DIRECT CLINICAL ANTI-CANCER ACTIVITY OF ZOL

In addition to the established use of N-BPs to preserve skeletal integrity, emerging preclinical and clinical evidence supports their anticancer activity. N-BPs may target several steps involved in the metastatic process, extracellular matrix, extravasation into distant tissues, angiogenesis and avoidance of immune surveillance [46]. Among BPs recent advances suggest that ZOL, beyond the strongest activity of anti-bone resorption, has direct anti-cancer effects. In fact, extensive *in vitro* and *in vivo* preclinical studies support that ZOL displays an antitumor activity, including direct antitumor effects (*in vitro* and animal models) such as inhibition of tumor cell adhesion to mineralized bone, invasion and proliferation and induction of tumor cell apoptosis [47]; effects on the metastatic process (animal models)[48]; effects on angiogenesis (*in vitro*, animal models and in humans) probably due to the modification of various angiogenic properties of endothelial cells [49]; stimulation of γ/δ T lymphocytes (*in vitro* and in humans) which play important roles in innate immunity against cancer [50]. One of the crucial mechanisms responsible for the antitumor activity of ZOL is the induction of tumor cell apoptosis. Chemical and biological characteristics of ZOL indicate the potential for *in vivo* growth inhibition and the mechanisms responsible for the observed anti-cancer effects are beginning to be elucidated [51].

In the preclinical setting ZOL has demonstrated synergistic anticancer activity when used in combination with a variety of anticancer agents including chemotherapeutic drugs, molecular targeted agents, and other biological agents, and clinical investigations to further explore this synergy are ongoing [46]. The preclinical data provide, in fact, a solid rationale that ZOL might prevent disease progression. Based on these potential anti-cancer properties, several clinical trials have been initiated to test the combination of ZOL and other agents. The accumulated encouraging evidence to date indicates that ZOL is an attractive anti-cancer agent that promises to be the next exciting therapy for patients with various cancers.

The first preliminary retrospective analysis on survival rate has been carried out on a subset of patients with multiple myeloma included in a prospective phase III randomized, controlled trial comparing the effect of ZOL with PAM [52]. Patients were stratified by baseline bone alkaline phosphatase (BALP) levels. The (OS) rate at 25 months was significantly higher in patients treated with ZOL compared with PAM (76% versus 63%; p = 0.038). Among patients with low baseline BALP level, the survival rates were similar for both treatment groups. However, among patients with a high baseline BALP level, ZOL treatment significantly improved survival compared with PAM (82% versus 55%; p = 0.048). It was interesting to observe that the highest impact on risk of death concerned a subset of patients (high BALP) with worse prognosis. This finding could indicate that tumors characterized by low sensibility to standard therapy were more responsive to ZOL therapy [52]. This represents the first evidence in literature demonstrating a positive impact on survival of BPs therapy in cancer patients. Moreover, although preliminary, the positive effect on survival was confirmed in a retrospective analysis of a phase III trial of ZOL in patients with bone metastasis from lung cancer and high baseline N-telopeptide levels (NTX) [53]. The results showed that the relative risk ratio was significantly reduced (35%) in patients who received ZOL compared with those received placebo. The relative risk ratios of death for patients who had both high baseline NTX and BALP levels were also significantly reduced (46%) in patients who received ZOL compared with placebo. No differences were detected comparing patients with normal BALP levels [53]. These findings suggest that treatment with ZOL may improve survival compared with placebo in patients with lung cancer who have high levels of bone metabolism. Another even if preliminary, retrospective analysis evaluated the reduced risk of disease progression in a subset of breast cancer patients with bone metastases treated with ZOL and compared with PAM [54]. The results supported a reduced risk of overall disease progression (24%, hazard ratio = 0.760; p = 0.021) in patients who developed bone metastasis more than 3 years from initial diagnosis [54].

A recent study examines the clinical impact of ZOL on lung cancer patients with bone metastases focusing on the survival and time to progression [55]. Patients (n= 144) were divided into 2 groups according to their bone pain symptoms. Eighty-seven of 144 (Group A) experienced bone pain and the remaining 57 (Group B) were asymptomatic. Patients belonging to group A received ZOL, 4 mg i.v. every 21 days, whereas the other 57 patients (Group B) did not received ZOL. All patients were treated with a combination chemotherapy consisting of docetaxel 100 mg/m^2 and carboplatin AUC = 6. It was found that Group A had a statistically significant longer survival when compared to Group B (578 days vs 384 days; p < 0.01). Median time to progression was 265 days for group A and was statistically significant higher in comparison to 150 days for Group B (p < 0.001). A statistically significant positive correlation was found between the number of cycles of therapy with ZOL and total patient survival (p < 0.01, Pearson correlation) and time to progression (p < 0.01). NTX levels in group A reduced from 447.29 before treatment in 204.85 after 3 months and was preserved, with little fluctuations, stable till the 12th month after the beginning of therapy [55]. The results of this suggested that the addition of ZOL increased in lung cancer patients with bone metastases. The longer was the period of receiving ZOL, the better was the effect on survival and time to progression.

Early clinical data show that ZOL can improve clinical outcomes in patients with prostate cancer. In a phase I clinical trial, 22 patients with castration-resistant prostate cancer and bone metastases received increasing doses of docetaxel (30, 40 and 50 mg/m every 14 days) in combination with a constant dose of ZOL (2 mg every 14 days) for a median of 6 cycles (12 weeks). Patients received either docetaxel first followed by ZOL the next day (sequence A, n= 10) or ZOL first followed by docetaxel the next day (sequence B, n= 12). For patients who received docetaxel followed by ZOL, 66.7% of patients had an objective response and stable disease. Furthermore, PSA (prostate specific antigen, normally present in small amounts, increases only in pathological cases, i.e. in the case of prostate cancer) levels decreased by 450% in four patients who received docetaxel followed by ZOL. No anticancer activity was observed in patients who received sequence B, ZOL followed by docetaxel, confirming the importance of sequencing observed in preclinical studies. This study also investigated the modulation of circulating cytokines involved in the processes of angiogenesis and bone metastatization. Low doses of ZOL induce an early, long-lasting and significant decrease of VEGF, marker able to predict time to first skeletal-related event, time to bone progression disease and time to worsening of performance status. Patients treated with sequence A showed a reduction of serum levels of intrleukin-8 (IL-8), matrix metalloproteases (MMP2) and (MMP9) [56]. IL-8 expression correlates with the angiogenesis, tumorigenicity and metastasis, while MMPs play a crucial role in tumor invasion and metastases.

Prospective studies were designed to evaluate the role of ZOL as adjuvant therapy in different tumors. Several large clinical trials in patients with breast cancer support the emerging role of ZOL as an anticancer agent and provide the rationale to continue investigations into this therapeutic potential.

A large trial program (Z-/ZO-/E-ZO-FAST, AZURE,ABCSG-12) is exploring the use of N-BPs as adjuvant therapy in patients with breast cancer. The 3 large randomized multicenter companion Zometa-Femara Adjuvant Synergy Trials—Z-FAST (n= 602 patients),ZO-FAST (n= 1065 patients), and E-ZO-FAST(n= 527 patients)—are similarly designed trials that compare the effects of immediate (initiated simultaneously with adjuvant treatment) vs. delayed [initiated only when a patient's bone mineral density (BMD) T-score decreased to<– 2.0 at either the lumbar spine (LS) or total hip (TH), or the patient experienced a nontraumatic fracture] treatment with ZOL (both at 4mg every 6 months) for preventing Aromatase inhibitor-associated bone loss (AIBL) in postmenopausal women with early-stage breast cancer [57-59]. Aromatase inhibitors (AIs) are widely used for the adjuvant treatment of postmenopausal women with hormone receptor–positive (HR+) early breast cancer because these agents are highly effective at lowering estrogen levels [60]. However, several large controlled studies have reported that adjuvant AI therapy is associated with a significantly higher fracture risk [61]. In all Zometa-Femara Adjuvant Synergy Trials, patients were stratified by BMD T-score and other risk factors and were scheduled to receive adjuvant letrozole – an Aromatase inhibitor- for 5 years. Data from the Z-FAST andZO-FAST studies, conducted primarily in North America and Europe, respectively, clearly demonstrated that early initiation ofZOL treatment improves clinical benefit in terms of prevention ofAIBL compared with delayed ZOL treatment in the respective study populations [57;58]. The Z-FAST and ZO-FAST trials demonstrated also improved survival in patients who received upfront ZOL compared with delayed ZOL[57;58]. The ZO-FAST trial showed a 41% improvement in disease-free survival (DFS) (p = 0.0314) and demonstrateda decrease in local and distant disease recurrence in and outside of bone at 36 months' median follow-up [58]. The DFS benefit with upfront ZOL versus delayed ZOL continued through 60 months of follow-up [62]. A similar trend was observed at the36-month update of the Z-FAST study. Furthermore, a24-month integrated analysis of the Z-/ZO-FAST trials (n= 1667) showed that upfront ZOL increased DFS by 43% (p = 0.0183) compared with delayed ZOL [63]. However these studies were conducted in relatively homogeneous populations, a validation of bone loss and preservation patterns in a global population was needed. The E-ZO-FAST trial sought to extend these results to a patient population recruited across abroader geographic region that included Europe, Latin America, Africa,Asia, and the Middle East [59]. A total of 527 patients with HR+ early breast cancer, in whom adjuvant letrozole treatment was initiated (2.5 mg/day for 5 years), were enrolled and randomized to immediate (263 patients) or delayed ZOL (264patients) treatment (both at 4 mg every 6 months). Patients were stratified by established or recent postmenopausal status, baseline T-scores, and adjuvant chemotherapy history. At 12 months, the LS BMD increased in the immediate ZOL group (+2.72%) but decreased in the delayed ZOL group (−2.71%); the absolute difference between groups was significant (5.43%; p=0.0001). Across all subgroups, patients receiving immediate ZOL had significantly increased LS and TH BMD vs. those who received delayed ZOL (p = 0.0001). Differences in fracture incidence or disease recurrence could not be ascertained because of early data cut off and low incidence of events. Anyhow, no patients in the immediate ZOL group experienced severe osteopenia or osteoporosis by 12 months compared with 11 patients (12.6%) in the delayed ZOL group who did them. Adverse events were generally mild, transient, and consistent with the known safety profiles of both agents [59]. Taken together, the data of the report from the E-ZO-FAST study confirm, in amore diverse study population, the results reported in the North American Z-FAST and predominantly European ZO-FAST studieson the benefits of immediate ZOL administration in preventing AIBL and maintaining bone health in post-menopausal women with breast cancer.Moreover, these data clearly suggest that initiation of ZOL and AI therapies should coincide.

A report from the neoadjuvant substudy (n= 205) of Adjuvant Zoledronic Acid to Reduce Recurrence (AZURE) provides additional evidence of the anticancer benefits of ZOL. In this study, patients receiving ZOL and chemotherapy had a mean 43% reduction in residual tumor volume (p = 0.006) and an approximate 2-fold improvement in complete pathologic response (6.9% vs. 11.7%; p = 0.146) compared with patients receiving chemotherapy alone [64]. In a more recent follow-up of the AZURE trial, an open-label phase III study, 3,360 patients were randomly assigned to receive standard adjuvant systemic therapy either with or without ZOL (administered every 3 to 4 weeks for 6 doses and then every 3 to 6 months to complete 5 years of treatment) [65]. The primary end point of the study was DFS, which was defined as an absence of distant recurrence, of any invasive locoregional recurrence, and of death from any cause without recurrence. The secondary end point was OS. Prespecified subgroup analyses were based on variables included in the randomization. At a median follow-up of 59 months, there was no significant between-group difference with respect to the primary end point (DFS of 77% in eachgroup). Disease recurrence or death occurred in 377 patients in the ZOL group and 375 of those in the control group. The numbers of deaths — 243 in the zoledronic acid group and 276 in the control group —were also similar, resulting in rates of 85.4% in the ZOL group and 83.1% in the control group (p = 0.07). However, a prospective protocol-defined subgroup analysis (n= 1,041) based on menopausal status, showed that ZOL significantly improved DFS (hazard ratio = 0.76; p <0.05) in patients who were 5 or more years postmenopausal at baseline. In addition, ZOL significantly improved OS in women of unknown postmenopausal status but age>60 years (hazardratio = 0.71; p =0.017; n= 1,101) [65]. These data suggest that ZOL may augment anticancer benefit in patients with low estrogen levels (relative to premenopausal women) at baseline.

In the Austrian Breast and Colorectal Cancer Study Group trial-12 (ABCSG-12), it was compared the effect of adding ZOL to a combination of either goserelin and tamoxifen or goserelin and anastrozole in premenopausal women with endocrine-responsive early breast cancer [66].1,803 patients were randomized to receive goserelin (3.6 mg given subcutaneously every 28 days) plus tamoxifen (20 mg per daygiven orally) or anastrozole (1 mg per day given orally) with or without ZOL (4 mg given intravenously every 6 months) for 3 years. The primary end point was DFS; secondary end points were recurrence-free survival and OS [66].

However, because patients in this trial had a good prognosis, there was an insufficient number of events to assess definitively the effects of individual treatments on OS or to examine benefits in informative patient subgroups. For example, there was a non-significant difference in favouring patients receiving tamoxifen versus patients receiving anastrozole [66], which is counter to previous reports of superior estrogen depletion in premenopausal women [67] and significant increase in DFS in postmenopausal patients with breast cancer treated with aromatase inhibitors versus tamoxifen [68].At a median follow-up of 62 months, more than 2 years after treatment completion, 186 DFS events had been reported (53 events in 450 patients on tamoxifen alone, 57 in 453 patients on anastrozole alone, 36 in 450 patients on tamoxifen plus ZOL, and 40 in 450 patients on anastrozole plus ZOL) [69]. ZOL was found to reduce risk of DFS events overall (hazard ratio = 0.68; p = 0.009), although the difference was not significant in the tamoxifen (hazard ratio = 0.67; p=0.067) and anastrozole arms (hazard ratio = 0.68; p=0.061) assessed separately. ZOL did not significantly affected risk of death (30 deaths with zoledronic acid vs 43 deaths without; hazard ratio = 0.67; p=0.09).

Moreover, there was no difference in DFS between patients on tamoxifen alone versus anastrozole alone (hazard ratio = 1.08; p=0.591), but was worse with anastrozole than with tamoxifen (46 vs 27 deaths; hazard ratio = 1.75; p=0.02). Treatments were generally well tolerated, with no reports of renal failure or osteonecrosis of the jaw [69].This follow-up was longer and substantially with more events than the correspondent earlier report; however, new analyses confirmed previous findings and showed that addition of ZOL (4 mg every 6 months) for 3 years in premenopausal women receiving ovarian function suppression with goserelin plus adjuvant endocrine therapy for low-or-moderate-risk, hormone-receptor-positive, early-stage breast cancer significantly improves DFS. These and several additional adjuvant trials showing extended DFS with ZOL are consistent with the idea that ZOL modifies the microenvironment surrounding cancer cells, making it less conducive to cancer-cellsurvival and seeding of disease recurrence. However,because ZOL has a wide range of anticancer activities and prefer entially targets bone, it might be especially effective in reduction of disseminated tumour cells. These results are, apparently, contrary to those of AZURE; nevertheless, from an endocrine perspective, the postmenopausal patients in AZURE study were similar to the goserelin-treated subgroup patients in the study ABCSG-12, who had low levels of reproductive hormones at study entry. On the basis of the interpretation that ZOL might be most effective in a low-estrogenic environment, AZURE results were scientifically consistent with ABCSG-12 data showing that the DFS benefit with ZOL seemed to be driven by the subgroup of patients who were older than 40 years of age. Although all patients in ABCSG-12 received ovarian function suppression plus endocrine therapy, those who were older than 40 years at baseline might have achieved more complete estrogen deprivation.

PHARMACOKINETIC CONCERNS THAT LIMIT THE ANTI-CANCER ACTIVITY OF ZOL

FPP synthase is a highly conserved, ubiquitous enzyme; therefore, N-BPs have the potential to affect any cell type *in vitro*. Inhibition of protein prenylation by N-BPs can be shown by measuring the incorporation of $[^{14}C]$ mevalonate intofarnesylated and geranylgeranylated proteins [70]. The most potent FPP synthase inhibitor, ZOL, almost completely inhibits protein prenylation in J774 cells at a concentration of 10 µmol/L, which is similar to the concentration that affects osteoclast viability *in vitro* [71] .Alternatively, the inhibitory effect of N-BPs on the mevalonate pathway can be shown by detecting accumulation of the unprenylated form of the small GTPase Rap1A, which acts asa surrogate marker for inhibition of FPP synthase and which accumulates in cells exposed to N-BPs. Roelofs et al. detected the unprenylated form of Rap1A in osteoclasts purified from ALN-treated rabbits using immunomagnetic beads, thereby showing that N-BPs inhibit protein prenylation *in vivo* [13]. Roelofs et al. also shown the ability of N-BPs to inhibit the prenylation of Rap1A in a wide range of cultures of different types of primary cells and cell linessuch as osteoclasts, osteoblasts, macrophages, epithelial and endothelial cells, and breast,myeloma, and prostate tumor cells [13].

Macrophages and osteoclasts were the most sensitive to low concentrations of N-BPs (1-10 µmol/L) *in vitro*. Moreover, treatment with 100 µmol/L N-BP caused a detectable accumulation of unprenylated Rap1A already after few hours. For myeloma cells were required longer times of treatment *in vitro* and higher concentrations to detect the unprenylated form of Rap1A [13]. The sensitivity of different cell types to N-BPs most likely depends largely on their ability to internalize sufficient amounts of N-BP to inhibit FPP synthase. Recent studies with a fluorescently labelled bisphosphonate have shown that macrophages and osteoclasts internalize bisphosphonates into membrane-bound vesicles by fluid-phaseendocytosis; endosomal acidification then seems to be absolutely required for exit of bisphosphonate from vesicles and entry into the cytosol [72]. This mechanism of uptake suggests that a large amounts ofN-BP is in intracellular vesicles but probably only very small amounts of bisphosphonate enter the cytosol or other organelles for inhibition of FPP synthase. Even though, the relatively poor uptake of bisphosphonates into the cell cytosolis overcome by their extremely potent inhibition of FPP synthase [4].Bisphosphonates are poorly absorbed in the intestine due to their negative charge hindering their transport across the lipophilic cell membrane; they are given mainly intravenously.A pharmacokinetic evaluation of ZOL for treatment of multiple myeloma and bone metastases, carried out by Ibrahim et al., exhibited a three compartment model [73]. The distribution half-life (α-$t_{1/2}$) was 14 min, followed by a β-phase of 1.9 h. A prolonged terminal phase, with a half-life of at least 146 h, might indicate a slow release of ZOL from the bone back into the plasma. ZOL pharmacokinetics was dose proportional from 2 to 16 mg based on peak plasma concentration (C_{max}) and area under the curve ($AUC_{24\,h}$).

ZOL dosed every 21days did not demonstrate significant plasma accumulation. *In vitro* studies indicated that 22% of ZOL is protein bound. The excretion of ZOL was primarily renal. Approximately40% of the radiolabeled ZOL dose was recovered in urine within 24 h. Only traces of ZOL were observed in the urine after two days, suggesting a prolonged period of ZOL binding to bone.

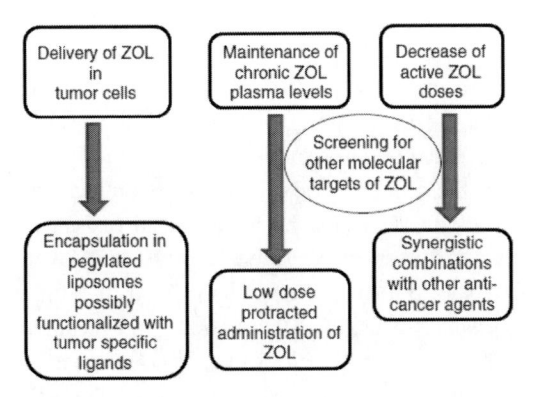

Figure 5. Description of strategies to improve the clinical activity of ZOL. The delivery of ZOL in tumor tissues and cells can be achieved through its encapsulation in PEGylated liposomes that can escape from the reticulo-endothelial system and transmigrate through fenestrated capillaries that are typical of tumor neoangiogenesis.The subsequent evolution of these devices is their functionalizing with peptides binding tumor-associated antigens (i.e., growth factor receptors). The maintenance of chronic ZOL plasma concentrations can be achieved through the administration of metronomic-like doses of ZOL (low doses over protracted time). The decrease of active doses of ZOL required for its antitumor effects can beachieved through the finding of synergistic conditions of interaction with other biological or cytotoxic agents. The screening for other molecular targets of ZOL can indicate other pharmacological combinations with agents specifically affecting these targets.

Population modeling described the ZOL clearance as a function of creatinine clearance. On the basis of a comparison of $AUC_{24\,h}$,patients with mild or moderate renal impairment had 15 and43% higher exposure, respectively, than patients with normal renal function. However, no significant relationship between ZOL exposure (AUC) and adverse events might be established. The use of ZOL in patients with severe renal failure was not recommended. *In vitro* studies showed no inhibition of or metabolism by cytochrome P-450 enzymes [73].

One of the most important limits of N-BPs, which makes the direct anti-cancer activity difficult to demonstrate *in vivo*, is just their pharmacokinetic profile. This issue is demonstrated by also other pharmacological studies performed on different N-BPs. In fact, after intravenous administration (4 mg over 15 min) of ZOL, an immediate increase of its concentration in peripheral blood was recorded, as shown by estimations of the early distribution and elimination of the drug, which resulted in plasma half-lives of the drug of about 15 min ($t_{1/2\alpha}$) and of 105 min($t_{1/2\beta}$) respectively. The maximum plasma concentration (C_{max}) of ZOL was about 1 µM; that was10- to 100-fold less than that required in *in vitro* studies to induce apoptosis and growth inhibition in tumour cell lines,while the concentrations required for anti-invasive effects were in the range of those achieved after *in vivo* administration. Moreover, approximately 55% of the initially administered dose of the drug was retained in the skeleton and was slowly released back into circulation, resulting in a terminal elimination half-life ($t_{1/2\gamma}$) of about 7 days [74;75]. Other studies performed on ALN demonstrate that N-BP concentration in non-calcified tissues declined rapidly at 1 h (5% of the initial concentration). On the other hand, its concentration in the bone continuously increased, reaching its peak at 1 h, demonstrating that a significant redistribution of the drug from non-calcified tissues to bone occurred. The drug was retained in bone tissue for a long time and was slowly released into plasma, with a terminal half-life of about 200 days [76]. Similar data were obtained with IBA and ZOL [74;77] demonstrating that long-lasting accumulation in bone is a common feature of N-BPs. The rapid redistribution of N-BPs results both in a short exposure of non-calcified tissues to the drug but also in a prolonged accumulation in bone where N-BPs can also reach higher and tumor icidal concentrations. These considerations explain the relative efficacy of N-BPs on tumours placed in bone tissues [17]. In biodistribution studies by Weiss et al. performed in rats and dogs administered with single or multiple intravenous doses of ^{14}C-labeled ZOL, its levels rapidly decreased in plasma and non calcified tissue, but higher levels persisted in bone and slowly diminished with a half-life of approximately 240 days. In contrast, the terminal half-lives (50 to 200 days) were similar in bone and non calcified tissues,consistent with ZOL rapidly but reversibly binding to bone, being rapidly cleared from the plasma, and then slowly released from bone surfaces back into circulation over a longer time. The results suggested that a fraction of ZOL is reversibly taken up by the skeleton, the elimination of drug is mainly by renal excretion,and the disposition in blood and noncalcified tissue is governed by extensive uptake into and slow release from bone [78]. It is important to consider that ZOL is not taken up by tumor cells but prevalently by cells with increased endocytosis processes such as osteoclasts and macrophages. However, owing to the intrinsic pharmacokinetics limitations of ZOL, more efforts were required to increase the anticancer activity of both this drug and the other members of N-BPs family. In the last decade the scientists have defined the following pharmacological and molecular strategies: i) the rational use of ZOL in combination with other target-based agents to overcome escape mechanism occurring in cancer cells; ii) the sequential combination of ZOL with conventional cytotoxic agents to strengthen their apoptotic and antiangiogenic potential; iii) the administration of ZOL in metronomic-like modality (low doses for protracted time); iv) the discovery and the targeting of new intracellular molecules found through the use of new advanced molecular technologies, such as DNA microarray;and v) the encapsulation of ZOL in suitable nanotechnological devices in order to selectively deliver ZOL in neoplastic tissue. These strategies are illustrated in Figure 5. Some possibility was represented by the design of rationale-based drug combinations and the improvement of the pharmacokinetic profile. Evidence from both *in vitro* and *in vivo* models indicated a synergistic antitumor activity of N-BPs when used in combination with either cytotoxic drugs or targeted molecular therapies [19]. The demonstration of these synergistic effects suggested that the low serum concentrations of N-BPs *in vivo* were still sufficient to exert anti-tumour actions in peripheral tissues. Based on the relevance of the farnesylation inhibitory effects on anti-tumour activity of N-BPs, the farnesyl transferase inhibitor (FTI) R115777 or Zarnestra ® was used together with PAM or ZOL and the effects of the combination treatment on growth inhibition and apoptosis were evaluated. N-BPs and FTI given in combination were strongly synergistic effects [20].

Notably, low concentrations of FTI induced a strong increase of Ras expression with only a moderate reduction of Ras activity that was, on the other hand, significantly reduced by the combined treatment [20]. These data suggested that escape mechanisms for the inhibition of isoprenylation of ras might be based on the geranylgeranylation or other prenylating processes [79]. The addition of farnesol to cells treated with the combination abolished the effects of the N-BPs/FTI combination on apoptosis and on the activity of the signaling molecules, suggesting that the synergistic growth-inhibitory and pro-apoptotic effects produced by the N-BPs/FTI combination involved the inhibition of both Erk and Akt survival pathways acting in these cells in a Ras-dependent fashion [20].

A synergistic interaction between R115777 and ZOL was also found on both androgen-independent PC3 and androgen-dependent LNCaP prostate cancer cell lines [20]. Moreover, ZOL/R115777 combination induced cooperative effects also *in vivo* on tumour growth inhibition of prostate cancer xenografts in nude mice with a significant survival increase [20]. These *in vivo* and *in vitro* effects were in both cases attributed to enhanced apoptosis and inactivation of Erk and Akt.

Several papers reported the significant cytostatic and cytotoxic effects of docetaxel (DTX) and ZOL on the hormone sensitive prostate cancer cell line, LNCaP [14;80-83] and in nude mice bearing LnCaP tumours [84]. In details, the highest inhibition of cell proliferation was observed after DTX exposure and was already evident at concentrations 200-fold lower than the plasma peak level. Fabbri et al. hypothesized the use of low DTX doses in concomitance with and followed by a prolonged ZOL exposure to reduce the prostatic tumour cell population and to rapidly induce eradication of hormone-resistant cells present in hormone-responsive tumours, without compromising the use of conventional-dose DTX for the first-line treatment for hormone-sensitive prostate cancer. The principal molecular mechanisms involved were found to be apoptosis and decreased pMEK and Mcl-1 expression. [85].On the basis of preliminary results about sequence-dependent synergistic effects of ZOL and DTX combination on growth inhibition and apoptosis of human prostate cancer cells, was designed a phase I clinical study on the combination between these two drugs metronomically administered in two different sequences in hormone-refractory advanced prostate cancer patients.

The aim of this study was to perform a pharmacodynamic evaluation of the effects of the two sequential combinations through the dosage of serum angiogenic, immunologic and bone factors and through the study of both lymphocyte sub-populations and modification of isoprenylation of intracellular proteins. Final endpoint of this study was the evaluation of information for further clinical development of this combination, such as toxicity, as well as information about the mechanism of action of the combination to be translated in the preclinical setting.

In patients with metastatic hormone refractory prostate cancer, the DTX and ZOL combination therapy decreased serum prostate-specific antigen levels by >50% and resulted in a concurrent improvement in symptoms [86]. In a phase II trial of estramustine, ZOL, and DTX in patients with metastatic androgen independent prostate cancer a PSA decrease of >50% for a duration of 5–63 weeks and a clinically notable reduction in pain was recorded, suggesting that this combination therapy might delay disease progression in this setting [87]. Finally, an orally available mTOR inhibitor RAD001 (Everolimus ®) that inhibits growth of prostate cancer in the bone, was found to increase its inhibitory effects by combination with DTX and ZOL[88].

The closely related taxane, paclitaxel (PTX), with a similar set of clinical uses to DTX, has showed synergistic inhibitory activity with ZOL in animal models for lung cancer. There was a trend towards differences in survival between the groups and survival was significantly longer for the PTX + ZOL group vs. vehicle. Compared with vehicle and ZOL alone, cancerous cells in the bone of mice treated with PTX + ZOL expressed higher levels of Bax and lower levels of Bcl-2 and Bcl-xl. Moreover, this drug combination produced a significant reduction in serum n-telopeptide of type I collagen which levels correlate with the rate of bone resorption. The results of this study indicated that ZOL enhanced the efficacy of PTX synergistically, by reducing the incidence of bone metastasis from lung cancer and prolonging survival in a mouse model of non-small cell lung cancerwith a high potential for metastasis to bone [89].

In addition, the treatment with ZOL after exposure to doxorubicin (DOX) elicited substantial antitumor effects in a mouse model of breast cancer. Interestingly, the treatment induced an increase in the number of caspase-3-positive cells paralleled by a decrease in the number of tumour cells positive for the proliferation marker Ki-67. Moreover, the sequential treatment with clinically relevant doses of DOX, followed by ZOL, reduced intraosseous but not extraosseous growth of breast tumours in mice injected with a clone of MDA-MB-231 [90].

The findings of synergy of interaction between ZOL and other agents could reduce the ZOL concentrations required for anti-tumour activity and then could allow the achievement of its effective *in vivo* levels, overcoming the limits associated with the pharmacokinetics of ZOL.

Another strategy to potentiate the antitumor effects of chemotherapy agents and ZOL could be also the administration of the drugs at repeated low doses ("metronomic" way). Daubinee et al. recently demonstrated that weekly administration of ZOL has higher antitumor effects as compared with conventional 3-weekly administration in nude mice xenografted with breast cancer cells, even ifthe total administered dose is the same [91]. Moreover, a single dose of 1 mg ZOL is able to induce a significant reduction of circulating VEGF in patients with bone metastases suggesting an *in vivo* biological activity of low ZOL concentrations in humans [92].

Similarly, metronomic administration of ZOL and taxotere combination in castration resistant prostate cancer patients was evaluated in ZANTEtrial, were the schedule of bi-weekly DTX given at day 1 followed by ZOL at day 2 resulted feasible, well tolerated and showed to induce a disease control in 66.7% of patients. Moreover, it was also recorded a strong down-regulation of circulating cytokines involved in the processes of angiogenesis and bone metastatization [56].

An additional strategy for the increase of ZOL anti-cancer activity is the interference of its molecular targets. DNA microarrays and proteomics represent, for this purpose, an attractive opportunity to analyze the post-transcriptional modifications induced by ZOL treatment, and to better understand the *in vivo* intratumor molecular pathways involved in the response to the drug.

Moreover, protein microarrays might allow discovery of new ZOL targets, identification of new biomarkers predictive of response, and analysis of specific molecular profiling related to the clinical response toN-BP-based therapy. Identification of critical interactions within the proteome network is a potential starting point for drug development, and will aid the design of individual tailored therapies or identification of either new molecular orgene profiles that are predictive of response to ZOL-based therapy [93].

The recent analysis - performed by cDNA microarray platform - of gene modulation induced by ZOL in androgen-resistant prostate PC3 cell line showed a significant dose- and time-dependent reduction of transcriptional activity of CYR61 after exposure to ZOL, as demonstrated by the reduction of the transcriptional activity of Cyr61 promoter [93]. This result is considered of interest in designing new therapeutical approaches in androgen-independent prostate cancer.

However, in recent years, the strategy of choice for the strengthening of ZOL antitumor effects is certainly its delivering in the tumor by encapsulation in nanoparticles.

NANOTECHNOLOGICAL MODIFICATIONS OF ABPS: ENCAPSULATION OF ABPS AND ZOL IN NANODEVICES

A method to increase the availability of BPs inextra-bone tissues and improve their plasma half-lives is their encapsulation in liposome vehicles [94]. The encapsulation of BPs (i.e. CLO) and N-BPs (i.e. PAM and ALN) in liposomes has been historically used for their ability to accumulatein the reticulo-endothelial system and in order to cause a depletion of macrophages for anti-inflammatory purposes [95;96].

The evidence that solid tumours are not only composed of malignant cells, but are complex organ-like structures comprising many cell types, including a wide variety of migratory haematopoietic and residentstromal cells [97] has opened the way for new developments in the search for innovative anticancer strategies. Migration of leucocyte into tumours was initially interpreted as evidence foran immunological response of the host against a growing tumour; more recently it became clear that tumours are largely recognised as self and lack strong antigens. Instead, they appear to have been selected to manipulate the host immune system to prevent rejection and to use it to facilitate their own growth and spread [98;99]. This led to the proposal that haematopoietic cell infiltrates composed of myeloid cells, neutrophils, dendritic cells (DCs), eosinophils, mastcells, lymphocytes and macrophages have a causal role in carcinogenesis. Clinical data collected from a wide range of solid tumours corroborated these findings given that high densities of leucocytic infiltrations, most notably macrophages, were linked with poor prognosis of the diseases [100;101]. Tumour-associated macrophages (TAMs) produce a vast number of factors that promote tumorigenesis such as basic fibroblast growth factor (bFGF), vascular endothelial growth factor (VEGF), platelet-derived growth factor (PDGF), transforming growth factor beta (TGFβ), the angiopoietins (Ang1 and Ang2), interleukins such as IL-1 and IL-8, tumour necrosis factor-α (TNF-α), thymidine phosphorylase (TP), the matrix metalloproteinases MMP-9 and MMP-2, nitric oxide (NO)and chemokines [97]. The coordinated expression of these molecules results in proliferation and migration of endothelial cells (ECs), remodelling of the extracellular matrix and formation of stabilised blood vessels. Macrophages are perfectly able to promote these processes, as their monocytic precursors migrate to specific locations such as hypoxic tumour tissues [102;103;97], where they differentiate and synthesize angiogenic molecules. It is well established the crucial role of angiogenesis for extensive tumour growth and metastasis by providing oxygen and nutrients and removal of waste products [104]. It was demonstrated that the encapsulation of the BP CLO into liposomes makes it an efficient reagent for the selective depletion of TAM [105]. In fact, after injection,liposomes are ingested and digested by macrophages followed by intracellular release and accumulation of CLO.At a certain intracellular concentration, CLO induces apoptosis of the macrophage. Through the creation of an animal model with macrophage depleted tissues or organs,functional aspects of macrophages might be studied *in vivo*. Recently, Zeisberger group has demonstrated that depletion of these stromal cell subsets, through the CLO encapsulated into liposomes (Clodrolip), presumably disrupted the cytokine network owing to an imbalance in the cells responsible to the production of tumour stimulatory chemokines and cytokines probably involved in tumour angiogenesis [105]. In their experiments, tumour-bearing mice were treated with Clodrolip as single therapy in comparison to free CLO and in combination with anti-VEGF single chain fragment antibodies (Abs),resulting in drastic tumour growth inhibition and exhaustion of TAM and tumor-associated dendritic cells (TADC) populations. Treatment with Clodrolip efficiently depleted phagocytic cells in the murine F9 teratocarcinoma and human A673 rhabdomyosarcoma mouse tumor models resulting in significant inhibition of tumor growth from 75 to 92%, depending on therapy and schedule. Tumor inhibition was accompanied by a drastic reduction of blood vessel density in the tumor tissue, and the strongest effects were obtained with the combination Clodrolip/VEGF neutralising antibody. Immunohistologic evaluation of the tumors showed significant depletion - reduction rates of 85 to 94%, even 9 days after the end of therapy - of both TAMsand TADCsin the A673 model. To assess the effect of the treatments on tumor vascularisation, it was analysed vessel density by CD31+ staining. At 3 days after the end of therapy (day 16), tumor blood vessels were virtually undetectable and significant reduction in vessel density was observed even 9 days later [105].These results validated Clodrolip therapy in combination with angiogenesis inhibitors as a promising novel strategy for an indirect cancer therapy and as a tool to study the role of tumor infiltrating cells, for example by gene expression profiling of TAM-depleted tumors.

Any premature discharge of the encapsulated drug from the liposome might reduce its bioactivity since less drug would be delivered to the phagocytic cell and might increase the possibility of untoward effects. Consequently, for the design of an optimal liposomal formulation in general, and for an anti-inflammatory effect in particular, it should be required careful consideration of the factors that contribute to their *in vitro* stability and *in vivo* integrity upon dilution in the blood after injection. The physicochemical properties of liposomes including size, charge, lipid composition, and cholesterol content are governing factors of stability, blood integrity and clearance rate from the circulation [106]. The study carried out by Epstein et al. was the first report that examined the disruption extent and rate of the vesicles in the circulation [107]. Moreover, liposomal ALN was prepared with an improved formulation by lyophilization, a modified thin lipid film hydration technique, followed by extrusion, resulting in relatively smaller size vesicles, narrow size distribution, and low drug to lipid ratio in comparison to the reverse phase evaporation method. In order to rule out premature leakage of the drug, the integrity of the vesicles was examined by means of size-exclusion chromatography *in vitro* and *in vivo*, with subsequent analysis of size, drug and lipid concentrations. Vesicles were found to be stable in serum, and intact liposomes were detected in the circulation 24 h following administration [107]. It was concluded that the new formulation resulted in increased stability (2.5 years)as determined by the insignificant changes in vesicle size, drug leakage, lipid and drug stability, *in vitro* bioactivity (macrophages inhibition), as well as *in vivo* in depleting circulating monocytes and inhibition of restenosis in rabbits. Moreover, the parallel results found between the *in vitro* and *in vivo* data on liposome integrity upon dilution in serum, provided a valuable new toolin assessing *in vivo* integrity of new liposomal formulations [107].

Infectious diseases caused by intracellular pathogens (i.e., HIV and Mycobacterium tuberculosis), being characterized by high morbidity and mortality, have resulted in a most serious global health problem. Particularly for these diseases, a strategy of intracellular drug delivery with a high degree of specificity, by reaching every single infected cell with the drug at therapeutic doses, could dramatically improve the efficacy of the therapy. FPP synthase inhibition by ZOLis also achieved at the level of monocytes,inducing the accumulation of molecules able to activate Vγ9Vδ2T cells, key effectors during infectious progression. Activated Vγ9Vδ2 T cells are able to proliferate and to exerta broad antimicrobial and antitumoral activity by both cytolytic andnon-cytolytic mechanisms. Hence, ZOL has recently been proposed as an effective adjuvant therapy in HIV infection [108] targeting Vγ9Vδ2 T cells; in addition to its suitability as molecular reporter, the potential of this substance as an effective payload for macrophage-targeted drug vectors, has prompted the design of niosomal drug delivery systems for encapsulation and release of ZOL. Niosomes are vesicular structures analogous to liposomes, made of nonionic surfactants that self-assemble in aqueous media, yielding closed bilayers. Similarly to liposomes, niosomes are able to entrap both hydrophilic molecules, within their aqueous core, and hydrophobic molecules by their partitioning into the hydrophobic domain of the bilayer [109]. Niosomes, however, show several advantages over liposomes: i) a greater versatility; ii) an increased stability, and iii) lower cost [110-112]. Multicompartment nanoscopic carriers can be easily assembled by inducing the aggregation of anionic "hybrid" niosomes by means of cationic biocompatible polyelectrolytes [i. e. ε -polylysine (ε -PLL)], forming stable finite-size clusters. The resulting vesicle clusters, whose size and overall net charge can be easily controlled by varying the polyelectrolyte-to-particle charge ratio, show an interesting potential for multidrug delivery. Cells of the immune system are devoted to the capture and destruction in tissues of mesoscopic "foreign particles" (cellulardebris and pathogens). However, when the vector-designed targets are the macrophages, this inconvenience turns into an advantage. In general, "large particles" of whatever nature can be considered cell-specific transporters of drugs against macrophage-specific infections, such as the chronically infected macrophages present in HIV. Reports by Agrati et al. on the interaction *in vitro* of hybrid niosomes, loaded with ZOL, with different leukocyte subsets combining characteristics of niosomes and the versatility of their ε -PLLinduced aggregates, provides a first and cleare vidence of a selective interaction of aggregates characterized by a well-defined size and charge with a subset of lymphocytes, the monocyte/macrophages. Interestingly, the monocyte/ macrophage-mediated activation of Tγδ lymphocytes induced by ZOL was enhanced by a factor 10^3 when ZOL was intracellularly delivered through these carriers [113].

Among N-BPs, neridronateis one of the least efficient ones, as compared to ZOL and RIS relatively to their ability for cellkilling, but it does not bear the consequent toxicity [114]. Therefore,it is a fairly good choice, in order to optimize its cell delivery,to use a neridronate liposomal formulation. This N-BP was tested *in vitro* on human breast cancer cells(MDA-MB-231) both in free and in liposomal formulations. Cell viability evaluation showed a drastically more effective action of the neridronate while entrapped in liposome. This result was confirmed using cell migration and cell invasion assays. Furthermore, MMPs expression was significantly reduced in the case of cell lines treated with liposomal neridronate and this was a rather good indication of the therapy efficiency [115]. However, in view of testing *in vivo* this delivery system and of making it suitable for anti-cancer therapy, chemical modifications or substitutions would be necessary to allow a better escape from reticulo-endothelial cells.

'Stealth' liposomes (PEGylated liposomes or second-generation liposomes) are, indeed, more useful for anti-tumour clinical practice because they escape the reticulo-endothelial system and, therefore, they are not internalized by macrophages such as the 'non-stealth' liposomes. They are characterized by very long circulation half-lives, favourable pharmacokinetic behaviour and specific accumulation in tumour tissues [116]. In fact, liposomes PEGylation is designed to avoid the internalization of liposomes by macrophages. Moreover, liposomes have a size that allows their diffusion only through fenestrated vessels that are typical of tumor neo-angiogenesis and, therefore, their biodistribution is limited above all in tumors and not in normal tissues. This effect reduces the toxicity of the delivered drug and, in general, allows a retargeting of the drug in the tumor (Figure 6). One of the first anti cancer drugs encapsulated in PEGylated liposomes and used in clinical trials was doxorubicin [117; 118]. The favourable pharmacokinetic properties of PEGylated liposomes could encourage their use as N-BPs vehicles in order to increase their uptake in tumour sites [17]. Since ZOL accumulates in the bone, there is a need to develop new N-BPs with a lower affinity for bone and a longer half-life in the circulation that would be potentially better at affecting peripheral tumours. A delivery system based on Glycol-coated (PEGylated) formulation of ZOL (LipoZOL) with lower affinity for bone was developed with the aim to increase its bioavailability in extraskeletal tumor sites through the enhanced permeability retention (EPR) effect [119]. The mean size of LipoZOL was in fact of about 200 and 240 nm, a size compatible with gaps present in the endothelia of tumor vessels. It has been investigated whether the LipoZOL fomulation increased antitumor properties in comparison with standard (free) ZOL, using both *in vitro* and *in vivo* models of two different human cancers. Compared to ZOL, LipoZOL induced a stronger inhibition of *in vitro* growth. It has been demonstrated that ZOL requires endocytosis to gain access into the cytoplasm [72], where its molecular targets are placed. The liposome intracellular uptake observed by confocal microscopy studies could contribute to increase the amount of ZOL that reaches its cytoplasmic targets. It was also found that LipoZOL caused significantly larger inhibition of tumor growth and increased the in murine models of human prostate cancer and multiple myeloma, in comparison with ZOL. Moreover, a strong inhibition of vasculogenetic events without evidence of necrosis in the tumor xenografts from prostate cancer was recorded after treatment with LipoZOL. In addition, it was demonstrated both antitumor activity and tolerability of LipoZOL in preclinical animal models of both solid and hematopoietic malignancies, providing a rationale for early exploration of use of LipoZOL as a potential anticancer agent in cancer patients [119].

Subsequently, it was designed a new carrier to deliver ZOL to tumors [120]. This new delivery system consisted in self-assembly PEGylated nanoparticles (NPs) based on calcium/phosphate (CaPZ) NPs and cationic liposomes [120]. CaP NPs had already been used by different authors to deliver nucleic acids [121;122], proteins [123:124], anti-cancer drugs [125] and antigens [126]. The use of calcium phosphate ceramics offered advantages such, low cost, biocompatibility and non-toxic degradation product [127].

PEGylation was achieved by two different strategies [120]. The preparation conditions were optimized in order to achieve NPs easily prepared before use, with colloidal dimensions and high ZOL loading. CaPZ NPs were covered with PEGylated liposomes (pre-PLCaPZ NPs); alternatively, CaPZ NPs were previously mixed with cationic liposomes and then PEGylated by post-insertion method (post-PLCaPZ NPs). Pre-PLCaPZ NPs showed the best technological characteristics, with a narrow size distribution and a high ZOL loading [120]. Studies on different cancer cell lines, showed that these NPs enhanced the antiproliferative effect of ZOL [120]. It was noteworthy that the maximal potentiation was observed in human breast cancer cell lines. In fact, as stated above, ZOL is presently indicated in the treatment of bone metastases from breast cancer and for the prevention of the skeletal related events. Moreover, the first clinical evidence of a direct anti-tumor effect of ZOL comes specifically from the treatment of early breast cancer in the adjuvant setting [66].

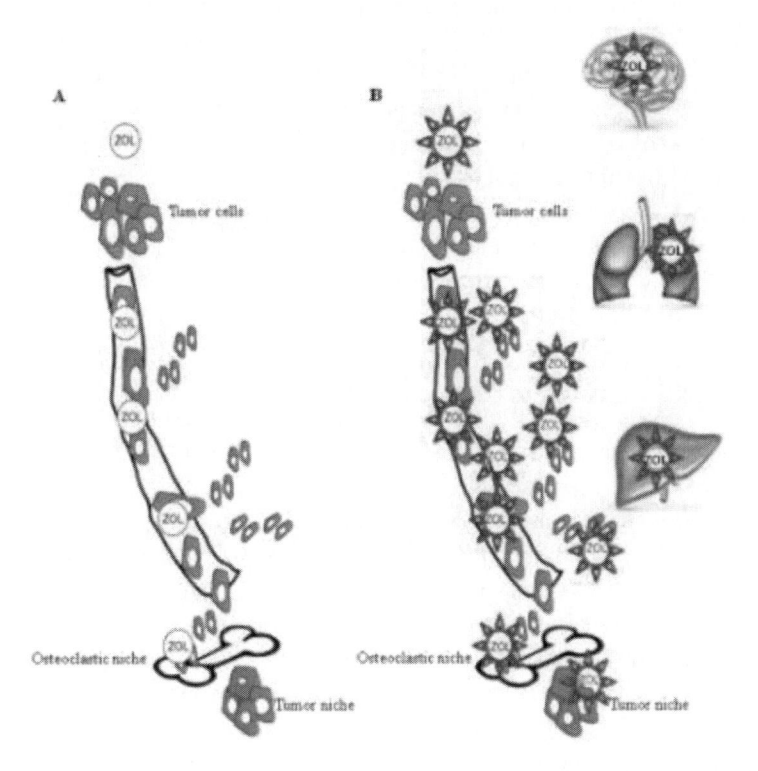

Figure 6. Liposome encapsulation strategy. The lack of ZOL antitumor effect outside bone is probably based on the almost exclusive localization and distribution of this agent in bone tissues and, above all, in the 'osteoid niche' (**A**) that is generally placed far from the 'tumor niche'. The delivery of ZOL in PEGylated liposomes (**B**) that escape from reticulo-endothelial system is able to overcome these limitations of ZOL allowing other cell types and tissues such as liver, lung, and brain to be reached.

Finally, in an animal model of prostate cancer, a significant reduction of tumor growth was achieved with pre-PLCaPZ NPs, while the tumor was unaffected by ZOL free in solution [120].

Recently, it was carried out a comparative study among the two developed nanotechnological strategies, LIPO-ZOL and ZOL-encapsulating self-assembly NPs, especially concerning their anti-cancer activity in a xenograft model of prostate adenocarcinoma [128]. It was found a higher anti-cancer activity of NPs in comparison with the one induced by LIPO-ZOL. In addition, NPs induced the complete remission of tumour xenografts and an increase of survival time higher than that one observed with LIPO-ZOL. It has also to be considered that PC3 tumour xenografts were almost completely resistant to the anti-cancer effects induced by free ZOL. Both nanotechnological products did not induce toxic effects not affecting the mice weight and not inducing deaths. Moreover, the histological examination of some vital organs such as liver, kidney and spleen did not find any changes in terms of necrotic effects or modifications in the inflammatory infiltrate. On the other hand, NPs but not LIPO-ZOL caused a statistically significant reduction of TAM in tumour xenografts. This effect was paralleled by a significant increase of both necroticand apoptotic indexes [128]. TAMs have been recently reported to be involved in the growth of prostate cancer cells in the bone, the main metastatic site of this cancer [129]. Moreover, the infiltration of TAMs in prostate biopsy specimens is predictive of disease progression after hormonal therapy for prostate cancer [130]. The effects of the NPs were also higher in terms of neo-angiogenesis inhibition. The more potent anti-cancer biological and clinical effects mediated by PLCaPZ NPs could be explained by the improved cell uptake of these NPs. It was hypothesized that the complexes between ZOL and CaP NPs/cationic lipids might actively enter into the cells by endocytotic mechanism. Moreover, the different surface characteristics of the two nanocarriers, close to the neutrality and positive for LIPO-ZOL and PLCaPZ NPs, respectively, might affect their uptake by TAM. It has been reported that both the degree of PEGylation and the presence of a net charge affect nanocarrier uptake by macrophages [131]. In particular, a high degree of PEGylation should hamper the adsorption of plasma proteins on the particles, thus hampering macrophage uptake. Moreover, nanocarriers with a zeta potential close to zero have been found to be less phagocytable in comparison with positively charged particles, probably due to the presence of negatively charged sialic acid on their surface [131].These results suggested the future preclinical development of ZOL-encapsulating NPs in the treatment of human cancer.

An additional recent application of BP exploits their exceptional affinity of BP for hydroxyl apatite (HAP)[132]. Since HAP is only present in 'hard' tissues like bone and teeth, it was considered a promising target for the selective drug delivery to bone. Henst et al. successfully reported liposomes incorporating with cholesteyl-trisoxyethylene bisphosphonicacid (CH-TOE-BP),a new tailor-made BP derivative, designed for bone targeting. CHOL-TOE-BP targeted liposomes were designed for the treatment of bone-related diseases to achieve prolonged local exposure to high concentrations of the bioactive compounds, thereby enhancing therapeutic efficacy and minimizing systemic side effects. The CHOL-TOE-BP-targeted liposomes were characterized regarding particle size and zeta potential. Moreover the bone targeting potential of these conjugates was studied through an *in vitro* HAP binding assay and the obtained data indicated that CHOL-TOE-BP was useful as targeting device for liposomal drug delivery to bone.

However, the desired HA affinity of these liposomes was been shown in *in vitro* tests with HA particles, and no *in vivo* studies were reported on their capability formineral-binding [132]. This is important considering that the protein-rich serum could compete for mineral binding under the physiological conditions.

Bone targeting of simple molecules by conjugation with bone-seeking ligands bisphosphonates has been achieved *in vivo* for various prodrug candidates such as estradiol

[133], cisplatin [134], prostaglandin E_2[135], and several model proteins [136-138]. Anada et al. synthesized an amphipathic molecule containing a BP head group, 4-N-(3,5-ditetradecyloxybenzoyl)-aminobutane-1-hydroxy-1,1-bisphosphonic acid disodium salt, which was subsequently formulated into liposomes along with distearoyl phosphotidylcholine (DSPC) and cholesterol (CH). The liposomes decorated with BP moieties were shown to display high affinity for pure HAparticles *in vitro* [139]. Unlike larger liposomes, micellar nanocarriers could be also advantageous for certain applications requiring smaller drug carriers.

A study by Wang et al.explored the feasibility of creating micellar and liposomal nanocarriers from building blocks that display bone mineral (HA) affinity. Towards this goal, they conjugated a thiol-containing BP, 2-(3-mercaptopropylsulfanyl)-ethyl-1, 1-bisphosphonic acid (thiolBP), with distearoylphosphoethanolamine-polyethylene glycol-maleimide (DSPE-PEG-MAL) to form a DSPE-PEG-thiolBP conjugate [140].The capacity of the prepared vehicles to encapsulate anticancer drug doxorubicin (DOX) and a model protein lysozyme (LYZ) was assessed. The mineral affinity of the vehicles was investigated using HA particles as well as a HA-embedded collagen scaffold that contains the major components of bone tissue. An effective mineral affinity was imparted to the prepared micelles and liposomes both *in vitro* and in an *in vivo* implant model, indicating that these HA-binding nanocarriers would facilitate a novel approach for drug delivery in treatment of bone diseases [140].

CONCLUSION

In vitro results have clearly demonstrated that bisphosphonates, in addition to inhibiting osteoclast-mediated bone resorption, can exert marked proapoptotic and antiproliferative effects on tumor cells, especially when combined with other standard antineoplastic therapy. *In vivo*, this antitumor effect appears to be better experienced in tumor cells of bone metastases, at least in the majority of experiments performed to date. This may be explained by the high local concentration of bisphosphonate in bone relative to the much lower one in other organs and plasma; this feature makes bisphosphonates the drugs of choice in the treatment of bone problems associated with malignancy. The goals of treatment for bone metastases are in fact to prevent disease-related skeletal complications, to palliate pain, and to maintain QoL.

Recently, large-scale clinical trials have investigated the benefit of bisphosphonate therapy in reducing the incidence of SRE in myeloma, in breast cancer metastases, in metastatic prostate cancer, in lung cancer, in renal cell carcinoma, and in other solid tumors. Many *in vivo* tumor models have demonstrated ZOL, PAM, CLO, and IBA antitumor efficacy compared with placebo.

In the preclinical setting ZOL has also demonstrated synergistic anticancer activity when used in combination with a variety of anticancer agents including chemotherapeutic drugs, molecularly targeted agents, and other biological agents. The preclinical data provide, in fact, a solid rationale that ZOL might prevent disease progression. The anti-cancer activity shown by ZOL includes inhibition of cancer cell proliferation,viability, motility, invasion and angiogenesis and induction of cancer cell apoptosis. Based on these potential anti-cancer properties, several clinical trials have been initiated to test the combination of ZOL and other agents. The accumulating encouraging evidence to date indicates that ZOL is an attractive anti-cancer agent that promises to be the next exciting therapy for patients with various cancers.

However, owing to the intrinsic pharmacokinetics limitations of ZOL, more efforts were required to increase the anticancer activity of both ZOL and the other members of N-BPs family.The optimization of anti-cancer activity of N-BPs and of ZOL above all seems to be now possible on the bases of several pre-clinical and clinical findings. Several strategies could be developed in the next future: i) the rational use of N-BPs in combination with other target-based agents in order to overcome escape mechanisms occurring in cancer cells; ii) the targeting of new intracellular molecules found through the use of new advanced molecular technologies, such as DNA microarray; iii) the discovery of new N-BP pharmacological formulations [ZOL-encapsulating PEGylated liposomes (LIPO-ZOL) and ZOL-encapsulating self-assembly PEGylated nanoparticles (NPs)] that can optimize the delivery and the homing of these agents in tumour cells.

REFERENCES

[1]   J. R.Ross, Y.Saunders, P. M.Edmonds, S.Patel, D.Wonderling, C.Normand and K.Broadley, *Health Technol. Assess.* 8, 1(2004).

[2]   R. G. Russell, *Pediatrics.*119, S150 (2007).

[3]   H .Fleisch, R. G. Russell and S.Bisaz, *Calcif. Tissue Res.* 2, 49 (1968).

[4]   J. E. Dunford, K. Thompson, F. P. Coxon, S.P. Luckman, F. M. Hahn, C. D. Poulter, F. H. Ebetino and M. J. Rogersjpet, *J. Pharmacol. Exp. Ther.* 296, 235 (2001).

[5]   J. R. Green. *Cancer.*97, 840 (2003).

[6]   L. I. Plotkin, R. S. Weinstein, A. M. Parfitt, P. K. Roberson, S. C. Manolagas and T.Bellido, *J. Clin. Invest.* 104, 1363 (1999).

[7]   M. J. Rogers, D. J. Watts, R. G. G. Russell, X.Ji, X. Xiong, G. M. Blackburn, A. V. Bayless and F. H. Ebetino, *J. Bone Miner. Res.* 9, 1029 (1994).

[8]   M. J. Rogers, *Calcif. Tissue Int.* 75, 451 (2004).

[9]   M. J. Rogers, R. J. Brown, V. Hodkin, R. G. G. Russell and D. J.Watts, *Biochem. Biophys. Res. Commun.* 224, 863 (1996).

[10]   J. C. Frith, J. Monkkonen, S. Auriola, H. Monkkonen and M. J. Rogers. *Arthritis Rheum.* 44, 2201 (2001).

[11]   P. P. Lehenkari, M. Kellinsalmi, J. J. J. P. Napankangas, K. V. Ylitalo, J. Mönkkönen, M. J. Rogers, A. Azhayev, H. K. Väänänen and I. E. Hassinen, *Mol. Pharmacol.* 61, 1255 (2002).

[12]   J. M. Halasy-Nagy, G. A. Rodan and A. A. Reszka, *Bone.* 29, 553 (2001).

[13]   J. Roelofs, K. Thompson, S. Gordon and M. J.Rogers, *Clin. Cancer Res.*12, 6222s (2006).

[14]   J. R. Berenson, *Curr. Opin. Support Palliat. Care.* 5, 233 (2011).

[15]   P. Carmeliet and R. K. Jain, *Nature.* 407, 249 (2000).

[16]   P. Carmeliet, *Nat. Med.* 9, 653 (2003).

[17] M. Caraglia, D. Santini, M. Marra, B. Vincenzi, G. Tonini and A. Budillon, *Endocr. Relat.Cancer.*13, 7 (2006).

[18] K. Kavanagh, K. Guo, J. E. Dunford, X. Wu, S. Knapp, F. H. Ebetino, M. J. Rogers, R. G. Russell and U. Oppermann, *Proc. Natl. Acad. Sci. U.S.A.*103, 7829 (2006).

[19] M. Marra, A. Abbruzzese, R. Addeo, S. Del Prete, P. Tassone, G. Tonini, P. Tagliaferri, D. Santini and M. Caraglia, *Curr. Cancer Drug Targets.*9, 791(2009).

[20] M. Caraglia, A. M. D'Alessandro, M. Marra, G. Giuberti, G. Vitale, C. Viscomi, A. Colao, S. D. Prete, P., Tagliaferri P. Tassone, A. Budillon, S. Venuta and A. Abbruzzese. *Oncogene.* 23, 6900 (2004).

[21] S. G. Senaratne, J. L. Mansi and K. W. Colston. *Br. J. Cancer.*86, 1479 (2002).

[22] L. Sewing, F. Steinberg, H. Schmidt and R. Göke. *Apoptosis.*13, 782(2008).

[23] M. Fujita, M. Tohi, K. Sawada, Y. Yamamoto, T. Nakamura, T. Yagami, M. Yamamori and N. Okamura, *Oncol.Rep.*27, 1371 (2012).

[24] L. M. Pickering and J. L. Mansi. *Proc. Am. Soc. Clin. Oncol.* 22, 863 (2003).

[25] J. Wood, K. Bonjean, S. Ruetz, A. Bellahcène, L. Devy, J. M. Foidart, V. Castronovo and J. R.Green. *J. Pharmacol. Exp. Ther.* 302, 1055 (2002).

[26] M. Caraglia, M. Marra, S. Naviglio, G. Botti, R. Addeo and A. Abbruzzese, *Expert Opin. Pharmacother.*11, 141 (2010).

[27] R. E. Coleman, *Cancer.*80, 1588 (1997).

[28] J. R. Ross, Y. Saunders, P. M. Edmonds, S. Patel, K. E. Broadley and S. R. D. Johnston, *BMJ.*327, 469 (2003).

[29] M. Marra, D. Santini, G. Tonini, G. Meo, S. Zappavigna, G. Facchini, A. Morabito, A. Abbruzzese, G. Cartenì, A. Budillon and M.Caraglia. *Eur.J. Cancer.* 6, 79 (2008).

[30] G. Facchini, M. Caraglia, D. Santini, G. Nasti, A. Ottaiano, S. Striano, P. Maiolino, M. Ruberto, F. Fiore, G. Tonini, A. Budillon, R. V. Iaffaioli and G. L. Zeppetella, *J. Exp. Clin. Cancer Res.* 26, 307 (2007).

[31] P. Major, A. Lortholary, J. Hon, E. Abdi, G. Mills, H. D. Menssen, F. Yunus, R. Bell, J. Body, E. Quebe-Fehling, J. Seaman, *J. Clin. Oncol.* 19, 558 (2001).

[32] J. R. Berenson, R.Vescio, L. S. Rosen, J. M. Von Teichert, M. Woo, R. Swift, A. Savage, E. Givant, M. Hupkes, H. Harvey and A. Lipton. A phase I dose-ranging trial of monthly infusions of zoledronic acid for the treatment of osteolytic bone metastases. *Cancer Res.*7, 478 (2001).

[33] J. R. Berenson, R. Vescio, K. Henick, C. Nishikubo, M. Rettig, R. A. Swift, F. Conde, J. M. Von Teichert. *Cancer.* 91, 144 (2001).

[34] L. S. Rosen, D. Gordon, N. S. Tchekmedyian, R. Yanagihara, V. Hirsh, M. Krzakowski, M. Pawlicki, P. De Souza, M. Zheng, G. Urbanowitz, D. Reitsma and J. Seaman, *Cancer.*100, 2613 (2004).

[35] C. Langer and V. Hirsh, *Lung Cancer.*67, 4 (2010).

[36] L. S. Rosen, D. H. Gordon, W. Dugan, P. Major, P. D. Eisenberg, L. Provencher, M. Kaminski, J. Simeone, J. Seaman, B. L. Chen, R. E. Coleman, *Cancer.*100, 36 (2004).

[37] F. Saad, D. M. Gleason, R. Murria,P. Venner , L. Lacombe , J. L. Chin , J. J. Vinholes , J. A. Goas , B. Chen and Zoledronic Acid Prostate Cancer Study Group. *J. Natl. Cancer Inst.* 94, 1458 (2002).

[38] Saad F, Gleason DM, Murria R, Tchekmedyian S, Venner P, Lacombe L, Chin JL, Vinholes JJ, Goas JA, Zheng M; Zoledronic Acid Prostate Cancer Study Group. Long-

term efficacy of zoledronic acid for the prevention of skeletal complications in patients with metastatic hormonerefractory prostate cancer. *J. Natl. Cancer. Inst*.96, 879 (2002).

[39] R. Gálvez, V.Ribera, J. R. González-Escalada, A. Souto, M. L. Cánovas, A. Castro, B. Herrero, M. de Los Angeles Maqueda, M. Castilforte, J. J. Marco-Martínez, C. Pérez, L. Vicente Fatela, C. N. Md, M. J. Orduña, A. Padrol, F.Reig. J,Carballido and J. M.Cózar, *Patient Prefer.Adherence*.2, 215 (2008).

[40] A.Berruti, L. Dogliotti, M. Tucci, R. Tarabuzzi, D. Fontana and A. Angeli, *J. Urol*. 166, 2023 (2001).

[41] H. Scher, *Cancer*. 97, 758 (2003).

[42] S. E.Papapoulos, N. A.Handy and G.Van der Pluijm, *Cancer*. 88, 3047 (2000).

[43] M. R. Smith, F. J. McGovern, A. L. Zietman, M. A. Fallon, D. L. Hayden, D. A.Schoenfeld, P. W. Kantoff and J. S. Finkelstein, *N. Engl. J. Med*. 345, 948 (2001).

[44] A. Lipton, M. Zheng and J.Seaman, *Cancer*.98, 962 (2003).

[45] J, Gralow and D.Tripathy, *J. Pain Symptom Manage*. 33, 462 (2007).

[46] H. K. Koul, S. Koul and R. B.Meacham, *Prostate Cancer Prostatic Dis*.15, 111 (2012).

[47] D. Santini, S. Galluzzo, B. Vincenzi, G. Schiavon, E. Fratto, F. Pantano and G.Tonini, *Ann. Oncol*.18, 164 (2007).

[48] P. Clezardin, *Semin. Oncol*.29, 33 (2002).

[49] P. I. Croucher, R. De Hendrik, M. J. Perry, A. Hijzen, C. M. Shipman, J. Lippitt, J. Green, E. Van Marck, B. Van Camp and K.Vanderkerken, *J. Bone Miner. Res*. 18, 482(2003).

[50] F. Dieli, N. Gebbia, F. Poccia, N.Caccamo, C.Montesano, F.Fulfaro, C. Arcara, M. R. Valerio, S. Meraviglia, C. Di Sano, G.Sireci and A. *Blood*. 102, 2310 (2003).

[51] T. Yuasa, S. Kimura, E. Ashihara, T. Habuchi and T.Maekawa, *Curr. Med. Chem*.14, 2126 (2007).

[52] M. Dimopoulos, J. Berenson, N. Shirina and Y. M. Chen, "Survival in patients with multiple myeloma receiving zoledronic acid: Stratification by baseline bone alkaline phosphatase levels", ASCO Annual Meeting, 2006 Abstract 7505.

[53] E. Matczak, V. Hirsh, A. Lipton, J. Cook, C. Langer, Y. J. Hei and P. Major, "Effects of zoledronic acid on survival in patients with lung cancer and high baseline N-telopeptide (NTX) levels: stratified by baseline bone alkaline phosphatase (BALP)", ASCO Annual Meeting 2006 Abstract 7228.

[54] Y. Hei, A. Lipton, N. Shirina, Y. M. Chen and T.Xie,"Effect of zoledronic acid (Zol) compared with pamidronate (Pam) on disease progression in breast cancer (BC) patients with bone metastases stratified by baseline characteristics", ASCO Annual Meeting 2006 Abstract 678.

[55] K. Zarogoulidis, E. Boutsikou, P. Zarogoulidis, E. Eleftheriadou, T. Kontakiotis, H. Lithoxopoulou, G. Tzanakakis, I. Kanakis, N. K. Karamanos, *Int. J. Cancer*.125, 1705 (2009).

[56] G. Facchini, M. Caraglia, A. Morabito, M. Marra M. C. Piccirillo, A. M. Bochicchio, S. Striano, L. Marra, G. Nasti , E. Ferrari, D. Leopardo, G. Vitale, D. Gentilini, A. Tortoriello, A. Catalano, A. Budillon, F. Perrone and R. V. Iaffaioli, *Cancer. Biol. Ther*.10, 543 (2010).

[57] A.M. Brufsky, L. D. Bosserman, R. R. Caradonna, B. B. Haley, C. M. Jones, H. C. Moore,L. Jin, G. M. Warsi, S. G. Ericson_and E. A.Perez,_*Clin. Breast Cancer*. 9, 77 (2009).

[58] H. Eidtmann, R. de Boer, N. Bundred, A. Llombart-Cussac, N. Davidson, P. Neven, G. von Minckwitz, J. Miller, N. Schenk, R. Coleman, *Ann. Oncol.* 21, 2188 (2010).

[59] A. Llombart, A. Frassoldati, O. Paija, H. P. Sleeboom, G. Jerusalem, J. Mebis, I. Deleu, J. Miller, N. Schenk and P.Neven, *Clin. Breast Cancer.*12, 40 (2012).

[60] S. Aebi, T. Davidson, G. Gruber, M. Castiglione and ESMO Guidelines Working Group, *Ann. Oncol.* 21, 9 (2010).

[61] A. Howell, J. Cuzick, M. Baum, A. Buzdar, M. Dowsett, J. F. Forbes, G. Hoctin-Boes, J. Houghton, G. Y. Locker, J. S. Tobias and ATAC Trialists' Group, *Lancet.*365, 60 (2005).

[62] R. de Boer, N. Bundred and H. Eidtmann,"The effect of zoledronic acid on aromatase inhibitor-associated bone loss in postmenopausal women with early breast cancer receiving adjuvant letrozole: The ZO-FAST study 5-year final follow-up", 33rd Annual San Antonio Breast Cancer Symposium, 8–12, Dec.2010 (San Antonio, TX) Poster P5-11-01.

[63] A. Frassoldati, A. Brufsky, N. Bundred, R. Lambert-Falls, P. Hadji and N. Schenk,"Effect of zoledronic acid in postmenopausal women with early breast cancer receiving adjuvant letrozole: a 24-month integrated follow-up of the Z-FAST/ZO-FAST trials", 11th International Conference on Primary Therapy of Early Breast Cancer,11–14 Mar. 2009 (St Gallen, Switzerland) Abstract 132.

[64] R. E. Coleman, M. C. Winter, D. Cameron, R. Bell, D. Dodwell, M. M. Keane, M. Gil, D. Ritchie, J. L. Passos-Coelho, D. Wheatley, R. Burkinshaw, S. J. Marshall, H. Thorpe and AZURE (BIG01/04) Investigators, *Br. J. Cancer.*102, 1099 (2010).

[65] R. E. Coleman, H. Marshall,D. Cameron, D. Dodwell, R. Burkinshaw, M. Keane, M. Gil, S. J. Houston, R. J. Grieve, P. J. Barrett-Lee, D. Ritchie, J. Pugh, C. Gaunt, U. Rea, J. Peterson,C. Davies, V. Hiley, W. Gregory, R. Bell and AZURE Investigators. BreastCancer. *N. Engl. J. Med.*365, 1396 (2011).

[66] M. Gnant, B. Mlineritsch, W. Schippinger, G. Luschin-Ebengreuth, S. Pöstlberger, C. Menzel, R. Jakesz, M. Seifert, M. Hubalek, V. Bjelic-Radisic, H. Samonigg, C. Tausch, H. Eidtmann, G. Steger, W. Kwasny, P. Dubsky, M. Fridrik, F. Fitzal, M. Stierer, E. Rücklinger, R. Greil, ABCSG-12 Trial Investigators and Marth C. *N. Engl. J. Med.* 360, 679 (2009).

[67] D. P. Forward, K. L. Cheung, L. Jackson and J. F. Robertson. *Br. J. Cancer.* 90, 590 (2004).

[68] BIG 1-98 Collaborative Group, H. Mouridsen, A. Giobbie-Hurder, A. Goldhirsch, B. Thürlimann, R. Paridaens, I. Smith, L. Mauriac, J. F. Forbes, K. N. Price, M. M. Regan, R. D. Gelber and A. S. Coates, *N. Engl. J. Med.*361, 766(2009).

[69] M. Gnant, B. Mlineritsch, H. Stoeger, G. Luschin-Ebengreuth, D. Heck, C. Menzel, R. Jakesz, M. Seifert, M. Hubalek, G.Pristauz, T. Bauernhofer, H. Eidtmann, W. Eiermann, G. Steger, W. Kwasny, P. Dubsky, G. Hochreiner, E. P. Forsthuber, C. Fesl, R. Greil and Austrian Breast and Colorectal Cancer Study Group, Vienna, Austria, *Lancet Oncol.*12, 631 (2011).

[70] H. L. Benford, J. C. Frith, S. Auriola, J. Monkkonen and M. J. Rogers, *Mol. Pharmacol.* 56, 131 (1999).

[71] F. P. Coxon, M. H. Helfrich, R. J. van 't Hof, S. Sebti, S. H. Ralston, A. Hamilton and M. J. Rogers, *J. Bone Miner. Res.*15, 1467 (2000).

[72] K. Thompson, M. J. Rogers, F. P.Coxon and J. C. Crockett, *Mol. Pharmacol.* 69, 1624 (2006).

[73] A. Ibrahim, N. Scher, G. Williams, R.Sridhara, N. Li, G. Chen, J. Leighton, B. Booth, J. V. Gobburu, A. Rahman, Y. Hsieh, R. Wood, D. Vause and R. Pazdur, *Clin. Cancer Res.* 9, 2394 (2003).

[74] T. Chen, J. Berenson, R. Vescio, R. Swift, A. Glichick, S. Goodin, P. LoRusso, P. Ma, C. Ravera, F. Deckert, H. Schran, J. Seaman and A. Skerjanec, *J. Clin. Pharmacol.* 42, 1228 (2002).

[75] A. Skerjanec, J. Berenson, C., Hsu, P. Major, W. H. Miller Jr, C. Ravera, H. Schran, J. Seaman and F. Waldmeier, *J. Clin. Pharmacol.* 43, 154 (2003).

[76] J. H. Lin, *Bone.* 18, 75 (1996).

[77] J. Barrett, E. Worth, F. Bauss and S. Epstein, *J. Clin. Pharmacol.* 44, 951 (2004).

[78] H. M. Weiss, U. Pfaar, A. Schweitzer, H. Wiegand, A. Skerjanec and, H. Schran, *Drug Metab.Dispos.* 36, 2043 (2008).

[79] G. Ferretti, A. Fabi, P. Carlini, P. Papaldo, P. Cordiali Fei, S. Di Cosimo, N. Salesi, D. Giannarelli, A. Alimonti, B. Di Cocco, G. D'Agosto, V. Bordignon, E.Trento and F.Cognetti, *Oncology.* 69, 35 (2005).

[80] R. S. Herbst and F.R. Khuri, *Cancer Treat. Rev.* 29, 407 (2003).

[81] A. Ullén, L. Lennartsson, U. Harmenberg, M. Hjelm-Eriksson, K. M. Kälkner, B. Lennernäs and S. Nilsson, *Acta Oncol.* 44, 644 (2005).

[82] C. Morgan, P. D. Lewis, R. M. Jones, G. Bertelli, G. A. Thomas, R. C. Leonard, *Acta Oncol.* 6, 669 (2007).

[83] B. Karabulut, C. Erten, M. K. Gul, E. Cengiz, B. Karaca, Y. Kucukzeybek, G. Gorumlu, H. Atmaca, S. Uzunoglu, U. A. Sanli, Y. Baran and R..Uslu, *Cell. Biol. Intl.* 33, 239 (2009).

[84] K. D. Brubaker, L. G. Brown, R. L. Vessella and E.Corey, *BMC Cancer.* 6, 15 (2006).

[85] F. Fabbri, G. Brigliadori, S. Carloni, P. Ulivi, I. Vannini, A. Tesei, R. Silvestrini, D. Amadori, W. Zoli, *J. Transl.Med.* 6, 43 (2008).

[86] D. Vordos, B. Paule, F. Vacherot, Y. Allory, L. Salomon, A. Hoznek, R. Yiou, D. Chopin, C. C., Abbouand A. de la Taille, *BJU Int.* 94, 524 (2004).

[87] J. G. Kattan, F. S. Farhat, G. Y. Chahine, F. L. Nasr, W. T. Moukadem, F. C. Younes, N. J. Yazbeck, M. G. Ghosn and Cancer Research Group, *Invest. New Drugs.* 26, 75 (2008).

[88] T. M. Morgan, T. E. Pitts, T. S. Gross, S. L. Poliachik, R. L. Vessella and E.Corey, *Prostate,*68, 861 (2008).

[89] S. Lu, J. Zhang, Z. Zhou, M. L. Liao, W. Z. He, X. Y. Zhou, Z. M. Li, J. Q. Xiang, J. J. Wang and H. Q. Chen, *Oncol. Rep.* 20, 581 (2008).

[90] P. D. Ottewell, ,B. Deux, H. Mönkkönen, S. Cross, R. E. Coleman, P. Clezardin and I. Holen, *Clin. Cancer Res.* 14, 4658 (2008).

[91] F. Daubiné, C. Le Gall, J. Gasser, J. Green and P. Clézardin, *J. Natl.Cancer Inst.* 994, 322 (2007).

[92] D. Santini, B. Vincenzi, S. Galluzzo, F. Battistoni, L. Rocci, O. Venditti, G. Schiavon, S. Angeletti, F. Uzzalli, M. Caraglia, G. Dicuonzo and G. Tonini, *Clin. Cancer Res.* 1315, 4482 (2007).

[93] M. Marra, D. Santini, G. Meo, B.Vincenzi, S.Zappavigna, A.Baldi, M. Rosolowski, G. Tonini, M. Loeffler, R. Lupu, S. R. Addeo, A. Abbruzzese, A. Budillon and M. Caraglia, *Int. J. Cancer.* 125, 2004 (2009).

[94] K. J. Harrington, K. N. Syrigos and R. G.Vile, *J. Pharm. Pharmacol.*54, 1573 (2002).

[95] N. van Rooijen and E. van Kesteren-Hendrikx, *J. Liposome Res.* 12, 81 (2002).

[96] H. D. Danenberg, G. Golomb, A. Groothuis, J. Gao, H. Epstein, R. V. Swaminathan, P. Seifert and E. R. Edelman, *Circulation.* 108, 2798 (2003).

[97] J. W. Pollard, *Nat. Rev. Cancer.* 4, 71 (2004).

[98] H. T. Khong and N. P. Restifo, *Nat. Immunol.* 3, 999 (2002).

[99] A. F. Ochsenbein, *Springer Semin. Immunol.* 27, 19 (2005).

[100] J. J. W. Chen, Y. C. Lin, P. L. Yao, A. Yuan, H. Y. Chen, C. T. Shun, M. F. Tsai, C. H. Chen and P. C. Yang, *J. Clin. Oncol.* 23, 953 (2005).

[101] J. A. Joyce, *Cancer Cell.* 7, 513 (2005).

[102] A. Mantovani, P. Allavena and A.Sica, *Eur.J. Cancer.* 40, 1660 (2004).

[103] C. Murdoch, A. Giannoudis and C. E. Lewis, *Blood.* 104, 2224 (2004).

[104] J. Folkman, *Curr. Mol. Med.* 3, 643 (2003).

[105] S. M. Zeisberger, B. Odermatt, C. Marty, A. H. M. Zehnder-Fja¨llman, K. Ballmer-Hofer and R. A. Schwendener. Clodronate liposome-mediated depletion of tumour-associated macrophages, a new and highly effective antiangiogenic therapy approach. *Br. J. Cancer.* 95, 272 (2006).

[106] H. Harashima, T. Hiraiwa, Y. Ochi and H. Kiwada, *J. Drug Target.* 3, 253 (1995).

[107] H. Epstein, D. Gutman, E. Cohen-Sela, E. Haber, O.Elmalak, N. Koroukhov, H. D. Danenberg and G. Golomb, *AAPS J.* 10, 505 (2008).

[108] F. Poccia, C. Gioia, F. Martini, A. Sacchi, P. Piacentini, M. Tempestilli, C.Agrati, A. Amendola, A. Abdeddaim, C. Vlassi, M. Malkovsky and G. D'Offizi, *AIDS.* 23, 555 (2009).

[109] F. Uchegbu, *Expert Opin. Drug Deliv.* 3, 639 (2006).

[110] T. Waku, M. Matsusaki, T. Kaneko and M. Akashi, *Macromolecules.* 40, 6385 (2007).

[111] Y. Huang, J. Chen, X. Chen, J. Gao and W. Liang, *J. Mater. Sci. Mater. Med.*19, 607 (2008).

[112] M. Hong, S. Zhu, Y. Jiang, G. Tang and Y. Pei, *J. Control Release.* 133, 96 (2009).

[113] C. Agrati, C.Marianecci, S.Sennato, M. Carafa, V. Bordoni, E. Cimini, M. Tempestilli, L. P. Pucillo, F. Turchi, F. Martini, G. Borioniand F. Bordi, *Nanomedicine.*7, 153(2011).

[114] C. K. Zacharis and P. D.Tzanavaras, *J. Pharm. Biomed. Anal.* 48, 483 (2008).

[115] I. Chebbi, E. Migianu-Griffoni, O. Sainte-Catherine, M. Lecouvey and O. Seksek, *Int. J. Pharm.*383, 116 (2010).

[116] L. Cattel, M. Ceruti and F. Dosio, *J. Chemother.* 16, 94 (2004).

[117] A. Gabizon, H. Shmeeda and Y. Barenholz, *Clin.Pharmacokinet.* 42,:419 (2003).

[118] M. Caraglia, R. Addeo, R. Costanzo, L. Montella, V. Faiola, M. Marra, A. Abbruzzese, G. Palmieri, A. Budillon, F. Grillone, S. Venuta, P. Tagliaferri and S. Del Prete, *Cancer Chemother. Pharmacol.* 57, 34 (2006).

[119] M. Marra, G. Salzano, C. Leonetti, P. Tassone, M. Scarsella, S. Zappavigna, T. Calimeri, R. Franco, G. Liguori, G. Cigliana, R. Ascani, M. I. La Rotonda, A. Abbruzzese, P. Tagliaferri, M. Caraglia and G. De Rosa, *Nanomedicine.*7, 955 (2011).

[120] G. Salzano, M. Marra, M. Porru, S. Zappavigna, A. Abbruzzese, M. I. La Rotonda, C. Leonetti, M. Caraglia and G. De Rosa, *Int. J. Pharm.* 403, 292 (2011).

[121] V. V. Sokolovaa, I. Radtkeb, R. Heumannb and M. Epple, *Biomaterials.* 27, 3147 (2006).

[122] C. E. Pedraza, D. C. Bassett, M. D. McKee, V. Nelea, U.G bureck and J. E.Barralet, *Biomaterials.* 29, 3384 (2008).

[123] M. J. Gorbunoff, *Anal. Biochem.* 136, 425 (1984).

[124] G. Spenlehauer, M. Vert, J. P. Benoit and A. Boddaert, 10, 557 (1989).

[125] A. Barroug, L. T. Kuhn, L. C. Gerstenfeld and M. J. Glimcher, *J. Orthop. Res.* 22, 703 (2004).

[126] Q. He, A. R. Mitchell, S. L. Johnson, C. Wagner-Bartak, T. Morcol and S. J. Bell, *Clin. Diagn. Lab. Immunol.* 7, 899 (2000).

[127] X. Cheng, L. Kuhn, *Int. J. Nanomed.* 2, 667 (2007).

[128] M. Marra, G. Salzano, C. Leonetti, M. Porru, R. Franco, S. Zappavigna, G. Liguori, G. Botti, P. Chieffi, M. Lamberti, G. Vitale, A. Abbruzzese, M. I. La Rotonda, G. De Rosa and M. Caraglia, *Biotechnol. Adv.*30, 302 (2012).

[129] S. W. Kim, J. S. Kim, J. Papadopoulos, H. J. Choi, J. He, M. Maya, R. R. Langley, D. Fan, I. J. Fidler and S. J.Kim, *Int.Immunopharmacol.* 11, 862 (2011).

[130] N. Nonomura, H. Takayama, M. Nakayama, Y. Nakai, A. Kawashima, M. Mukai, A. Nagahara, K. Aozasa and A. *BJU Int.* 107, 1918 (2010).

[131] F. Chellat, Y. Merhi, A. Moreau and L. Yahia, *Biomaterials.* 26, 7260 (2005).

[132] V. Hengst, C. Oussoren, T. Kissel and G. Storm, *Int. J. Pharm.*331, 224 (2007).

[133] F. Bauss, A. Esswein, K. Reiff, G. Sponer and B. Muller-Beckmann, *Calcif. Tissue Int.*59, 168 (1996).

[134] T. Klenner, P. Valenzuela-Paz, B. K. Keppler, G. Angres, H. R. Scherf, F. Wingen, F. Amelung and D. Schmahl, *Cancer Treat. Rev.* 17, 253 (1990).

[135] L. Gil, Y. Han, E. E. Opas, G. A. Rodan, R. Ruel, J. G. Seedor, P. C. Tyler and R. N. Young, *Bioorg. Med. Chem.* 7, 901 (1999).

[136] H. Uludag, N. Kousinioris, T. Gao and D. Kantoci, *Biotechnol. Prog.*16, 258 (2000).

[137] H. Uludag and J.Yang, *Biotechnol. Prog.* 18, 604 (2002).

[138] S. A. Gittens, G. Bansal, R. F. Zernicke and H. Uludag, *Adv. Drug Deliv. Rev.* 57, 1011 (2005).

[139] T. Anada, Y. Takeda, Y. Honda, K. Sakurai and O. Suzuki, *Bioorg. Med. Chem. Lett.* 19, 4148 (2009).

[140] G. Wang, N. Z. Mostafa, V.Incani, C.Kucharski and H. Uludağ, *J Biomed. Mater. Res. A.*100, 684 (2012).

In: Bone Tumors: Symptoms, Diagnosis and Treatment   ISBN: 978-1-62618-190-8
Editor: Moncef Berhouma   © 2013 Nova Science Publishers, Inc.

Chapter 7

MALIGNANT TRANSFORMATION OF BENIGN BONE TUMORS WITH SPECIAL REFERENCE TO GIANT-CELL TUMOR AND GIANT-CELL–CONTAINING LESIONS

Tsuyoshi Saito

Department of Human Pathology, Juntendo University, School of Medicine, Japan

ABSTRACT

Malignant transformation of benign bone tumors is sometimes encountered. Malignant transformation of giant-cell tumor of bone is a well-known phenomenon that occurs in 1%–2% of conventional giant-cell tumors. In addition, extremely rare cases of primary giant-cell tumor have been reported. The histological diagnosis of conventional giant-cell tumors may include necrosis, and some mitotic activity. These features can lead to a diagnosis of definite malignancy in certain tumors; however, a definite diagnosis often cannot be made because of a lack of diagnostic criteria for malignant transformation of giant-cell tumors. Other benign bone tumors, especially those with secondary changes such as fibrohistiocytic and aneurysmal bone cyst-like change, are known to share resembling histological features with conventional giant-cell tumors, although their malignant counterpart has rarely been reported for most of these benign bone tumors. Furthermore, a confusing term, "pseudosarcomatous (pseudoanaplastic) lesion," exists. For such cases, the patient's prognosis often tells us the true diagnosis. In this chapter, factors that may relate to the prolapse of a giant-cell tumor and that may influence the malignant transformation of giant-cell tumor of bone and related lesions are discussed.

INTRODUCTION

Giant-cell tumor of bone (GCTB) often exhibits secondary changes such as fibrohistiocytic and cystic changes, bleeding, and aneurysmal bone cyst (ABC)-like appearance. Thus, 2 giant-cell–containing lesions, neoplastic and reactive, frequently coexist in this tumor, and the latter can overshadow the underlying neoplastic lesion, leading to misdiagnosis. These reactive secondary changes masquerade as giant-cell–containing reactive lesions, such as giant-cell reparative granuloma, and benign fibrohistiocytic lesions such as benign fibrous histiocytoma and non-ossifying fibroma. A diagnosis of secondary malignant transformation is sometimes difficult even for experts in bone tumor pathology, as the secondary reactive change in benign giant-cell tumor can mimic malignant transformation. In addition, pseudoanaplastic bone tumors with benign clinical courses have been demonstrated. In this chapter, the malignant transformation of benign bone tumors is described with special emphasis on that of giant-cell tumor of bone.

CONVENTIONAL GIANT-CELL TUMOR OF BONE

Giant-cell tumors mainly affect the epiphyseal and metaphyseal region of the long bones in skeletally matured young adults, particularly around the knee and the wrist, comprising only 5% of all benign and malignant bone tumors and approximately 20% of all benign bone tumors. Conventional GCTB is a distinct, locally aggressive tumor composed of mononuclear histiocyte-like cells and uniformly scattered osteoclast-type multinucleated giant cells. Under the Enneking staging system, benign tumors are divided into 3 groups: latent (Stage 1), active (Stage 2), and aggressive (Stage 3) [1]. Latent tumors are usually discovered incidentally, having reached their non-growth stage by the time of discovery. Active tumors are histologically benign, slow-growing neoplasms that may cause mild symptoms. They grow steadily over a prolonged period. Aggressive tumors, despite being histologically benign, are locally invasive and may metastasize. According to this staging system, giant-cell tumors of bone are categorized from Stage 1 to Stage 3.

Conventional GCTB is an essentially benign tumor that tends to recur frequently. The local relapse rate within 2 years has been described to be 40%–50%. Malignant transformation of giant-cell tumor of bone is a well-known phenomenon that occurs in 1%–2% of conventional giant-cell tumors. Metastasis can develop from both benign and malignant giant-cell tumors.

HISTOLOGY OF GIANT-CELL TUMOR OF BONE

Histologically, a giant-cell tumor of bone is composed of a proliferation of oval to plump mononuclear cells comprising uniformly distributed, multinucleated osteoclast-type giant cells in the background of partially vascularized fibrous stroma (Figure 1). Stromal bleeding is frequently encountered. The mononuclear stromal cells can sometimes be spindle-shaped and fibroblast-like in appearance. The nuclei of stromal and giant cells are essentially the same, with regular outlines and prominent nucleoli, and it has been suggested that mononuclear cells transit into multinucleated giant cells. The presence of mixed-type of mononuclear stromal cells can give rise to the impression of pleomorphism, though true pleomorphism should not be seen in giant-cell tumor of bone. The mitosis of mononuclear stromal cells can be encountered quite commonly; however, atypical mitoses would not be observed. These basic histologic features of giant-cell tumor of bone are frequently modified by secondary reactive changes such as hemorrhage, necrosis, fibrohistiocytic change, and aneurysmal bone cyst-like formation (Figures 2 and 3). Hemorrhage and necrosis usually result from fracture or mechanical compression. Nuclear pyknosis and increased nuclear variability can be seen associated with these necrotic changes. The aneurysmal bone cyst-like change can be frequently observed, becoming predominant in some cases and leading to its misinterpretation as a primary ABC.

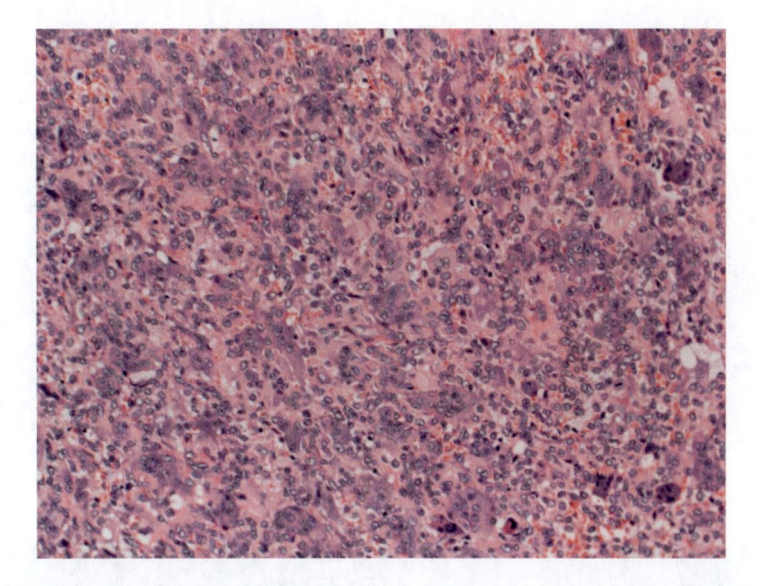

Figure 1. Histology of conventional giant-cell tumor of bone. Proliferation of mononuclear cells with scattered multinucleated giant cells.

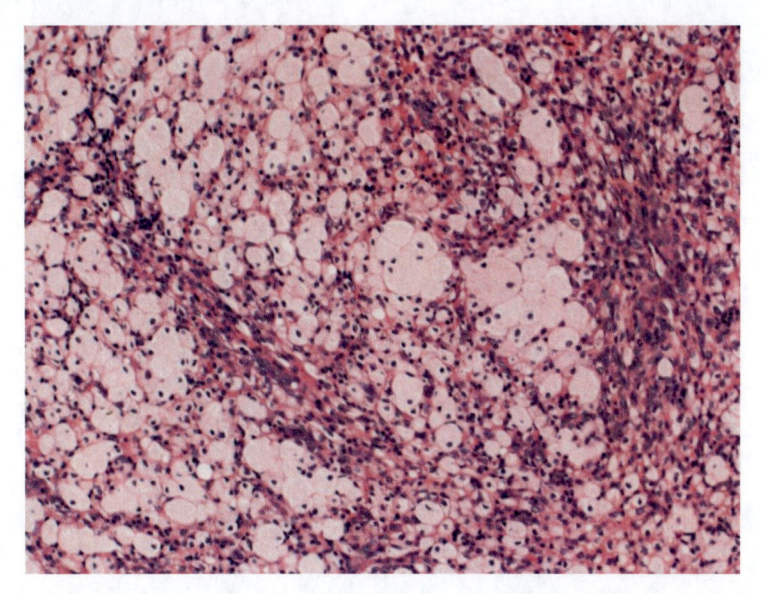

Figure 2. Secondary change in GCTB. Lymphocytic infiltration with aggregates of macrophages is prominent.

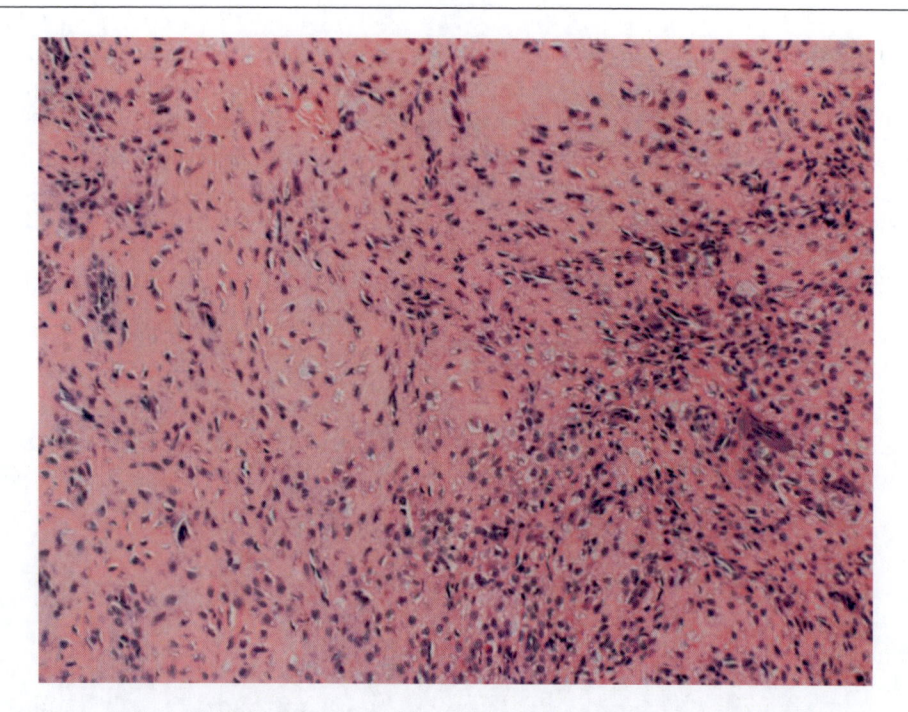

Figure 3. Stromal fibrosis is also prominent in another area in GCTB.

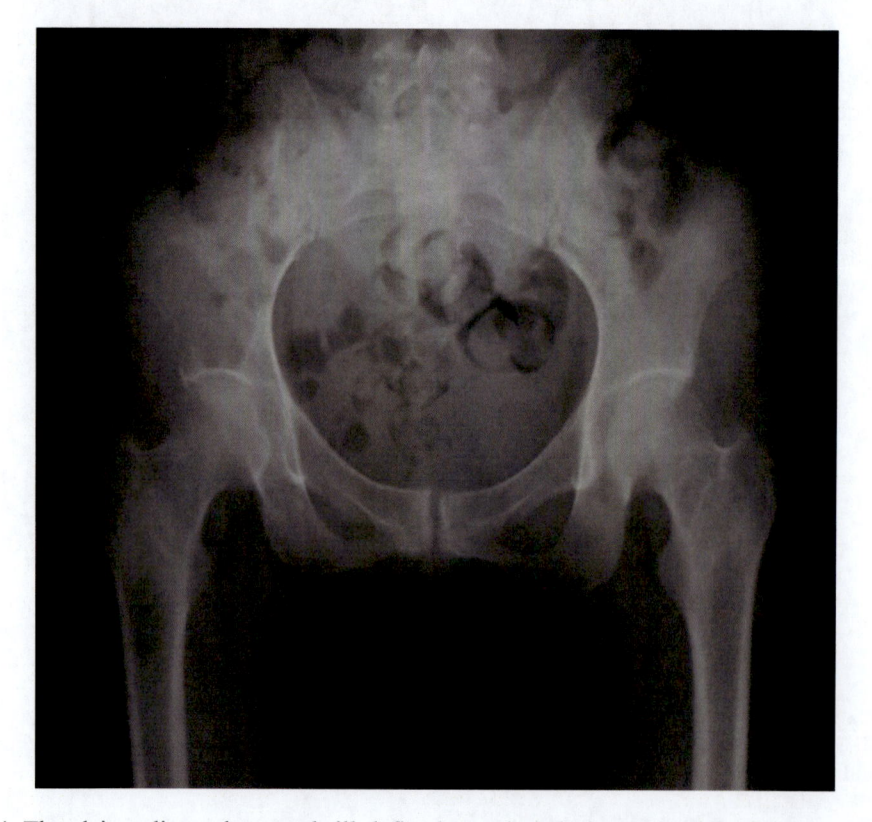

Figure 4. The plain radiography reveals ill-defined osteolytic lesion at the right ileum.

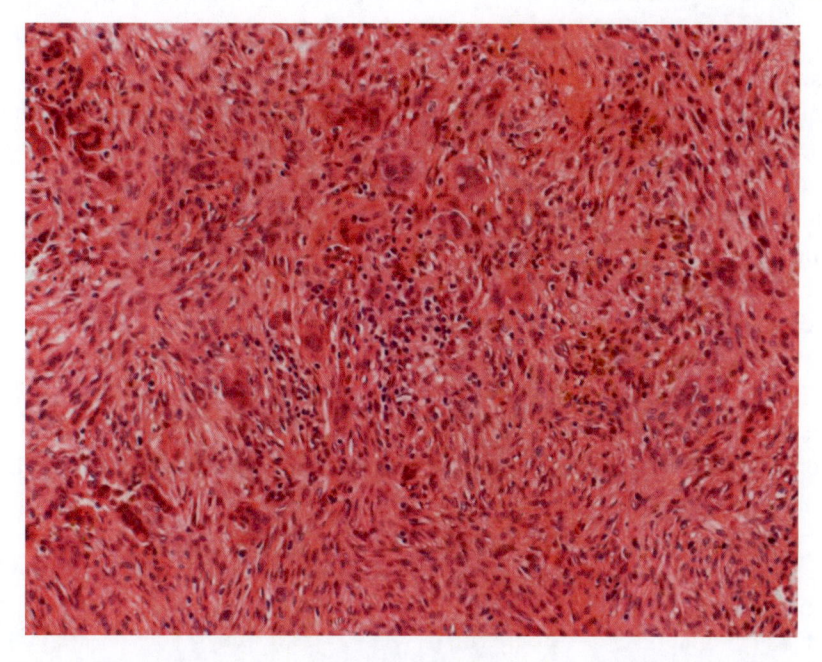

Figure 5. A biopsy specimen shows a proliferation of plump to spindle-shaped mononuclear cells with scattered multinucleated giant cells. Lymphocytic infiltration and hemosiderin deposits are also noted.

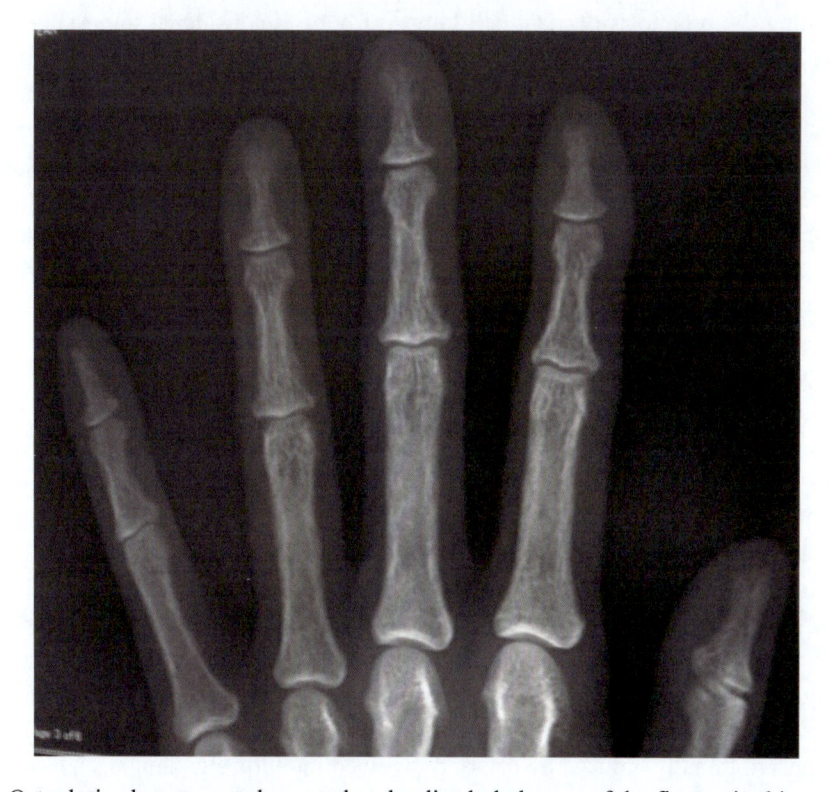

Figure 6. Osteolytic changes are also noted at the distal phalanxes of the fingers in this patient.

The reactive fibrohistiocytic changes, with a storiform pattern of fibroblast-like cells and xanthogranulomatous reaction, can also be frequently observed. These changes are also accompanied by reactive bone formation associated with pathological fracture or mechanical stress.

The fibrohistiocytic reaction sometimes replaces the preexisting underlying tumor, and the lesion masquerades as benign fibrohistiocytic lesions such as nonossifying fibroma or benign fibrous histiocytoma. A case of Brown tumor associated with hyperparathyroidism in 29y.o. female is presented here as one of the giant-cell containing reactive lesions, that need to be distinguished from giant-cell tumor of bone. This patient admitted to our hospital complaining her right coxalgia. A plain radiography revealed an ill-defined osteolytic lesion at the right ileum (Figure 4). A biopsy from this lesion showed a proliferation of plump to spindle-shaped mononuclear cells with scattered multinucleated giant cells.

Lymphocytic infiltration and hemosiderin deposits are also noted (Figure 5). In addition, further examination revealed bone absorption was evident in the distal phalanxes of fingers in this patient (Figure 6). This tumor is histologically indistinguishable from giant-cell reparative granuloma. It is necessary to take into consideration the laboratory data for accurate diagnosis.

FACTORS THAT AFFECT LOCAL RELAPSE OF CONVENTIONAL GIANT-CELL TUMORS

Predicting the prognosis of giant-cell tumor of bone is considered impossible. The local recurrence rate reported in the literature ranges 12%–49% [2-5]. The relapse of giant-cell tumor is related to many factors, though especially to the methods of tumor treatment such as en bloc wide resection or curettage, the extent and location of the tumor, and involvement into the adjacent soft tissue. Curettage is generally associated with a high rate of local recurrence than wide resection [6]. Extensive curettage, which consists of curettage of the lesion, burring of the surrounding normal cancellous and cortical bones, and removal of the soft tissue capsule over the tumor cortex, has been shown to have a significantly lower local recurrence rate than simple curettage [7]. In addition, cryosurgery is recommended as an adjuvant to curettage for giant-cell tumor of bone to improve the clinical outcome [8]. It has been shown that clinicoradiological staging and tumor size demonstrate a degree of correlation with giant-cell tumor of bone recurrence [9]. Possible biomarkers related to the progression of giant-cell tumor of bone are as follows: increased expression of human telomerase reverse transcriptase (hTERT) [10, 11], p53 [12], glutathione peroxidase 1 (GPX-1) [13], epithelial growth factor receptor (EGFR) [14], c-myc [15], matrix metalloproteinases (MMPs) [16, 17], c-met [18] and vascular endothelial growth factor (VEGF) [17, 19], high mitotic index [20-22], and DNA aneuploidy [22]. Nuclear staining of hTERT (>10%) correlates with recurrence-free survival [10]. Giant-cell tumors with p53 expression have a high potential for lung metastasis and recurrence [23], whereas a recent study using microarray and proteomics analyses determined that p53 failed to emerge as a biomarker for local recurrence and metastasis [13]. Proteomics analysis identified GPX-1, an antioxidant enzyme transcriptionally induced by p53 and involved in redox signaling, as a biomarker that relates to lung metastasis and local relapse [13]. It exerts negative control over the production of reactive oxygen species after oxidative stress, thereby protecting cells against DNA-damaging insults. EGFR expression is restricted to neoplastic mononuclear cells and is frequently observed in recurrent tumors [14]. c-Met expression is constantly positive in recurrent or locally aggressive tumors [18]. High levels of VEGF gene expression but not microvessel density correlate with advanced-stage tumors [19]. The expressions of VEGF and MMP-9 at both the mRNA and protein levels are higher in advanced tumors (Stage 2 and 3) than in Stage 1 tumors [17]. Cytogenetic analysis revealed that the vast majority of recurrent aberrations are telomeric associations, observed in approximately 70% of clonally abnormal tumors, whereas any association was found between cytogenetic features and adverse clinical outcome [24]. On the other hand, ploidy determination combined with FISH analysis may help to predict the recurrence potential of giant-cell tumor of bone, and chromosomal abnormalities superimposed on telomeric associations could be responsible for an aggressive clinical course [25].

MALIGNANCY IN GIANT-CELL TUMOR OF BONE

Malignant transformation of giant-cell tumor of bone is sometimes encountered. Malignant giant-cell tumors of bone, either primary or secondary, are extremely rare. A study of a Swedish population-based national cancer registry comprising 75 malignant giant-cell tumors revealed an average annual incidence of 0.63 per million from 1958 to 1968 [26]. In addition, in a recent study of the epidemiology of giant-cell tumor of bone, analysis of data from the Surveillance, Epidemiology, and End Results (SEER) program described the estimated annual incidence of giant-cell tumor of bone in the United States as 1.6 per 10,000,000 persons [27]. Most malignant GCTB are typically diagnosed in the third and fourth decades of life.

Most of the recurrent disease of giant-cell tumor of bone clinically manifests within 5 years after surgery, and recurrence of the tumor after this period implies the suspicion of malignant transformation. The histology of conventional giant-cell tumors may feature necrosis and even a high rate of mitotic activity. These features can lead to a diagnosis of definite malignancies in certain tumors; however, a definite diagnosis often cannot be made due to the lack of diagnostic criteria for malignant transformation of giant-cell tumors. The diagnostic criteria for secondary malignant giant-cell tumors have not been described so far, though essentially, the following needs to be fulfilled: (1) history of conventional giant-cell tumor of bone, (2) malignant area consists of pleomorphic tumor cells adjacent to the conventional giant-cell tumor area. The key microscopic features in diagnosing malignant change in giant-cell tumor of bone are the presence of atypical mitoses and true nuclear pleomorphism in a spindle cell component that is beside or intermingled with a conventional giant-cell tumor. A sarcomatous change in a pre-existing benign giant-cell tumor may occur without a history of irradiation, though it is more common after it. It has been reported that 156 postradiation sarcomas of bone comprised 89 cases of osteosarcoma, 45 cases of fibrosarcoma, 13 cases of malignant fibrous histiocytoma, 5 cases of chondrosarcoma, 2 cases of hemangioendothelioma, and a single case of Ewing's sarcoma and malignant lymphoma, respectively [28]. The interval between irradiation and the diagnosis of sarcoma has also been shown to vary from 1 year to 55 years, being less than 5 years in only 12 patients and more than 20 years in 46 patients [28]. All sarcomas arising after surgical intervention or therapeutic irradiation of benign GCTB are classified as secondary malignant GCTB, usually exhibiting the histology of osteosarcoma, malignant fibrous histiocytoma, or fibrosarcoma. In patients with giant-cell tumor of bone treated by surgery alone, the time for malignant transformation ranges 1–3 years, and their tumors are mostly well-differentiated, low-grade malignant types. On the other hand, the period of malignant conversion for patients treated only by radiation ranges 3–20 years, and most of the secondary malignant tumors exhibit high-grade, malignant anaplastic features [29], in line with the abovementioned general findings in postradiation sarcomas [28]. An inverse phenomenon has also been reported regarding the average latent period between diagnosis of giant-cell tumor and diagnosis of malignant transformation; being 9 years (range, 3–15 years) for patients with irradiation and 19 years (range, 7–28 years) for patients with spontaneous transformation [30].

Malignant transformation itself is a phenomenon of "dedifferentiation"; therefore, as with other dedifferentiated sarcomas, e.g., dedifferentiated chondrosarcoma, the dedifferentiated area can be observed histologically as being clearly separated by fibrous septa in the background of conventional GCTB. However, this is not always the case, and rather more predominant are the problematic cases where the malignant nature is obscure, with little cellular atypia [31].

Extremely rare cases of primary giant-cell tumor have also been reported. A primary, de novo malignant GCTB is defined as a newly arisen sarcoma in which, synchronously, a histologically identifiable typical benign giant-cell tumor component is present. It frequently occurs in typical anatomical sites involved by conventional GCTB. The microscopic feature is that of high-grade pleomorphic sarcoma without osteoid production. In case of any evidence of osteoid production, it is referred to as giant-cell–rich osteosarcoma.

Curettage with cryosurgery and en bloc resection are the favorable treatments for malignant GCTB [32]. In contrast to the poor overall survival in patients with secondary malignant GCTB, patients with primary de novo giant-cell tumors exhibit a more favorable prognosis [33], although poor prognosis is also reported in primary malignant GCTB [34]. Older age and metastatic disease at diagnosis are associated with poor survival, as seen with other carcinomas [27].

METASTASIZING BENIGN GIANT-CELL TUMOR OF BONE

There are many reports describing lung metastases of benign GCTB. Approximately 2%–3% of giant-cell tumor of bone is known to metastasize to the lung [7]. Pulmonary metastases (also termed benign implantations) of histologically benign GCTB are considered secondary to the iatrogenic seeding of tumor cells into vessels or lymphatics by vigorous curettage. This hypothesis can be explained by the observation of the self-limited growth potential of the metastasized tumors, which maintain the same size without excision, and the long-term benign clinical course of the patients. This hypothesis is also consistent with the findings that the mechanisms of metastasis may be unrelated to cell proliferative ability in giant-cell tumors, as hTERT staining does not correlate with metastasis-free survival [10, 11]. Pulmonary metastases in histologically benign GCTB usually occur within 3 years after the initial surgical treatment [35].

However, they can sometimes be detected at diagnosis of the primary tumor in patients who had not received prior surgical treatment, and can even occur at a substantially later stage after the removal of the primary tumor [36]. Some metastatic tumors may even spontaneously regress, and the patient has relatively good prognosis. Unusually, lung metastases can behave in a more aggressive fashion, and the patient may die due to the unresectable multiple pulmonary metastases [37].

In such cases, chemotherapy is indicated [37]. Although the overall survival in patients with pulmonary implants is much better than that of pulmonary metastasis of other malignancies, approximately 25% of patients die of the disease [38]. Giant-cell tumors may also metastasize to soft tissue, especially with the presence of lung implantation.

FACTORS THAT MAY RELATE TO MALIGNANT TRANSFORMATION IN GIANT-CELL TUMOR OF BONE

More than 100 cases of secondary malignant giant-cell tumors have been reported in the English literature. However, immunohistochemical and genetic analysis that could characterize the nature of the malignant giant-cell tumor has not yet been carried out adequately. Immunohistochemical analysis revealed that diffuse and strong p53 expression in the transformed tumor than the primary GCT [39].

On the other hand, the molecular genesis of malignant transformation remains unclear. Genetic alterations observed in secondary malignant GCTB so far are mutations of *p53* [40, 41], *H-ras* [41], loss of *p53* heterozygosity [31], and amplification of *CNND1* and *met* [42], although these reports described only single or a few cases. We observed that degradation-resistant mutated p53 might have association with malignant transformation of giant-cell tumor of bone as well as lung metastasis and local relapse through overexpression of GPX-1 transcriptionally induced by p53 [Okubo, Saito et al., unpublished findings].

SECONDARY MALIGNANT GIANT-CELL TUMOR OF BONE

We present 2 cases of malignant GCTB that we recently encountered. The first case (Case 1) was a 46-year-old man who had primary giant-cell tumor that had been treated with curettage and bone grafting at the age of 24 years. He experienced malignant GCTB after 4 times of local recurrence at the right distal femur. The first 3 instances of local recurrences had occurred at the ages of 26, 27, and 30 years, respectively, and had been treated with curettage and bone grafting. He had been disease-free for 16 years after the last treatment; however, the fourth local recurrence was detected when he was 46 years old, and was treated by en bloc resection and reconstruction with prosthesis. Pathologically, the fourth recurrent tumor did not contain any apparent malignant component; however, 6 months after this treatment, a solitary metastatic tumor of the lung as well as a metastatic tumor of the right lower leg was discovered. The fifth recurrent tumor contained a malignant area composed of a proliferation of spindle-shaped cells in fascicular fashion without giant-cells clearly separated by fibrous septa in the background of an otherwise benign giant-cell tumor (Figures 7-9).

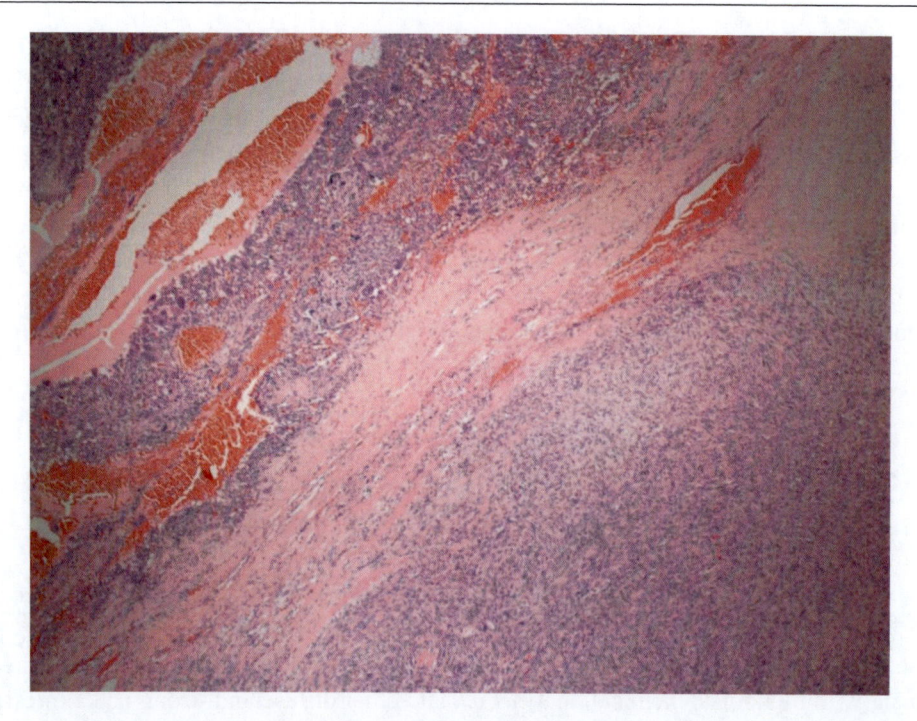

Figure 7. Transition area between malignant area (right below) and otherwise conventional GCT area (left upper). Both areas are clearly separated by fibrous septa.

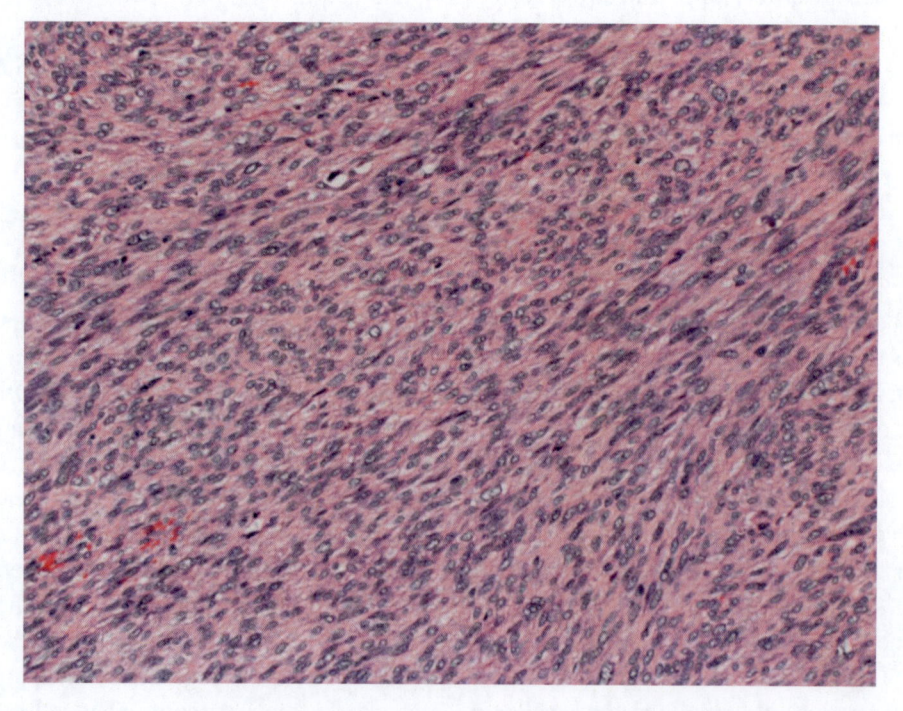

Figure 8. Malignant area is composed of a proliferation of spindle-shaped cells in fascicular fashion without giant-cells.

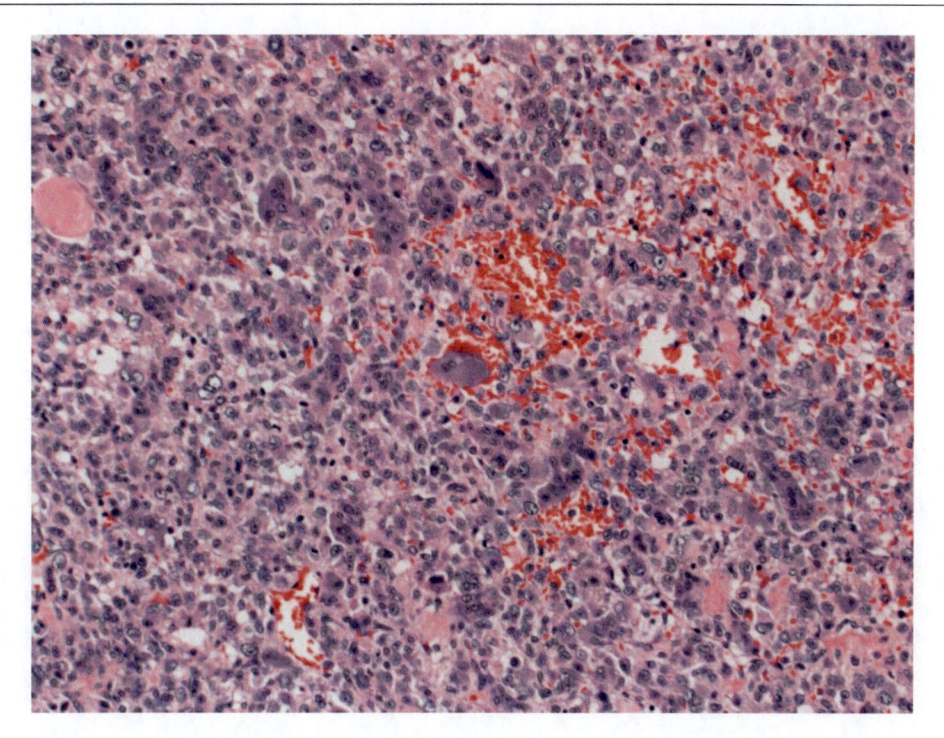

Figure 9. Otherwise conventional GCT area is composed of a proliferation of mononuclear stromal cells with evenly scattered multinucleated giant cells. Cellular and nuclear atypia is not evident in both mononuclear cells and giant cells. Mutation of the p53 gene was also detected in this area, thereby this lesion should be also regarded as malignant GCT.

The recurrent malignant tumor of the right leg was proven to contain a *p53* mutation. In addition, the lung metastatic lesion did not exhibit histologically sarcomatous transformation, though the metastatic lung tumor harbored the same type of *p53* mutation observed in the transformed tumor of the right leg. Histologically and clinically, this was a typical case of secondary malignant GCTB. A late development of malignant transformation as seen in this case has also been reported [43].

The second case (Case 2) was a 19-year-old woman admitted to the hospital with a complaint of right wrist pain [31]. Plain radiograph revealed a well-demarcated osteolytic lesion in the right distal radius. Surgical treatment with curettage and bone grafting was performed, and the pathological diagnosis was conventional GCTB.

However, local recurrence was detected 6 months after the treatment, and curettage with bone graft was performed again. The histology of the recurrent tumor was malignant giant-cell tumor composed of highly atypical stromal cells and tumor giant cells (Figure 10).

The patient received systemic chemotherapy along with curettage and cryosurgery using liquid nitrogen. A retrospective review of the primary tumor revealed a small focus of pleomorphic cells within the otherwise conventional giant-cell tumor, which was histologically almost similar to that seen in the recurrent malignant tumor (Figures 11-13). Further analysis showed that p53 overexpression and LOH of *p53* were present only in the recurrent tumor, suggesting the possibility that this genetic alteration occurred during the 6 months between the first and the second surgical treatments, thus a diagnosis of secondary malignant giant-cell tumor was made.

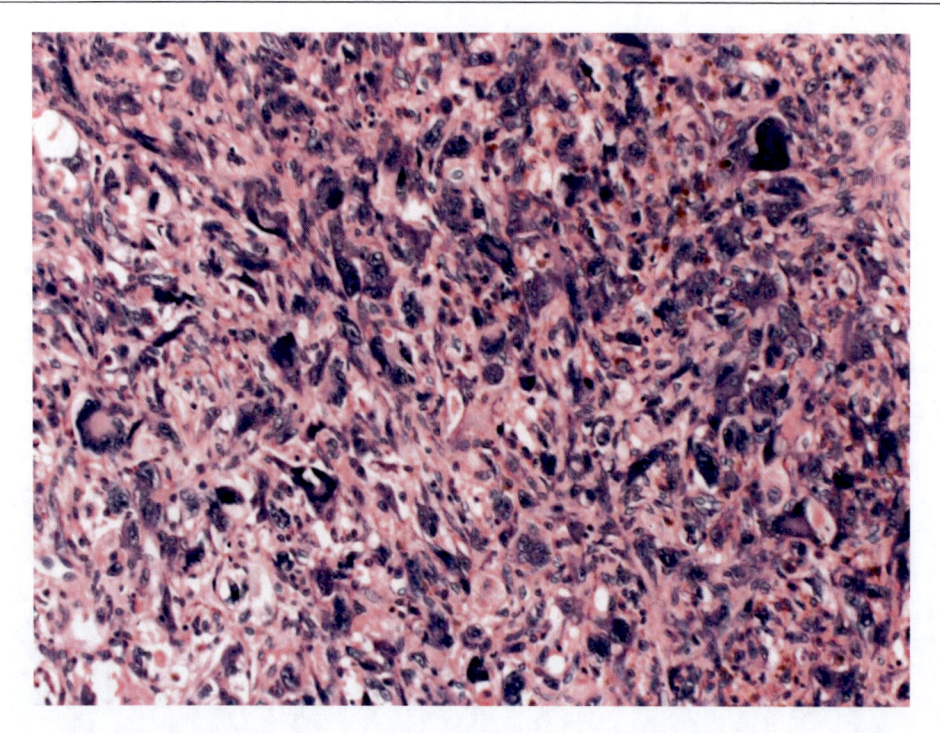

Figure 10. The histology of the recurrent tumor was malignant giant-cell tumor composed of highly atypical stromal cells and tumor giant cells.

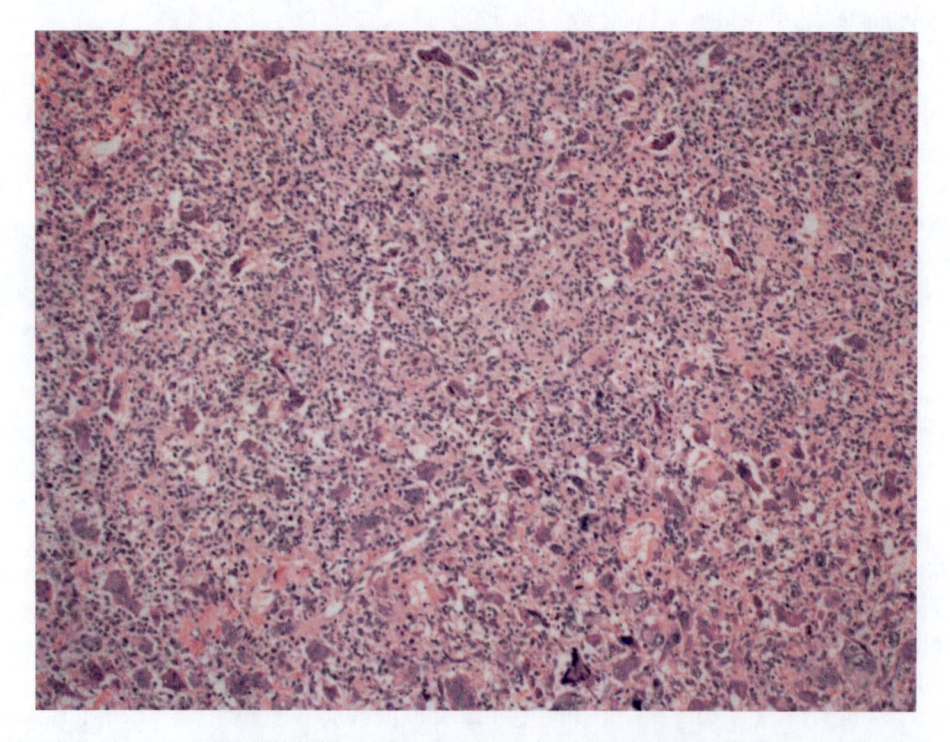

Figure 11. Low power view shows transition area between pleomorphic area (below) and otherwise conventional GCT in the primary tumor.

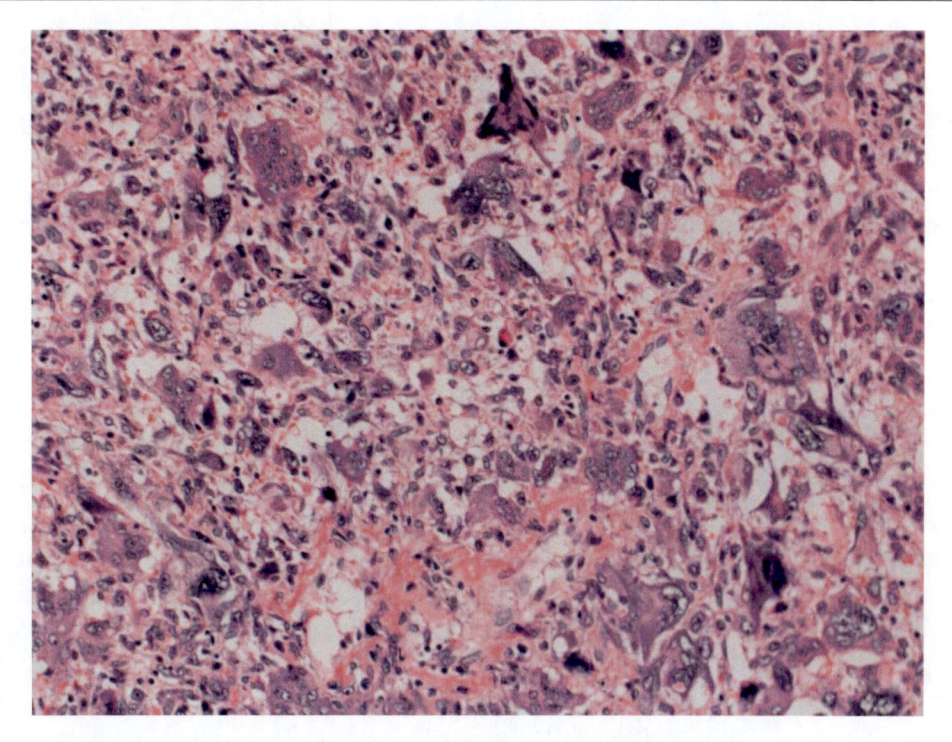

Figure 12. Pleomorphic area observed as a tiny area in the primary tumor.

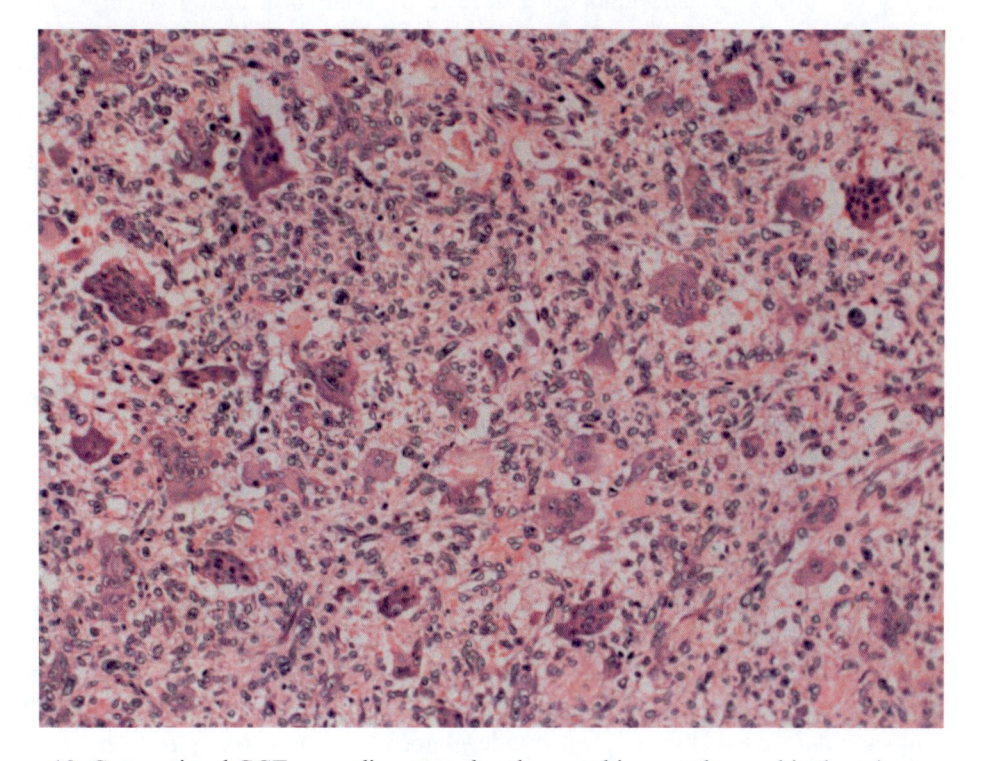

Figure 13. Conventional GCT area adjacent to the pleomorphic area observed in the primary tumor.

Apart from the phenomenon of malignant transformation in this tumor, the pleomorphic atypical cells observed in the primary tumor might be better understood as pseudoanaplasia, although if it were linked to the malignant recurrent tumor, the term "pseudoanaplasia" would be inappropriate (see below).

In this patient, no radiologic features of aggressiveness such as soft tissue involvement was observed in the recurrent tumor, although the absorption of grafting bone was evident. As observed in this case, the radiologic features of aggressiveness in giant-cell tumor of bone did not correlate with the histologic criteria of malignancy or with metastatic potential.

MALIGNANT TRANSFORMATION VS. PRIMARY MALIGNANCY IN OTHER BONE TUMORS

This is a major issue in which much room for debate remains, even among pathologists specializing in bone tumors. Giant-cell tumors of bone often exhibit secondary ABC-like change. Sometimes, areas with aneurysmal bone cyst-like change gain predominance, and the preexisting GCTB becomes obscure histologically. In such cases, aneurysmal bone cyst might also be considered a differential diagnosis for giant-cell tumor of bone. Primary ABC had been originally considered a tumor-like lesion. However, recurrent chromosomal translocation has recently been identified in primary ABC [44-47]; thus, primary ABC is considered a neoplastic lesion, different from secondary ABC.

One of the most important tumors that need to be distinguished from aneurysmal bone cyst is telangiectatic osteosarcoma. It might be possible today to distinguish primary ABC from telangiectatic osteosarcoma based on the aforementioned chromosomal translocation, though some cases that had initially been diagnosed as primary ABC eventually progressed to high-grade telangiectatic osteosarcoma [48]. Whether these lesions are purely malignant tumors at initial or secondary malignancy requires careful discussion. One of the most important points that need to be stressed is that we should never overlook a faint sign of malignancy.

A few atypical fibroblastic cells in the primary lesion revealed the true nature of the lesion in a case of malignant bone tumor that initially had been diagnosed as primary ABC [48]. Giant-cell reparative granuloma in extragnathic sites could be considered a reactive process that develops in intraosseous hemorrhagic lesions either in normal bone or within preexisting conditions such as hyperparathyroidism.

It has been argued that the entity of solid ABC is a manifestation of giant-cell reparative granuloma, and that whether it is a distinct lesion is controversial. Evidence favors the premise that this is a true neoplastic lesion, because a translocation involving USP6 was recently reported in a case of a solid variant of aneurysmal bone cyst, though the translocation partner for USP6 remained unclear [49]. Here, we describe 2 cases (Case 3 and 4, respectively) where initial diagnoses of malignant tumors were not possible.

Case 3: A 60-year-old man visited our hospital due to right hip pain. Plain radiography revealed an osteolytic lesion at the right greater trochanter (Figure 14). A biopsy specimen revealed a proliferation of less atypical spindle-shaped cells in a fascicular fashion (Figure 15). Hemosiderin deposition and a mild degree of lymphocytic infiltration were also noted.

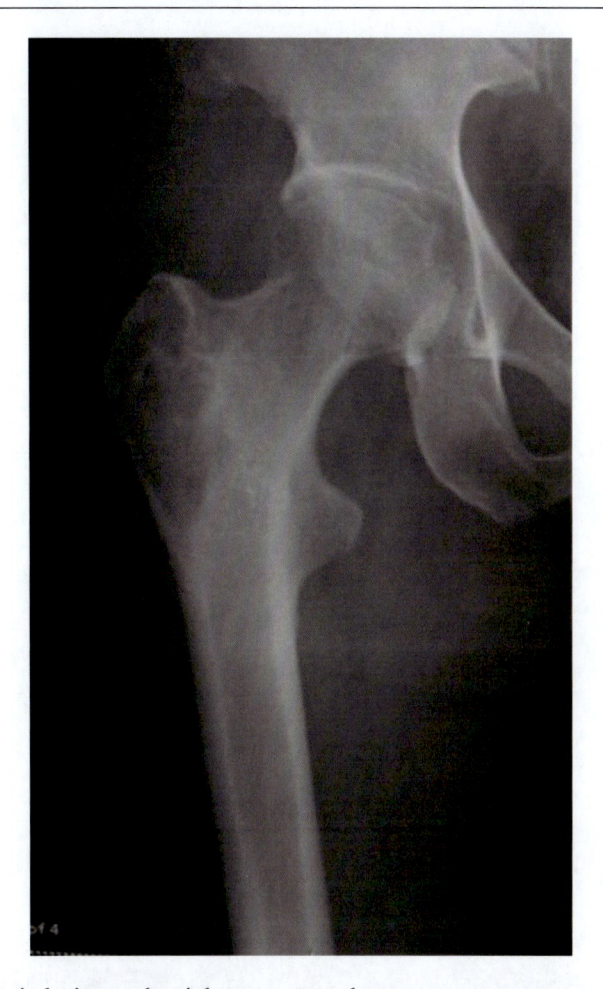

Figure 14. An osteolytic lesion at the right greater trochanter.

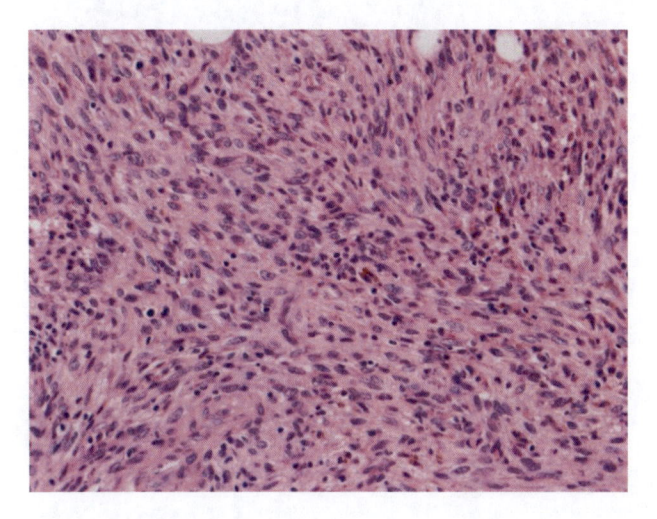

Figure 15. Histology from the initial biopsy specimen. Proliferation of less atypical spindle-shaped cells in a fascicular fashion. Hemosiderin deposition and a mild degree of lymphocytic infiltration were also noted.

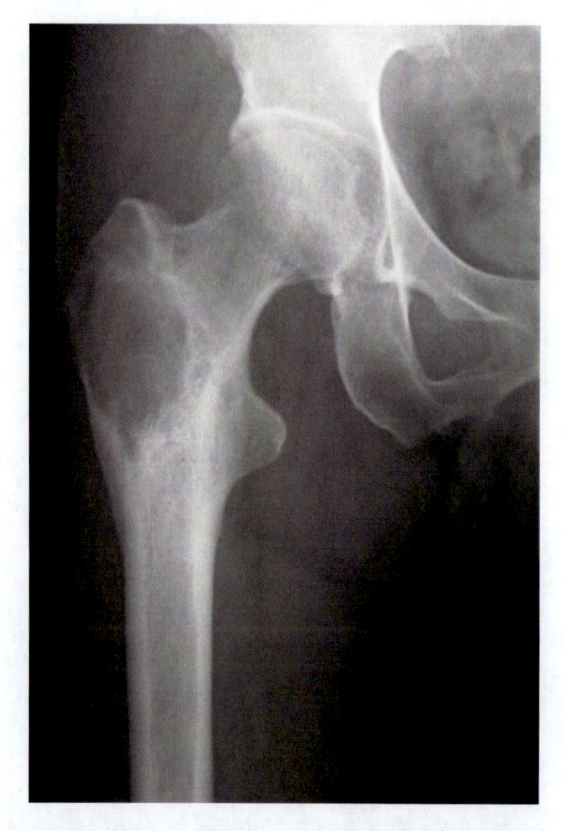

Figure 16. Approximately 1 year after the biopsy, the expansive osteolytic lesion had grown larger.

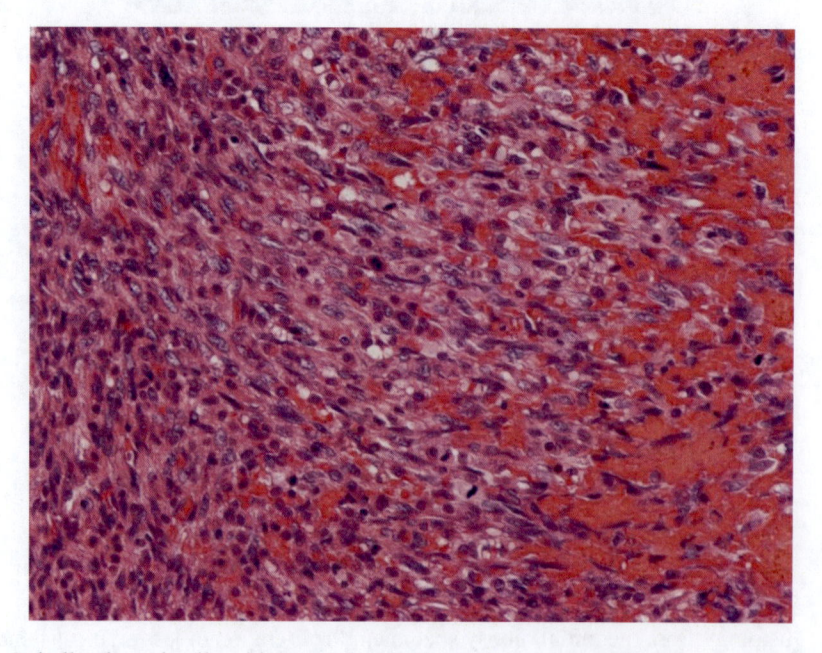

Figure 17. Spindle-shaped cells with hyperchromatic nuclei were proliferating in storiform fashion with stromal bleeding.

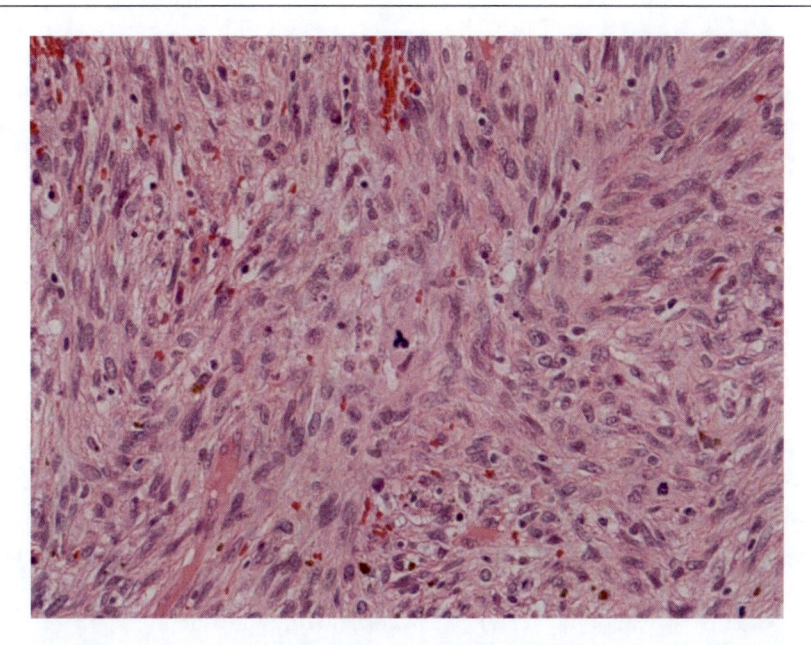

Figure 18. Atypical mitosis was also noted indicating that this tumor is malignant.

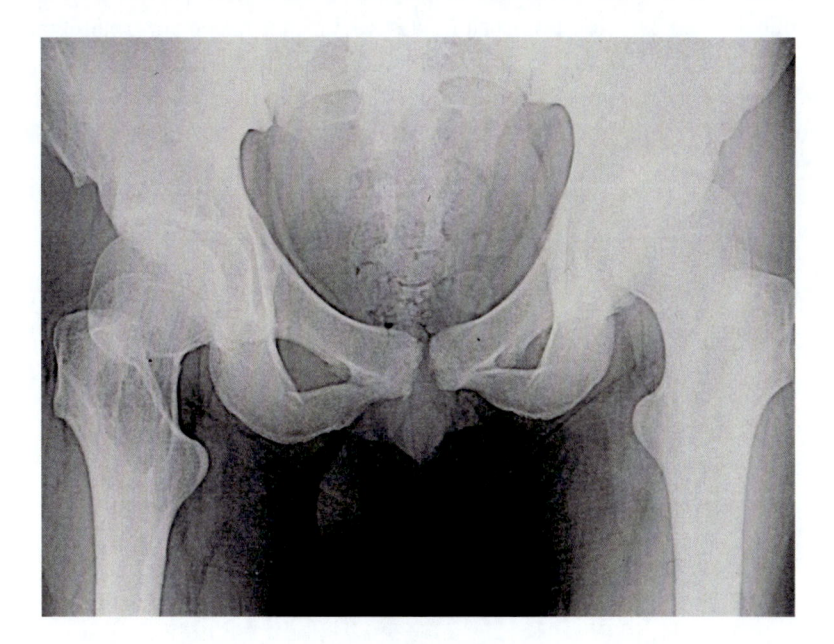

Figure 19. Plain radiograph of the patient at the time of presentation. Plain radiography reveals an osteolytic lesion of his right proximal femur, but without cortical destruction.

Although a few mitoses without atypical mitoses were observed, an initial diagnosis of benign fibrous histiocytoma was made, and a giant-cell tumor with secondary histiocytic change was considered as one of the differential diagnoses underlying this lesion. The patient was followed-up regularly and the lesion had remained at almost the same size. However, approximately 1 year after the biopsy, plain radiography revealed that the lesion had grown larger (Figure 16). Therefore, wide resection of the tumor was performed. The surgical specimen exhibited a proliferation of highly atypical spindle cells in storiform fashion without apparent osteoid production (Figures 17 and 18). A final diagnosis of malignant fibrous histiocytoma of bone was made. Obtaining additional biopsy samples when an accurate diagnosis is impossible is generally recommended. In fact, biopsies were performed twice in this case, though the malignant component leading to the diagnosis of malignant fibrous histiocytoma could not be obtained.

Case 4: A 21-year-old man visited a hospital with a 10-day history of right coxalgia. Plain radiography revealed a well-defined osteolytic lesion of his right proximal femur without cortical destruction (Figure 19)

Curettage with bone grafting was performed under a clinical diagnosis of aneurysmal bone cyst. A histologic section from the curettage material revealed membranous septa composed of collagenous tissue and plump, spindle-shaped cells (Figure 20). A high-power view of the septum revealed scattered large and bizarre cells with hyperchromatic nuclei in the stroma; however, neither mitosis nor neoplastic osteoid formation was detected (Figure 21). A diagnosis of pseudosarcomatous ABC was rendered. The first local recurrence was observed 4 years and 8 months after the initial treatment. A plain radiography at this time revealed an expansive osteolytic lesion with cortical thinning at the right proximal femur (Figure 22). Magnetic resonance imaging showed a multilocular low-intensity lesion on the T1-weighted image and a high-intensity lesion on the T2-weighted image (Figures 23 and 24). The clinical diagnosis for this lesion was recurrence of aneurysmal bone cyst, and curettage with bone grafting and internal fixation was again performed. At the time of surgery, the cystic space contained bloody fluid. The histological section of the first recurrent lesion was extensive granulation tissue with scattered, bizarre cells containing enlarged nuclei (Figure 25).

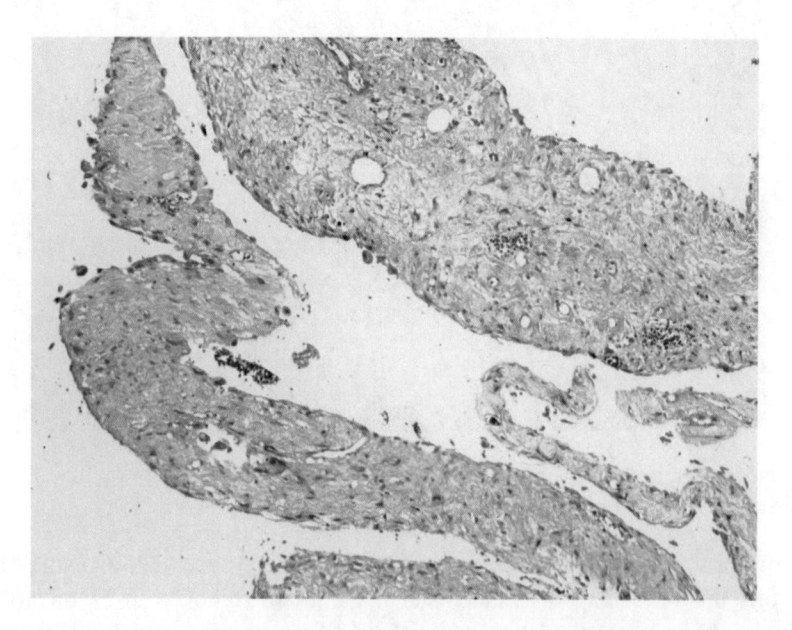

Figure 20. Histological section obtained from the curettage specimen shows cystic spaces separated by membranous septa of collagenous tissue with plump spindle[-]shaped cells. A small amount of erythrocytes are observed within the spaces. The features are quite similar to those seen in aneurysmal bone cyst.

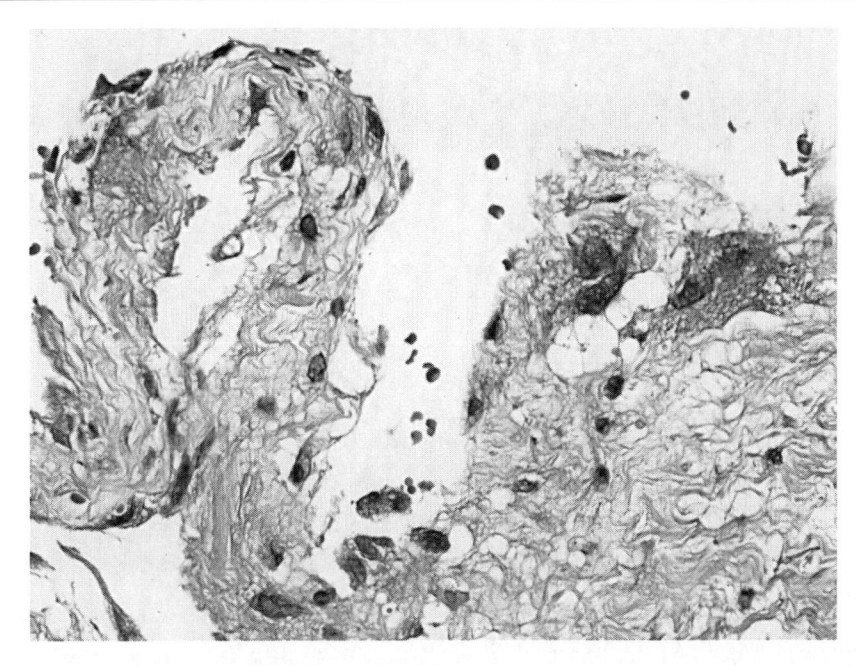

Figure 21. High-power magnification of the section shows some large and bizarre cells with hyperchromatic nuclei in the membranous septa, but neither mitosis nor neoplastic osteoid is detected in this specimen.

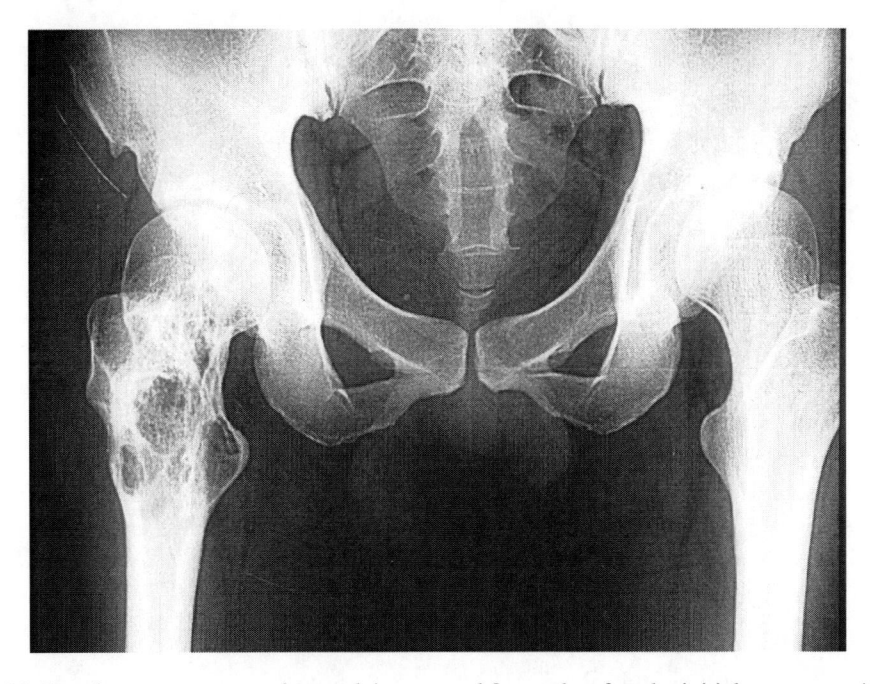

Figure 22. Local recurrence was observed 4 years and 8 months after the initial treatment. An expansile osteolytic lesion with cortical thinning[] but without cortical destruction is recognized at the right proximal femur by the plain radiograph.

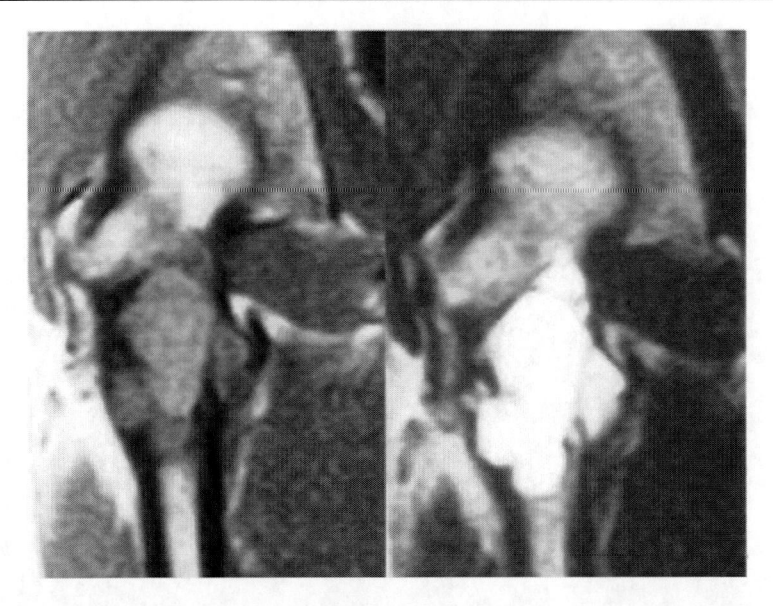

Figures 23 (left: T1) and 24 (right: T2). On MRI, the lesion shows low intensity on T1-weighted image and high intensity on T2-weighted image.

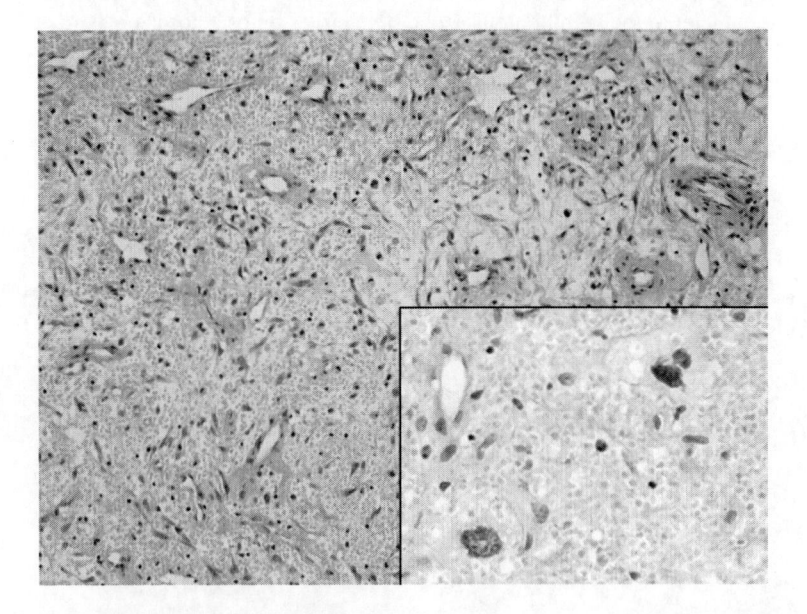

Figure 25. The histologic section from the first local recurrent tumor showed extensive granulation tissue with occasional bizarre cells with large nuclei (inset). Neither mitosis nor neoplastic osteoid is observed in this specimen.

The pathologic diagnosis of pseudosarcomatous ABC with extensive granulation tissue was again made for this lesion.

Further local recurrence was detected 8 months after the second surgery. On plain Xp, the lesser trochanter of the right femur had been completely destroyed, and an eggshell-like rim of reactive bone could not be observed (Figures 26 and 27). A clinical diagnosis of malignant tumor was made because of the rapid growth of the local recurrence. Wide resection of the tumor (Figure 28) and reconstruction by Kotz prosthesis was performed. The histology of the resected specimen exhibited a cystic wall composed of pleomorphic stromal cells bordering blood-filled spaces (Figure 29). High-power viewing revealed nuclear pleomorphism and frequent mitoses, including atypical mitoses (Figure 30). Neoplastic osteoid formation was also noted (Figure 31), leading to a diagnosis of telangiectatic osteosarcoma. This case was finally diagnosed as primary telangiectatic osteosarcoma [48], although malignant transformation of aneurysmal bone cysts have also been reported in at least 7 cases so far [50]. Molecular testing for the chimeric genes identified in primary ABC may be useful, although the presence of the aforementioned chimeric genes had not been tested in these cases.

In addition, 3 cases in total of osteosarcoma arising from desmoplastic fibroma have been reported in the literature and textbooks [28, 51, 52]. We have also encountered a similar case for which a few differential diagnoses were suggested, and we present it here as Case 5. This case was a bone tumor arising in a 50-year-old woman. She had felt pain in the right knee for almost 2 years. She had been admitted to our hospital due to her knee pain. She had a past history of thyroid carcinoma. Upon clinical examination, a tumor was identified on the right distal femur. X-ray and CT revealed a bone tumor of the distal femur with cortical thinning, partially destroying the cortex and invading into the surrounding soft tissue (Figures 32 and 33). Biopsy specimens were obtained from both the intraosseous lesion and the soft tissue mass. Histology of the intraosseous lesion revealed a hypocellular area with spindle-shaped cells in dense collagen fibers mimicking desmoplastic fibroma (Figure 34); however, the specimen from the soft tissue mass exhibited a relatively hypercellular area containing a proliferation of atypical spindle-shaped cells, raising the possibility of high-grade sarcoma (Figure 35).

Thus, the possibility of desmoplastic fibroma, low-grade fibrosarcoma, and high-grade sarcoma was considered based on the biopsy. Surgical resection was performed under the clinical and pathological diagnosis of malignant bone tumor. The histological features comprised a proliferation of spindle-shaped tumor cells with abundant collagenous fibers (Figure 36).

Some of the spindle-shaped tumor cells contained enlarged atypical nuclei (Figure 37). Immuno-histochemically, the tumor cells were positive for vimentin, SMA (quite focally), and M-actin, and negative for S-100 protein (Figure 38). We diagnosed this case as low-grade myofibroblastic sarcoma of bone, because the abundant collagenous fibers in this tumor that could have otherwise been observed in desmoplastic fibroma would have been somewhat unusual for leiomyo-sarcoma. It is important to detect even scant atypical cells to differentiate low-grade fibrosarcoma from desmoplastic fibroma of bone [53].

PSEUDOSARCOMATOUS CHANGE (PSEUDOANAPLASIA/PSEUDOMALIGNANT)

Pseudoanaplastic bone tumors, which can sometimes be mistaken for sarcoma even by pathology experts, are well described by Bahk and Mirra [54].

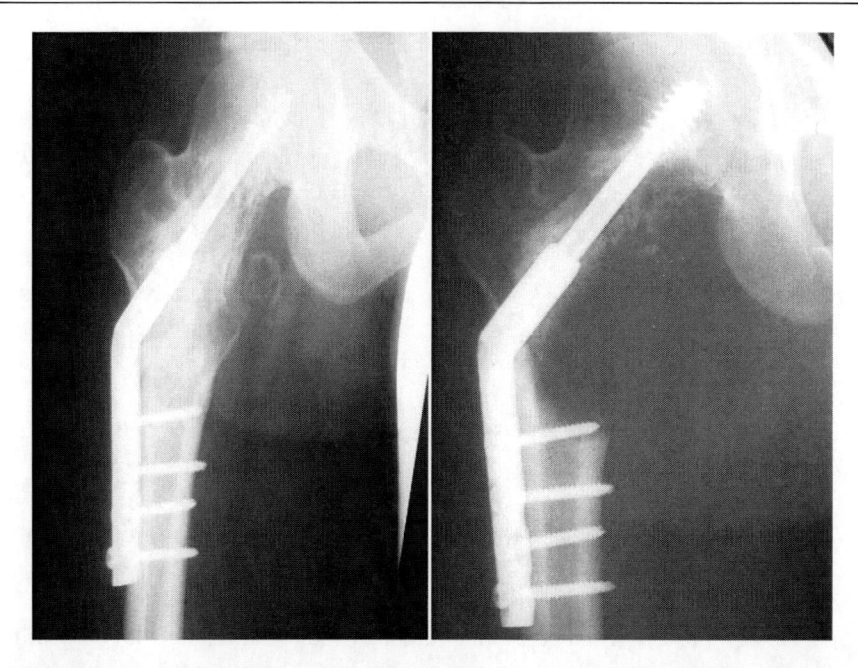

Figures 26 (left) and 27 (right). Plain radiograph at 2 months after the second operation (26). Plain radiograph at 11 months after the second operation (27). The lesser trochanter of the right femur disappeared and an eggshell-like rim of reactive bone could not be observed.

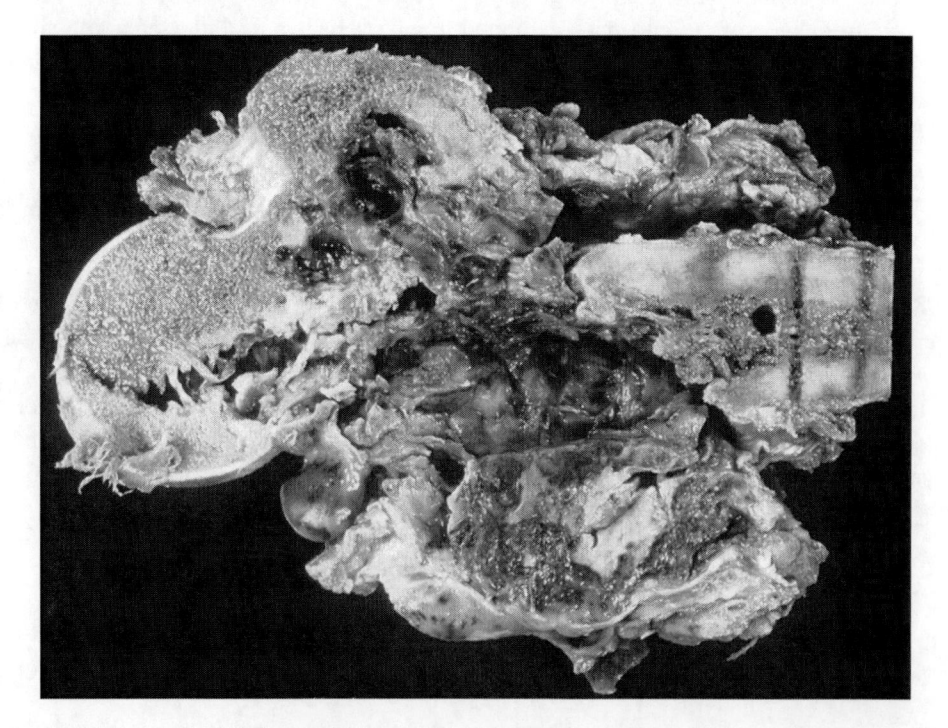

Figure 28. Gross section of the surgical specime shows destruction of the lesser trochanter with a soft tissue mass. The cystic lesion of the lesser trochanter contained a large amount of bloody fluid.

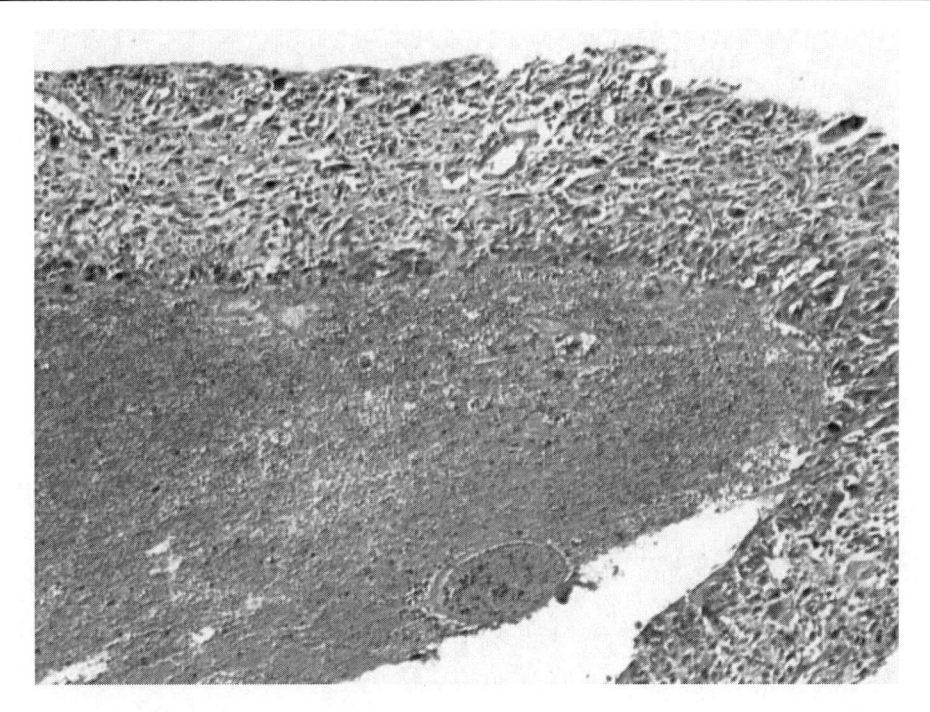

Figure 29. The histological section of the second local recurrence showed septa composed of pleomorphic stromal cells bordering blood-filled space.

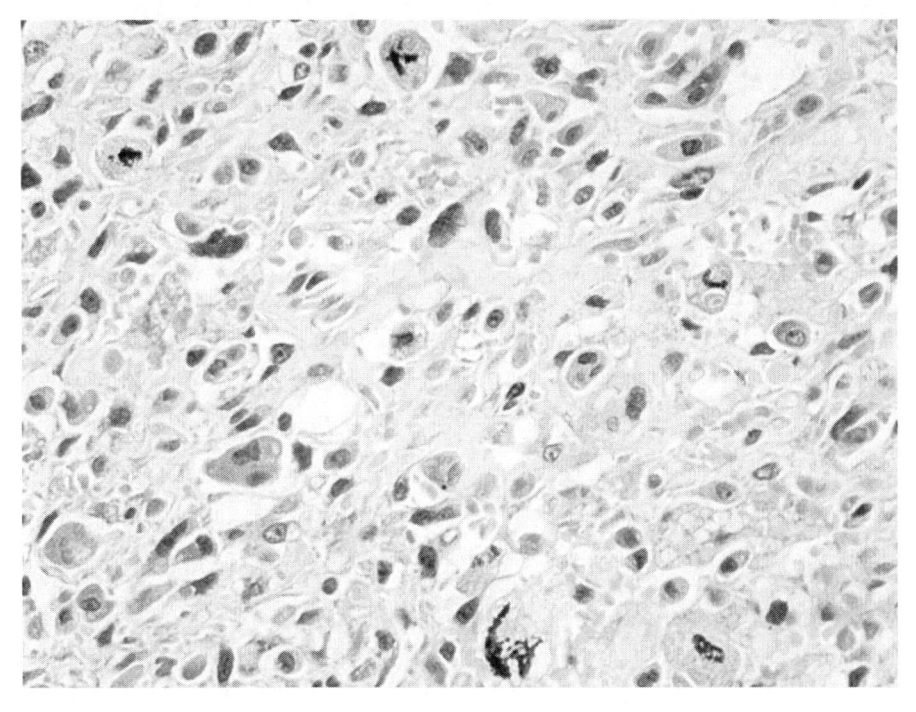

Figure 30. Higher magnification showed nuclear pleomorphism and frequent mitoses including atypical ones.

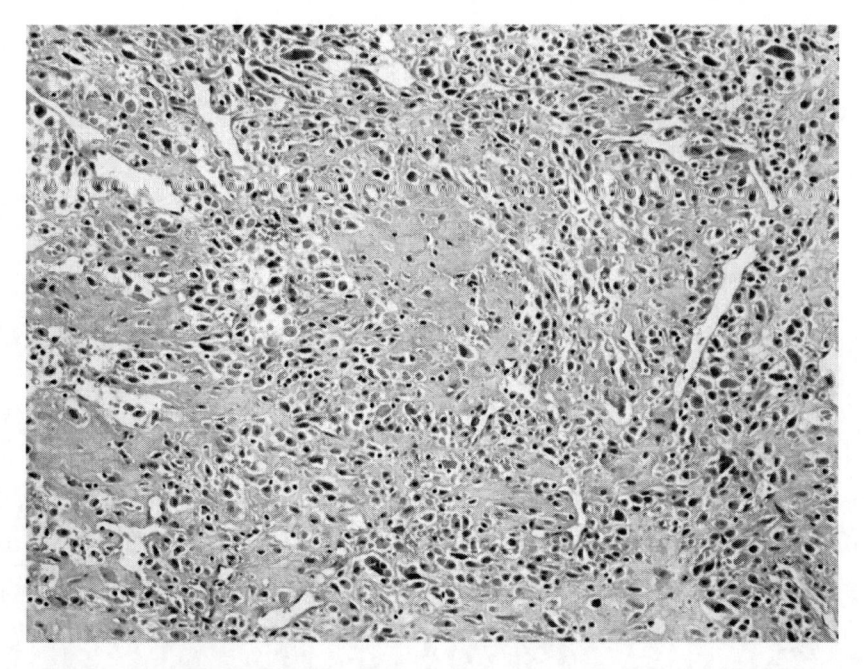

Figure 31. Neoplastic osteoid formation was also noted.

Their diagnostic criteria for pseudoanaplastic bone tumor are: (a) bizarre nuclear aberrations, including marked pleomorphism and hyperchromatism with absent to rare mitoses and no atypical mitoses; (b) a benign-looking radiographic picture in keeping with benign clinical manifestations; and (c) absence of metastasis or loss of life or limb from aggressive or cancerous local recurrence of the tumor [54]. They retrospectively reviewed a database containing 4262 cases of benign bone tumors, and found 15 cases of pseudoanaplastic bone tumors using the abovementioned criteria [54]. Pseudoanaplasia can be seen in giant-cell tumor of bone, chondromyxoid fibroma, osteoblastoma, aneurysmal bone cyst, fibrous dysplasia, fibrous cortical defect, and non-ossifying fibroma [54]. The patients were followed-up for at least 3 years and up to 7 years after surgical treatment. All patients, except a case of pseudoanaplastic ABC, were described as being well and living, with no evidence of local recurrence or metastasis. Interestingly, the single case of pseudoanaplastic ABC described in their findings is quite similar to the case of telangiectatic osteosarcoma described as Case 2 in the previous section. The ages of the 2 patients and the locations of their tumors are almost the same, and both tumors recurred 3–4 years after the initial treatments of curettage and bone grafting. In both cases, the recurrent tumors were re-curetted.

Atypical bizarre cells featuring nuclear pleomorphism were observed in histological sections from both cases, and even a single mitosis, which was not observed in the telangiectatic osteosarcoma case discussed earlier, was found in the pseudoanaplastic ABC case. Although the clinical settings of both cases, including the absence of significant soft tissue mass in the recurrent tumors and the absence of lung metastasis, were also similar, no evidence remained of local recurrence or metastasis 4 years after the simple re-curettage in the pseudoanaplastic ABC case.

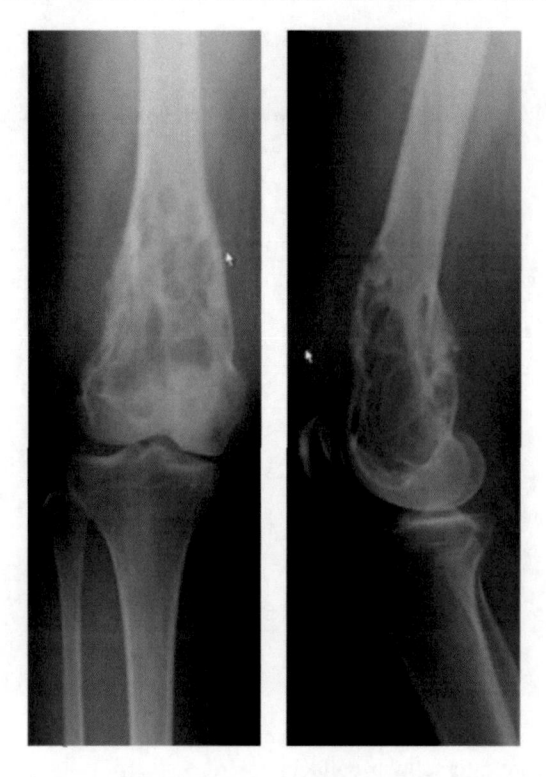

Figure 32. Plain radiography reveals honeycombed lucent lesion at the right distal femur.

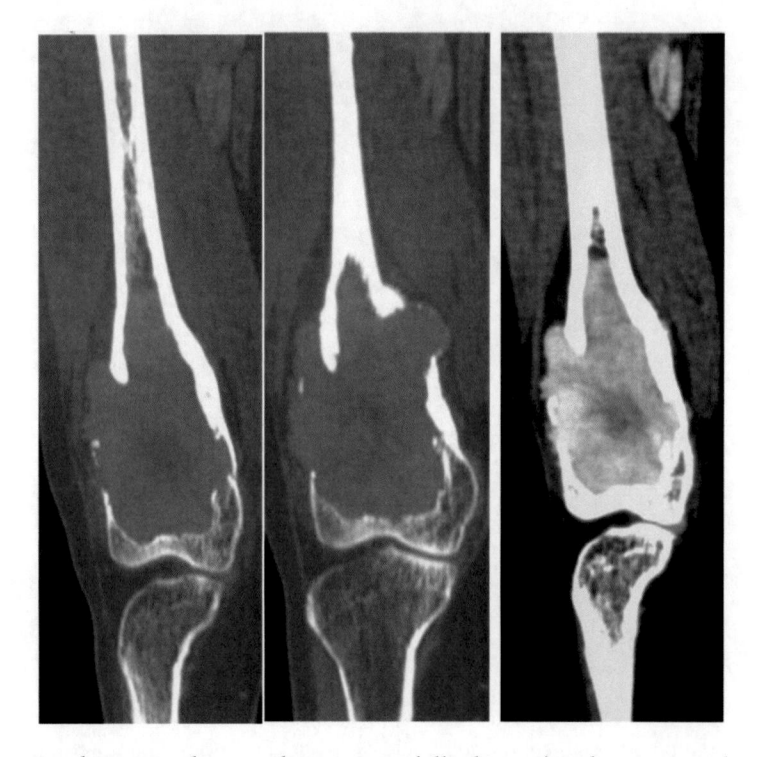

Figure 33. Computed tomography reveals tumor partially destroying the cortex and extending into the surrounding soft tissue.

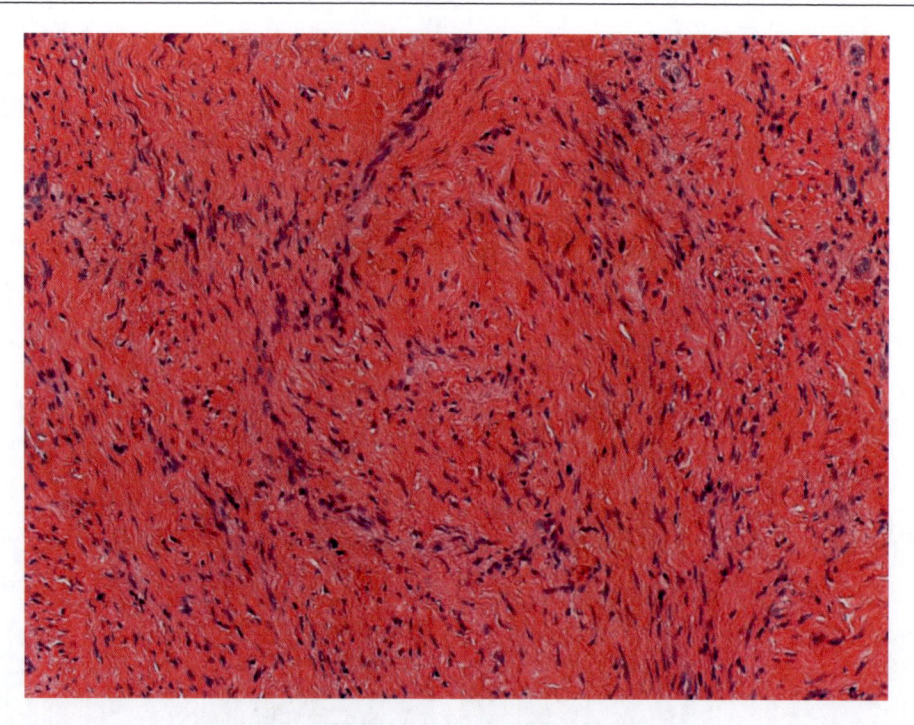

Figure 34. A biopsy from intra-osseous lesion shows hypocellular area with a proliferation of spindle cells with abundant intercellular collagen.

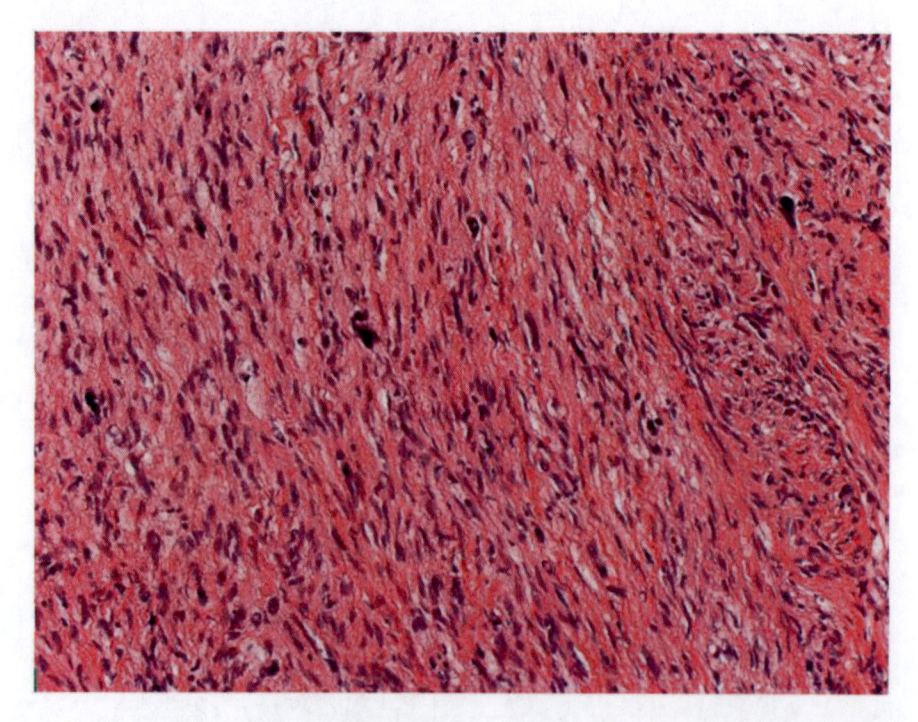

Figure 35. A biopsy from extra-osseous lesion shows a hypercellular area with a proliferation of spindle cells with hyperchromatic enlarged nuclei in a background of abundant intercellular collagen.

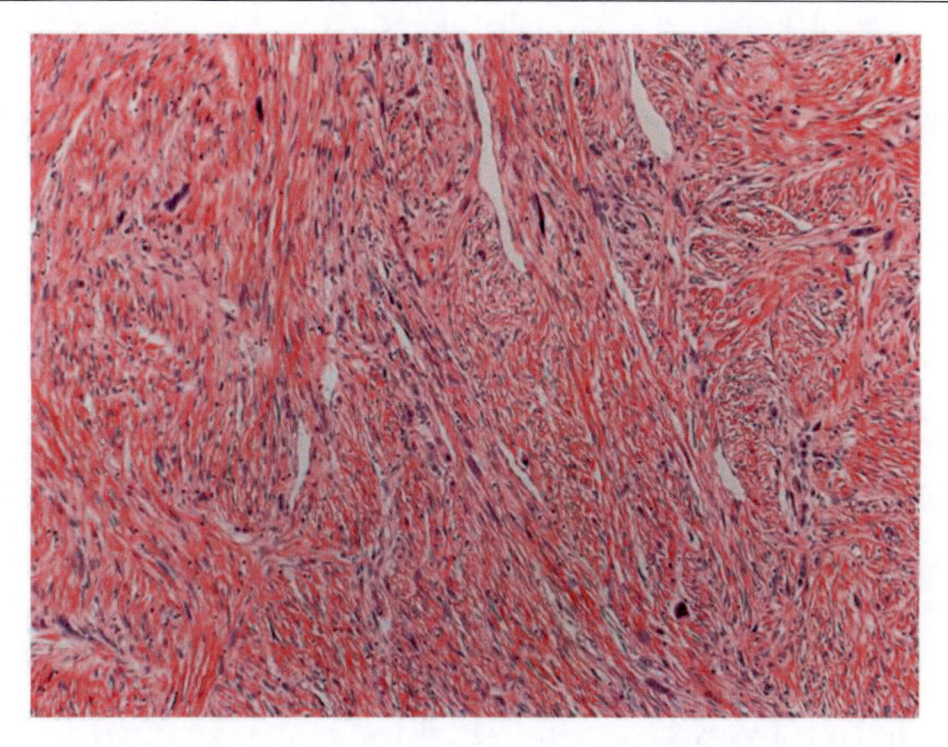

Figure 36. Low-power view from extra-osseous lesion of the surgical specimen shows a proliferation of spindle cells with hyperchromatic enlarged nuclei and eosinophilic cytoplasm.

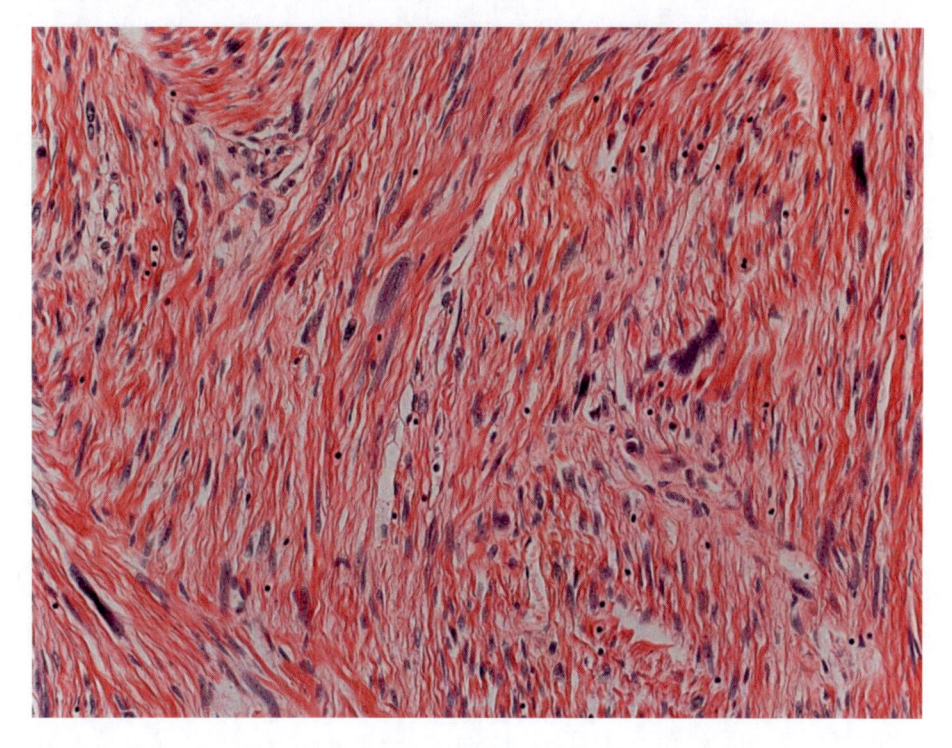

Figure 37. Atypical cells with enlarged nuclei are frequently observed.

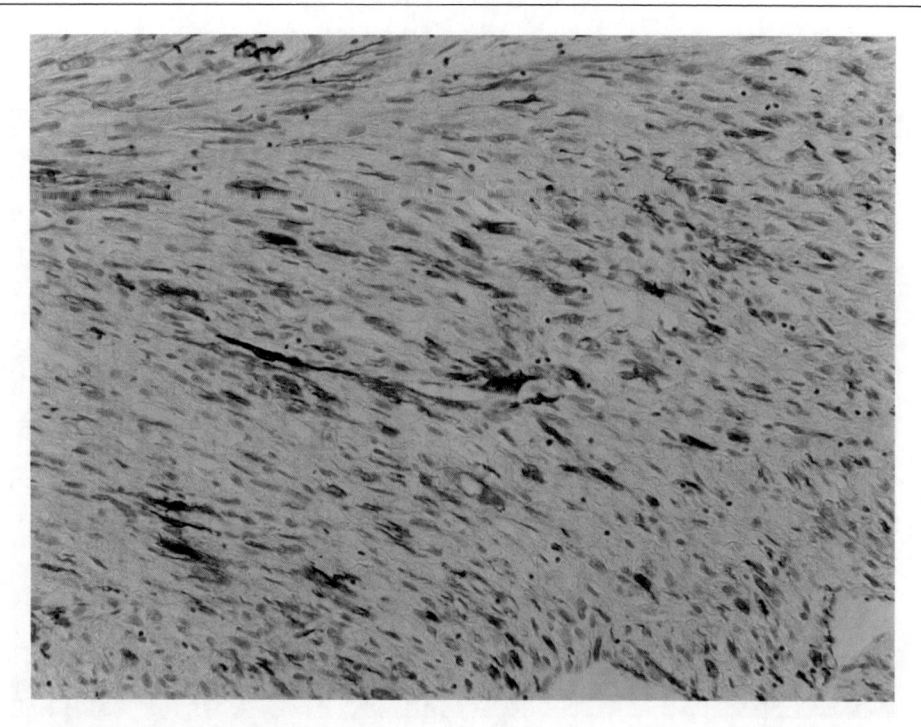

Figure 38. Tumor cells are positive for SMA.

Highly malignant pleomorphic tumor cells often exist only in the small portion of the thin cystic wall in telangiectatic osteosarcoma with massive secondary fibrohistiocytic change.

Inadequate curettage sometimes does not reach the true nature of the telangiectatic osteosarcoma. Atypical bizarre cells can be seen in reactive fibrohistiocytic lesions after surgical treatment or even after biopsy, and in the lesion, manifested by the mechanical stress. The bizarre cells observed in pathological sections of recurrent pseudoanaplastic ABC might be obscured by the initial surgical treatment. The presence of atypical bizarre cells observed in the primary sample may reflect the malignant nature in the case of telangiectatic osteosarcoma initially mistaken for aneurysmal bone cyst presented as Case 4 in this chapter.

REFERENCES

[1]   Enneking WF. A system of staging musculoskeletal neoplasms. *Clin. Ortho. Relat. Res.* 1986, 204:9-24.

[2]   Arbeitsgemeinschaft K, Becker WT, Dohle J, Bernd L, Braun A, Cserhati M, Enderle A, Hovy L, Matejovsky Z, Szendroi M, Trieb K, Tunn PU. Local recurrence of giant cell tumor of bone after intralesional treatment with and without adjuvant therapy. *J. Bone Joint Surg. Am.* 2008, 90:1060-1067.

[3]   Waldram MA, Sneath RS. Is bone graft necessary? Analysis of twenty cases of giant cell tumor of bone treated by curettage without graft. *Int. Orthop.* 1990, 14:129-133.

[4]   Vult von Steyern F, Bauer HC, Trovik C, Kivioja A, Bergh P, Holmberg Jogensen P, Folleras G, Rydholm A; Scandinavian Sarcoma Group. Treatment of local recurrences

of giant cell tumour in long bones after curettage and cementing. A Scandinavian Sarcoma Group study. *J. Bone Joint Surg. Br.* 2006, 88:531-535.

[5]   Saiz P, Virkus W, Piasecki P, Templeton A, Shott S, Gitelis S. Results of giant cell tumor of bone treated with intralesional excision. *Clin. Orthop. Relat. Res.* 2004, 424:221-226.

[6]   Chanchairujira K, Jiranantanakorn T, Phimolsarnti R, Asavamongkolkul A, Waikakul S. Factors of local recurrence of giant cell tumor of long bone after treatment: plain radiographs, pathology and surgical procedures. *J. Med. Assoc. Thai.* 2011, 94:1230-1237.

[7]   Niu X, Zhang Q, Hao L, Ding Y, Li Y, Xu H, Liu W. Giant cell tumor of the extremity: retrospective analysis of 621 Chinese patients from one institution. *J. Bone Joint Surg. Am.* 2012, 94:461-467.

[8]   Malawer MM, Bickels J, Meller I, Buch RG, Henshaw RM, Kollender Y. Cryosurgery in the treatment of giant cell tumor. A long-term followup study. *Clin. Orthop. Relat. Res.* 1999, 359:176-188.

[9]   Szendroi M. Giant cell tumor of bone. *J. Bone Joint Surg.* 2004, 86:5-12.

[10]   Horvai AE, Kramer MJ, Garcia JJ, O'Donnell RJ. Distribution and prognostic significance of human telomerase reverse transcriptase (hTERT) expression in giant cell tumor of bone. *Mod. Pathol.* 2008, 21:432-430.

[11]   Matsuo T, Hiyama E, Sugita T, Shimose S, Kubo T, Mochizuki Y, Adachi N, Kojima K, Sharman P, Ochi M. Telomerase activity in giant cell tumor of bone. *Ann. Surg. Oncol.* 2007, 14:2896-2902.

[12]   Masui F, Ushigome S, Fujii K. Giant cell tumor of bone: an immunohistochemical comparative study. *Pathol. Int.* 1998, 48:355-361.

[13]   Conti A, Rodriguez GC, Chiechi A, Blazquez RM, Barbado V, Krenacs T, Novello C, Pazzaglia L, Quattrini I, Zanella L, Picci P, De Alava E, Benassi MS. Identification of potential biomarkers for giant cell tumor of bone using comparative proteomics analysis. *Am. J. Pathol.* 2011, 178:88-97.

[14]   Balla P, Moskovszky L, Sapi Z, Forsyth R, Knowles H, Athanasou NA, Szendroi M, Kopper L, Rajnai H, Pinter F, Petak I, Benassi MS, Picci P, Conti A, Krenacs T. Epidermal growth factor receptor signalling contributes to osteoblastic stromal cell proliferation, osteoclastogenesis and disease progression in giant cell tumour of bone. *Histopathology.* 2011, 59:376-389.

[15]   Gamberi G, Benassi MS, Bohling T, Ragazzini P, Molendini L, Sollazzo MR, Merli M, Ferrari C, Magagnoli G, Bertoni F, Picci P. Prognostic relevance of C-myc gene expression in giant-cell tumor of bone. *J. Orthop. Res.* 1998, 16:1-7.

[16]   Schoedel KE, Greco MA, Stetler-Stevenson WG, Ohori NP, Goswami S, Present D, Steiner GC. Expression of metalloproteinases and tissue inhibitors of metalloproteinases in giant cell tumor of bone: an immunohistochemical study with clinical correlation. *Human Pathol.* 1996, 27:1144-1148.

[17]   Kumta SM, Huang L, Cheng YY, Chow LT, Lee KM, Zheng MH. Expression of VEGF and MMP-9 in giant cell tumor of bone and other osteolytic lesions. *Life Sci.* 2003, 73:1427-1436.

[18]   Ferracini R, Scotlandi K, Cagliero E, Acquarone F, Olivero M, Wunder J, Baldini N. The expression of Met/hepatocyte growth factor receptor gene in giant cell tumors of bone and other benign musculoskeletal tumors. *J. Cell Physiol.* 2000, 184:191-196.

[19] Zheng MH, Xu J, Robbins P, Pavlos N, Wysocki S, Kumta SM, Wood DJ, Papadimitriou JM. Gene expression of vascular endothelial growth factor in giant cell tumors of bone. *Human Pathol.* 2000, 31:804-812.

[20] Sanerkin NG. Malignancy, aggressiveness, and recurrence in giant cell tumor of bone. *Cancer.* 1980, 46:1641-1649,

[21] Fornasier VL, Protzner K, Zhang I, Mason L. The prognostic significance of histomorphometry and immunohistochemistry in giant cell tumors of bone. *Human Pathol.* 1996, 27:754-760.

[22] Antal I, Sápi Z, Szendröi M. The prognostic significance of DNA cytophotometry and proliferation index (Ki-67) in giant cell tumors of bone. *Int. Orthop.* 1999, 23:315-319.

[23] Masui F, Ushigome S, Fujii K. Giant-cell tumor of bone: a clinicopathologic study of prognostic factors. *Pathol. Int.* 1998, 48:723-729.

[24] Gorunova L, von Steyern FV, Storlazzi CT, Bjerkehagen B, Folleras G, Heim S, Mandahl N, Mertens F. Cytogenetic analysis of 101 giant cell tumors of bone: Nonrandom patterns of telomeric associations and other structural aberrations. *Genes Chromosomes Cancer.* 2009, 48:583-602.

[25] Moskovszky L, Szuhai K, Krenács T, Hogendoorn PC, Szendroi M, Benassi MS, Kopper L, Füle T, Sápi Z. Genomic instability in giant cell tumor of bone. A study of 52 cases using DNA ploidy, relocalization FISH, and array-CGH analysis. *Genes Chromosomes Cancer.* 2009, 48:468-479.

[26] Larsson SE, Lorentzon R, Boquist L. Giant-cell tumor of bone. A demographic, clinical, and histopathological study of all cases recorded in the Swedish Cancer Registry for the years 1958 through 1968. *J. Bone Joint Surg. Am.* 1975, 57:167-173.

[27] Beebe-Dimmer JL, Cetin K, Fryzek JP, Schuetze SM, Schwartz K. The epidemiology of malignant giant cell tumors of bone: an analysis of data from the Surveillance, Epidemiology and End Results Program (1975-2004). Rare Tumors. 2009, 1:e52.

[28] Unni KK. Dahlin's bone tumors. 5th edn. New York: Lippincott-Raven; 1996. P.206-210.

[29] Hutter RV, Worcester JN Jr., Francis KC, Foote FW Jr. Stewart FW. Benign and malignant giant cell tumor of bone. A clinicopathological analysis of the natural history of the disease. *Cancer.* 1962, 15:653-690.

[30] Bertoni F, Bacchini P, Staals EL. Malignancy in giant cell tumor of bone. *Cancer.* 2003, 97:2520-2529.

[31] Saito T, Mitomi H, Suehara Y, Okubo T, Torigoe T, Takagi T, Kaneko K, Yao T. A case of de novo secondary malignant giant-cell tumor of bone with loss of heterozygosity of p53 gene that transformed within a short-term follow-up. *Pathol. Res. Pract.* 2011, 207:664-669.

[32] Torigoe T, Tomita Y, Iwase Y, Aritomi K, Suehara Y, Oukubo T, Sakurai A, Terakado A, Tatsuya T, Kaneko K, Saito T, Yazawa Y. Pedicle freezing with liquid nitrogen for malignant bone tumour in the radius: a new technique of osteotomy of the ulna. *J. Orthop. Surg.* 2012, 20:98-102.

[33] Domovitov SV, Healey JH. Primary malignant giant-cell tumor of bone has high survival rate. *Ann. Surg. Oncol.* 2010, 17:694-701.

[34] Kapoor SK, Jain V, Agrawal M, Singh S, Mandal AK. Primary malignant giant cell tumor of bone: a series of three rare cases. *J. Surg. Orthop. Adv.* 2007, 16:89-92.

[35] Maloney WJ, Vaughan LM, Jones HH, Ross J, Nagel DA. Benign metastasizing giant-cell tumor of bone. Report of three cases and review of the literature. *Clin. Orthop. Relat. Res.* 1989, 243:208-215.

[36] Wray CC, Macdonald AW, Richardson RA. Benign giant cell tumour with metastases to bone and lung. One case studied over 20 years. *J. Bone Joint Surg. Br.* 1990, 72B:486-489.

[37] Moon JC, Kim SR, Chung MJ, Lee YC. Multiple pulmonary metastases from giant cell tumor of a hand. *Am. J. Med. Sci.* 2012, 343:171-173.

[38] Rock MG, Sim FH, Unni KK, Witrak GA, Frassica FJ, Schray MF, Beabout JW, Dahlin DC. Secondary malignant giant-cell tumor of bone. Clinicopathological assessment of nineteen patients. *J. Bone Joint Surg. Am.* 1986, 68A:1073-1079.

[39] Gong L, Liu W, Sun X, Sajdik C, Tian X, Niu X, Huang XY. Histological and clinical characteristics of malignant giant cell tumor of bone. *Virchows Arch.* 2012, 460:327-334.

[40] Saito T, Mitomi H, Izumi H, Suehara Y, Okubo T, Torigoe T, Takagi T, Kaneko K, Sato K, Matsumoto T, Yao T. A case of secondary malignant giant-cell tumor of bone with p53 mutation after long-term follow-up. *Human Pathol.* 2011, 42:727-733.

[41] Oda Y, Sakamoto A, Saito T, Matsuda S, Tanaka K, Iwamoto Y, Tsuneyoshi M. Secondary malignant giant-cell tumour of bone: molecular abnormalities of p53 and H-ras gene correlated with malignant transformation. *Histopathology.* 2001, 39:629-637.

[42] Saada E, Peoc'h M, Decouvelaere AV, Collard O, Peyron AC, Pedeutour F. CCND1 and MET genomic amplification during malignant transformation of a giant cell tumor of bone. *J. Clin. Oncol.* 2011, 29:e86-89.

[43] Muramatsu K, Ihara K, Miyoshi T, Kawakami Y, Nakashima D, Taguchi T. Late development of malignant fibrous histiocytoma at the site of a giant cell tumour 38 years after initial surgery. *Acta Orthop. Belg.* 2012, 78:279-284.

[44] Oliveira AM, Perez-Atayde AR, Cin PD, Gebhardt MC, Chen C-J, Neff JR, Demetri GD, Rosenberg AE, Bridge JA, Fletcher JA. Aneurysmal bone cyst variant translocations upregulate USP6 transcription by promoter swapping with the ZNF9, COL1A1, TRAP150, and OMD genes. *Oncogene.* 2005, 24:3419-3426.

[45] Oliveira AM, His B-L, Weremowicz S, Rosenberg AE, Cin PD, Joseph N, Bridge JA, Perez-Atayde AR, Fletcher JA. USP6(Tre2) fusion oncogenes in aneurysmal bone cyst. *Cancer Res.* 2004, 64:1920-1923.

[46] Oliveira AM, Perez-Atayde AR, Inwards CY, Medeiros F, Derr V, His B-L, Gebhardt MC, Rosenberg AE, Cin PD, Fletcher JA. USP6 and CDH11 oncogenes identify the neoplastic cell in primary aneurysmal bone cysts and are absent in so-called secondary aneurysmal bone cysts. *Am. J. Pathol.* 2004, 165:1773-1780.

[47] Panagopoulos I, Mertens F, Lofvenberg R, Mandahl N. Fusion of the COL1A1 and USP6 genes in a benign bone tumor. *Cancer Genetics Cytogenetics.* 2008, 180:70-73.

[48] Saito T, Oda Y, Kawaguchi K, Tanaka K, Matsuda S, Sakamoto A, Iwamoto Y, Tsuneyoshi M. Five-year evolution of a telangiectatic osteosarcoma initially managed as an aneurysmal bone cyst. *Skeletal Radiol.* 2005, 34:290-294.

[49] Geiersbach K, Rector LS, Sederberg M, Hooker A, Randall RL, Schiffman JD, South ST. Unknown partner for USP6 and unusual SS18 rearrangement detected in fluorescence in situ hybridization in a solid aneurysmal bone cyst. *Cancer Genet.* 2011, 204:195-202.

[50] Brindley GW, Greene JF Jr., Frankel LS. Case reports: malignant transformation of aneurysmal bone cysts. *Clin. Orthop. Relat. Res*. 2005, 438:282-287.

[51] Takazawa K, Tsuchiya H, Yamamoto N, Nonomura A, Suzuki M, Taki J, Tomita K. Osteosarcoma arising from desmoplastic fibroma treated 16 years earlier: a case report. *J. Orthop. Sci*. 2003, 8:864-868.

[52] Abdelwahab IF, Klein MJ, Hermann G, Steiner GC, Yang DC. Osteosarcoma arising in a desmoplastic fibroma of the proximal tibia. *AJR Am. J. Roentgenol*. 2002, 178:613-615.

[53] Saito T, Oda Y, Tanaka K, Matsuda S, Sakamoto A, Yamamoto H, Iwamoto Y, Tsuneyoshi M. Low-grade fibrosarcoma of the proximal humerus. *Pathol. Int*. 2003, 53:115-120.

[54] Bahk W-J, Mirra JM. Pseudoanaplastic tumors of bone. *Skeletal Radiol*. 2004, 33:641-648.

In: Bone Tumors: Symptoms, Diagnosis and Treatment   ISBN: 978-1-62618-190-8
Editor: Moncef Berhouma   © 2013 Nova Science Publishers, Inc.

Chapter 8

CALVARIAL LESIONS: CLASSIFICATION AND MANAGEMENT

Mahmoud Messerer[1] and Julie Dubourg[2]

[1]Department of Clinical Neurosciences, Department of Neurosurgery,
Centre Hospitalier Universitaire Vaudois, Lausanne, Switzerland
[2]Research and Education Unit of Medicine, Claude Bernard University Lyon 1, France

ABSTRACT

The calvarium is a common site of lesions that may arise from bony structures or from invasion of the skin or brain based lesions into bony structures. Calvarial lesions (CL) can be classified in benign and malignant, or as tumoral, congenital, inflammatory, or traumatic, or as primary and metastatic. This wide variety of calvarial lesions is mostly identifiable as incidental findings on neuroimaging or palpable masses. Neuro-imaging (CT-scan, MR imaging) is mandatory to determine the possible etiology of CL. Such examination allows identifying lytic and sclerotic lesions, or defects in calvarium. Solitary lytic lesions may orientate to epidermoid and dermoid, eosinophilic granuloma, osteoblastoma, hemangioma, lipoma and aneurysmal bone cyst. Multiple lytic lesions may be considered as metastases or multiple myeloma, particularly in older patients. Defects in calvarium can be due to cephalocele, leptomeningeal cyst, pseudomeningocele, or sinus pericranii. Finally sclerotic lesions can evoke fibrous dysplasia, osteoma, Paget's disease, or osteosarcoma. However the wide variety of CL makes the exact imaging-based diagnosis tricky and therefore requires patient's clinical history. Achieving an accurate diagnosis is required to choose the adequate management although surgical resection remains a treatment of choice for most of these lesions, mostly benign. In this chapter, we provide a synthetic classification of common calvarial lesions both in children and adults, their diagnosis and specific management.

INTRODUCTION

The calvarium consists of part of the frontal, parietal, temporal and occipital bones and forms the convexity of the skull. It consists of inner and outer tables separated by the diploe containing red marrow. The calvarium can be affected by a variety of benign and malignant lesions. These lesions are frequently asymptomatic and discovered incidentally. They may cause focal scalp tenderness but the typical symptom is a painless palpable mass. In cases of erosion of inner table, lesions can apply pressure effect or invade brain parenchyma and adjacent structures causing specific symptoms. Neuroimaging and clinical history are mandatory to determine the etiology. This specific diagnosis is required to determine the treatment of choice.

BENIGN LESIONS

Aneurysmal Bone Cyst

Definition – Epidemiology. Aneurysmal bone cysts are benign lesions with rapid growing within the diploe. They may be due to the development of local hemodynamic alteration with secondary venous hypotension. They usually occur in the two first decades of life. The calvarium is a rare location (3% - 6 %) of aneurysmal bone cysts. Many cases of these lesions seem to occur secondarily in fibrous dysplasia [1, 2].

Clinical presentation. Scalp palpable mass.

Imaging. They are eccentric expansible osteolytic lesions with a narrow zone of transition. On plain X rays, lesions are a "Blow-out" appearance [3-5] and it may be possible to see a peripheral sclerosis. CT and MR imaging show multiloculation of the cyst [6].

Differential diagnostic. Fibrous dysplasia; osteoblastoma; metastases; infection

Treatment. Surgical total removal is recommended, as these lesions tend to recur. Others management modalities are: arterial embolization, injection slcerotherapy, cryotherapy, and radiotherapy.

Cephalocele

Definition – Epidemiology. Cephalocele are herniations of brain (encephalocele) or meninges (cranial meningocele) through a defect along the mid line of the calvarium occurring in 1 to 4 per 10 000 births [7]. They belong to neural tube defects. However, cephalocele are far less common that spinal dysraphism. The most common location is occipital (75%). There is a high risk of mortality during the first days of life and newborns with large cephalocele risk to be physically and intellectually disabled.

Clinical presentation. Scalp palpable mass.

Imaging. Ultrasonography can detect these types of lesions and prenatal diagnosis is possible. CT allows the visualization of internal and external bony defect. On MRI, the herniated contents within the sac can be visualized and may also help in detecting other brain anomaly [8].

Differential diagnostic. Cystic hygroma; teratoma; branchial cleft cyst; scalp edema; epidermal scalp cyst;

Treatment. Surgery is recommended soon after birth in order to replace brain back into the skull, remove any dysplastic brain tissue and close the defect. The main potential complications of such procedure are: cerebrospinal fluid leakage in cases of large cephalocele, postoperative hydrocephalus and infection

Epidermoid and Dermoid

Definition – Epidemiology. Dermoid and epidermoid are ectodermal inclusion cysts. They are due to early embryonic displacements of epithelial nests associated with the neural tube closure and the viscerocranium clefts. The difference between dermoid and epidermoid is histologic. Epidermoid arise from epidermal origin and contain pure ceratoid material. Dermoid may also contain follicle, sebaceous glands, fatty material and fairs. These lesions both have the potential to growth because of the accumulation of material but they rarely grow and if it is the case, the progression is very slow. It is always benign lesion. These cysts can be seen on different locations of the skull and neck [9, 10]. In the skull, they are located in the diploe. They are the most common calvarial lesions. Epidermoid and dermoid of the calvarium are separate entities and have specific features [11, 12]. They are most often epidermoid and seen in the early infancy. However epidermoid can also be seen in the parietal and temporal bones of adults aged from 20 to 50 years.

Clinical Presentation. The diagnosis is made early in the infancy because of the existence of an elevation from the convexity adherent to the calvarium.

Imaging. They are lytic lesions with sclerotic borders. Plain X rays that allow showing a typical round lytic lesion with a sclerotic rim can make diagnostic. However, to avoid unnecessary radiation to newborns or infants, ultrasonography may be use [13]. On MR imaging, lesions are hypointense en T1 weighted images and hyperintense on T2 weighted images. Contrast enhancement is inconstant.

Differential diagnostic. Eosinophilic granuloma.

Treatment. Surgery is the preferred treatment option as it allows to histologically confirming the diagnosis.

Eosinophilic Granuloma (Histiocytosis X)

Definition – Epidemiology. Histiocytosis X is a disease of unknown etiology characterized by an abnormal proliferation of histiocytes with a variable granulomatous and inflammatory component [14-16]. The calvarium is one of the most common location [17] of this lesion located in the diploe. It is seen in patients of 5 to 15 years old. Despite it is a benign lesion, it has often a rapid and aggressive course but the exact mechanism of the invasion is unclear.

Clinical Presentation. Painless palpable scalp mass.

Imaging. Figure 1. The characteristic imaging feature is an osteolytic lesion of the calvarial bone. It is possible to see residual bone tissue within the lesion called button sequestrum. In MR imaging, the typical feature is a hypointense mass within bone in T1-weighted images and heterogeneously hyperintense mass in T2 weighted images. After contrast administration, the lesion enhances homogeneously. Some compression or invasion on dura matter may be seen.

Differential diagnostic. Epidermoid-dermoid cyst; osteoblastoma; meningioma [18].

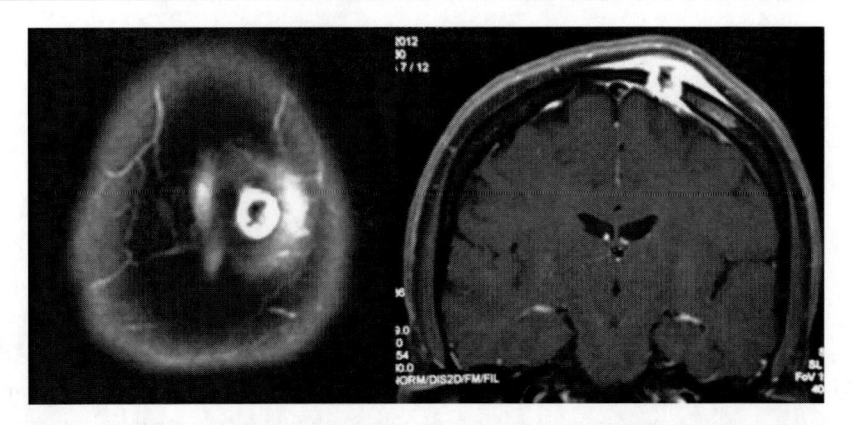

Figure 1. Histiocytosis X. T1 weighted MR imaging (left: axial plane; right: coronal plane) with gadolinium administration showing an osteolytic lesion of the calvarial bone enhancing homogeneously. A "button sequestrum" is seen within the lesion centre.

Treatment. Conservative treatment with a follow-up CT is recommended because spontaneous resolution is relatively common.

Fibrous Dysplasia

Definition – Epidemiology. Fibrous dysplasia is characterized by an abnormal proliferation of immature woven bone and fibrous tissue in replacement of normal bone [19]. It approximately represents 7.5 % of all benign bone neoplasms. It usually occurs during the three first decades of life with the same frequency in each sex [20, 21]. There are three different type of fibrous dysplasia: the most common (70 %) is the single bone involvement (monostotic), multiple bone involvement (polyostotic) (30 %) and McCuneAlbright syndrome or Mazabraud syndrome. The most common lesion is the monostotic fibrous dysplasia of the orbital region [22, 23]. This is a benign lesion but it may be complicated of pathologic fracture and rarely by malignant degeneration [24].

Clinical presentation. Palpable scalp mass. Patients may present with potentially clinical symptoms resulting from the mass effect exerted by the fibrous dysplasia.

Imaging. Lesions are a typical "ground glass" appearance. CT is the gold standard for evaluation of this pathology. On MR imaging, lesion are hypointense on T1 weighted images and heterogeneous and variable intensity on T2 weighted images. Contrast enhancement is inconstant. There is a characteristic black ring corresponding to the sclerotic border.

Differential diagnostic. Paget's disease;

Treatment. Treatment options are clinical and radiological follow-up, medical management and surgical intervention. Surgical intervention is mostly recommended in cases of pressure exerted by the lesion.

Hemangioma

Definition – Epidemiology. Hemangiomas of the calvarium approximately represent 0.2 % of all bone neoplasms. These benign lesions can be seen in all age ranges but they are predominant in women [25, 26]. These lesions can be sessile or more rarely globular and are composed of dilated blood vessels contained within the bony trabeculae. They are most seen in the frontal and parietal regions. There are multiple lesions in 15% of patients [27].

Clinical presentation. Painless palpable scalp mas.

Imaging. They are osteolytic lesions. Pain X rays allow visualizing an appearance of a honeycomb or sunburst pattern of bony spicules radiating from the center of a radiolucent round. A reactive sclerosis is present in approximately 30 % of cases. On MR imaging, hemangioma appears as a mottled isointense lesion within the diploe with scattered hypointensity due to iron storage and hyperintensity due to fatty tissue in T1 weighted images. Lesion is hyperintense on T2 weighted images due to the iron storage [28]. Contrast enhancement is characteristic with enhancement in focal areas during the early phase and diffusion of contrast during le later phase eventually with enhancement of adjacent meninges.

Differential diagnostic. Eosinophilic granuloma in cases of small hemangioma.

Treatment. These lesions are typically not treated. However, surgical resection is possible.

Leptomeningeal Cyst

Definition – Epidemiology. Leptomeningeal cysts usually occur after 0.6 % of skull fractures and they are most frequent in children less than 3 years old and almost never after 8 years old [29]. The mechanism is the traumatic laceration of the dura that is exposed to the pulsations of the cerebrospinal fluid. These pulses then gradually widen the fracture line.

Clinical presentation. Patients present with a progressive, commonly pulsatile, scalp mass appearing after head trauma history. These lesions may induce progressive neurological deficit due to atrophy of underlying cerebral tissue during the growing of the fracture.

Imaging. On plain X Rays a fracture line is seen. On CT, they are hypodense lesions near a fracture site.

Differential diagnostic. Eosinophilic granuloma; infection disease.

Treatment. Surgical management is required in order to avoid the risk of neurological deterioration and seizure disorder.

Meningioma

Definition – Epidemiology. Meningioma of the calvarium results from the invasion of meningothelial cells within the bone resulting in hyperostosis. They are rare compared to "classic" intracranial meningiomas and represent 1% to 2% of all meningiomas [30, 31]. They are typically benign lesions but potentially malignant. Unlike classic meningiomas, they occur with the same frequency in each sex especially during the second decade [32]. The most common locations are the frontoparietal and orbital regions.

Clinical presentation. Painless sclap palapable masse.

Imaging. Figure 2. There are lytic lesions. On CT, lesions have uniform enhancement but the features can be atypical in 10 % to 15 % of case. On MR imaging, lesions are typically hypointense in T1 weighted images and hyperintense in T2 weighted images. Sometimes, there is a dural tail sign corresponding to peritumoral enhancement.

Differential diagnostic. Lytic metastasis; epidermoid; dermoid; eosinophilic granuloma; fibrous dysplasia; hemangiopericytoma; hemangioma.

Treatment. The treatment of choice remains the surgical removal of the lesion followed by cranial reconstruction. Adjuvant radiotherapy is recommended in patients with symptomatic residue and/or evidence of progression [33]. In all cases, follow-up imaging is of paramount importance.

Osteoma

Definition – Epidemiology. Osteomas are slowly-growing benign tumors reprensentig 5% of calvarial lesions.

Clinical presentation. It is a painless mass. There are potential symptoms in function of the location of the lesions: sinusitis, nasal discharge, headache, and loss of smell, exophthalmos, diplopia and loss of vision.

Imaging. On plain X rays, there are intensely homogeneous dense oval lesions, typically inferior to 1 cm. On CT, lesions have variable density. On MR imaging, lesions are homogeneously hypointense on T1 weighted images and heterogeneously hyperintense on T2 weighted images. No contrast enhancement. No change in the diploe.

Differential diagnostic. Osseous meningioma.

Treatment. These lesions are potentially locally aggressive and may cause possible intracranial complication so surgical removal is recommended.

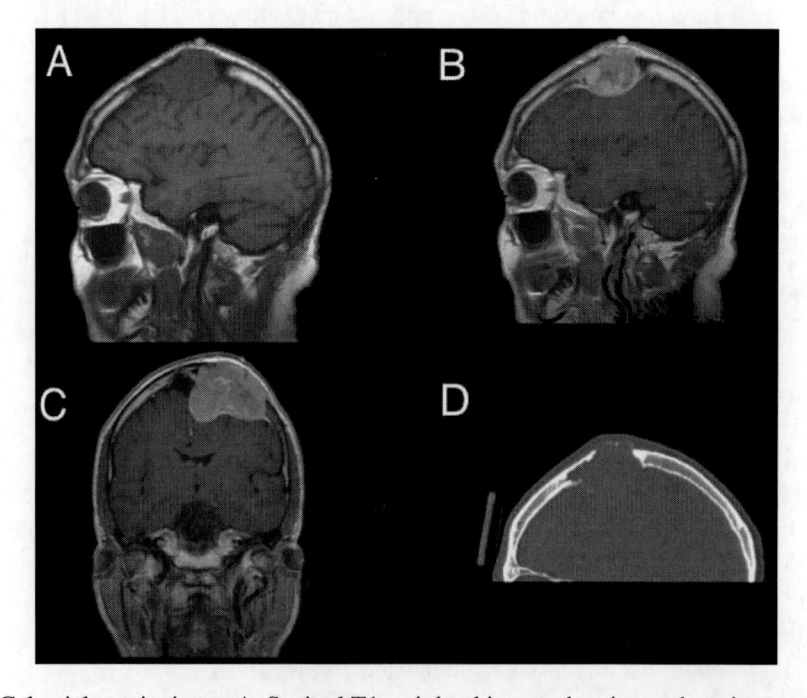

Figure 2. Calvarial meningioma. A: Sagittal T1 weighted image showing an hypointense lesion involving the calvarial bone with enhancement after gadolinium administration (B and C); D: CT-scan showing lytic lesion of the calvarial bone.

Paget's Disease and Paget's Sarcoma

Definition – Epidemiology. Paget's disease typically occurs after the fourth decade of life. The skull is involved in around 50 % of cases. This disease typically progresses in three stages: osteolytic, mixed and osteosclerotic. This disease may rarely degenerate in a sarcomatous neoplasm.

Clinical presentation. The majority of patients are asymptomatic but the main potential symptoms are: localized pain, increased local temperature; mass lesion; symptoms related to eventual intracranial compression.

Imaging. There are 3 stages in Paget's disease: there are lytic lesions eroding the outer table named "osteoporosis circumscripta" during the osteolytic stage; there are loss of differentiation between the inner and outer tables and enlargement of the diploe during the osteosclerotic stage; there are irregular areas of the sclerosis with a cotton-wool appearance during the mixed stage. On MR imaging, there are enlargement of the diploe and heterogeneous signal intensity.

Differential diagnostic. Fibrous dysplasia; hyperostosis frontalis interna.

Treatment. Medical treatment is recommended such as calcitonin, diphosphonate and mithramycin.

Single Plasmocytoma

Definition – Epidemiology. Solitary calvarial plasmocytoma is not the result of extension from extracranial myeloma and is not associated with plasmacytosis [34]. It occurs at a younger age that multiple myeloma. There are two subsets: those arising from the bone and those arising from the dura mater.

Clinical presentation. The main potential symptoms are: local pain and headache.

Imaging. On CT and plan X-rays, there are osteolytic lesion without sclerotic rim. On CT, contrast enhancement is homogeneous. On MR imaging, lesions are iso or hyperintense on T1 weighted images with homogeneous contrast enhancement.

Differential diagnostic. Intraosseous meningioma.

Treatment. The treatment of choice is the surgical removal followed by postoperative radiotherapy.

Sinus Pericranii

Definition – Epidemiology. Sinus pericranii is an abnormal communication between the intracranial dural sinuses and the dilated epicranial veins. It usually occurs in the pediatric age group.

Clinical presentation. It appears as a soft fluctuant mass located near intracranial sinus. It varies in size according to intracranial pressure. It is usually asymptomatic but potential symptoms are: headache, local pain, vertigo, and feelings of fullness.

Imaging. The gold standard diagnostic tool is angiography that makes in evidence the sinus pericranii in the venous phase. MR imaging shows a signal void [35].

Differential diagnostic. Arteriovenous malformation; epicranial varix; cavernoma; leptomeningeal cyst; eosinophilic granuloma; epidermoid and dermoid; cephalocele.

Treatment. Surgical management is recommended for sinus removal and blocking the communicating veins. The main potential complications are: bleeding, air embolism.

PRIMARY MALIGNANT LESIONS

Hemangiopericytoma

Definition – Epidemiology. Hemangiopericytomas are low-grade malignant neoplasm accounting for less than 1 % of all central nervous system tumors and occurs in young people [36]. They are vascular tumors composed of angular pericytes. They are a high rate of recurrence and metastasize extracranially. They occur at the same site of meningiomas.

Clinical presentation. There are deep soft tissue masses.

Imaging. There are extraaxial heterogeneously enhancing masses with usually neither hyperostosis nor calcification

Differential diagnostic. Malignant meningiomas.

Treatment. Total gross removal of lesions is recommended to improve survival rate. Both chemotherapy and radiotherapy are effective and are recommended in cases of tumoral residue or invasive tumors.

Multiple Myeloma

Definition – Epidemiology. Multiple myeloma represents the disseminated form of a disease that is characterized by monoclonal proliferation of immunoglobulin-secreting plasma cells.

Clinical presentation. The typical symptom is local pain.

Imaging. They are multiple small, roundship osteolytic lesions with sharp, non-sclerotic margins of uniforms size. On CT, some lesions invisible on plain X rays may be revealed. On MR imaging, signal intensity is similar with those of metastases.

Differential diagnostic. Metastases.

Treatment. The management of multiple myeloma is complex and include in majority chemotherapy, corticosteroids and stem cell transplantation.

Osteosarcoma

Definition – Epidemiology. Osteosarcomas are malignant neoplasm consisting in a proliferation of immature bone. These lesions that occur preferentially in adolescents and young adults rarely affect the calvarium. Affected older adults usually have pre-existing benign disease such as Paget's disease. They are three types: osteoblastic that is the most frequent, fibroblastic and telangiectatic.

Clinical presentation. Painless palpable mass.

Imaging. On MR imaging, the lesion is hypointense on T1 weighted images and is of heteregenous intensity on T2 weighted images. Contrast enhancement is heterogeneous.

Differential diagnostic.

Treatment. Surgery is the main stay of the therapy. Adjuvant treatment are chemotherapy and/or radiotherapy.

Secondary Malignant Lesions

Metastases

Definition – Epidemiology.

Clinical presentation. They are often asymptomatic but they may cause pain due to an irritation of the periosteum. The most frequent primary cancer responsible for such metastases are: breast, lung, prostate, renal, thyroid and melanoma. They are typically diagnosed on the course of malignancy but they may be the mode of revelation.

Imaging. On plain X rays and CT, these ingle or multiple lesions are osteolytic with ill defined margins. To be noted that metastases of prostate and osteosarcoma are osteoblastic. Contrast enhancement with or without bone destruction, compression of adjacent structures. On MR imaging, they appear hypointense to the background marrow on T1 weighted images and hyperintense on T2 weighted images in cases of osteolytic lesions and hypointense is case of osteoblastic metastases.

Differential diagnostic. Osteoma; dermoid; epidermoid; fibrous dysplasia; eosinophilic granuloma.

Treatment. Treatment decision is based on the stage of the cancer, the number of lesions and the performance status of the patient. Treatment modalities regroup: surgery, radiosurgery, radiotherapy and chemotherapy.

Conclusion

The specific diagnosis of calvarial lesions is very challenging solely on characteristics imaging. However, this diagnosis may be helped by careful examination of patient history and clinical characteristic to improve the specificity of diagnosis and patient management.

References

[1]   Branch CL, Jr., Challa VR, Kelly DL, Jr. Aneurysmal bone cyst with fibrous dysplasia of the parietal bone. Report of two cases. *Journal of neurosurgery.* 1986;64(2):331-5. Epub 1986/02/01.

[2]   Som PM, Schatz CJ, Flaum EG, Lanman TH. Aneurysmal bone cyst of the paranasal sinuses associated with fibrous dysplasia: CT and MR findings. *Journal of computer assisted tomography.* 1991;15(3):513-5. Epub 1991/05/01.

[3]   Cacdac MA, Malis LI, Anderson PJ. Aneurysmal parietal bone cyst. Case report. *Journal of neurosurgery.* 1972;37(2):237-41. Epub 1972/08/01.

[4]   O'Gorman AM, Kirkham TH. Aneurysmal bone cyst of the orbit with unusual angiographic features. *AJR American journal of roentgenology.* 1976;126(4):896-9. Epub 1976/04/01.

[5]   Chalapati Rao KV, Rao BS, Reddy CP, Sundareshwar B, Reddy CR. Aneurysmal bone cyst of the skull. Case report. *Journal of neurosurgery.* 1977;47(4):633-6. Epub 1977/10/01.

[6]   Revel MP, Vanel D, Sigal R, Luboinski B, Michel G, Legrand I, et al. Aneurysmal bone cysts of the jaws: CT and MR findings. *Journal of computer assisted tomography.* 1992;16(1):84-6. Epub 1992/01/01.

[7]   McLone DG. Congenital malformations of the central nervous system. *Clinical neurosurgery.* 2000;47:346-77. Epub 2001/02/24.

[8]   Naidich TP, Altman NR, Braffman BH, McLone DG, Zimmerman RA. Cephaloceles and related malformations. *AJNR American journal of neuroradiology.* 1992;13(2):655-90. Epub 1992/03/01.

[9]   Pryor SG, Lewis JE, Weaver AL, Orvidas LJ. Pediatric dermoid cysts of the head and neck. Otolaryngology--head and neck surgery : *official journal of American Academy of Otolaryngology-Head and Neck Surgery.* 2005;132(6):938-42. Epub 2005/06/10.

[10] Ruge JR, Tomita T, Naidich TP, Hahn YS, McLone DG. Scalp and calvarial masses of infants and children. *Neurosurgery.* 1988;22(6 Pt 1):1037-42. Epub 1988/06/01.

[11] Holthusen W, Lassrich MA, Steiner C. Epidermoids and dermoids of the calvarian bones in early childhood: their behaviour in the growing skull. *Pediatric radiology.* 1983;13(4):189-94. Epub 1983/01/01.

[12] McAvoy JM, Zuckerbraun L. Dermoid cysts of the head and neck in children. *Archives of otolaryngology* (Chicago, Ill : 1960). 1976; 102 (9): 529-31. Epub 1976/09/01.

[13] Riebel T, David S, Thomale UW. Calvarial dermoids and epidermoids in infants and children: sonographic spectrum and follow-up. Child's nervous system : *ChNS : official journal of the International Society for Pediatric Neurosurgery.* 2008;24(11):1327-32. Epub 2008/06/19.

[14] Angeli SI, Alcalde J, Hoffman HT, Smith RJ. Langerhans' cell histiocytosis of the head and neck in children. *The Annals of otology, rhinology, and laryngology.* 1995;104(3):173-80. Epub 1995/03/01.

[15] Brabencova E, Tazi A, Lorenzato M, Bonay M, Kambouchner M, Emile JF, et al. Langerhans cells in Langerhans cell granulomatosis are not actively proliferating cells. *The American journal of pathology.* 1998; 152(5): 1143-9. Epub 1998/05/20.

[16] Murayama S, Numaguchi Y, Robinson AE, Richardson DE. Magnetic resonance imaging of calvarial eosinophilic granuloma. *The Journal of computed tomography.* 1988;12(4):251-2. Epub 1988/10/01.

[17] Kilpatrick SE, Wenger DE, Gilchrist GS, Shives TC, Wollan PC, Unni KK. Langerhans' cell histiocytosis (histiocytosis X) of bone. A clinicopathologic analysis of 263 pediatric and adult cases. *Cancer.* 1995; 76(12): 2471-84. Epub 1995/12/15.

[18] Okamoto K, Ito J, Furusawa T, Sakai K, Tokiguchi S. Imaging of calvarial eosinophil granuloma. *Neuroradiology.* 1999;41(10):723-8. Epub 1999/11/07.

[19] Megerian CA, Sofferman RA, McKenna MJ, Eavey RD, Nadol JB, Jr. Fibrous dysplasia of the temporal bone: ten new cases demonstrating the spectrum of otologic sequelae. *The American journal of otology.* 1995; 16(4):408-19. Epub 1995/07/01.

[20] Ricalde P, Horswell BB. Craniofacial fibrous dysplasia of the fronto-orbital region: a case series and literature review. *Journal of oral and maxillofacial surgery : official journal of the American Association of Oral and Maxillofacial Surgeons.* 2001;59(2):157-67; discussion 67-8. Epub 2001/02/24.

[21] Finney HL, Roberts TS. Fibrous dysplasia of the skull with progressive cranial nerve involvement. *Surgical neurology.* 1976;6(6):341-3. Epub 1976/12/01.

[22] Lustig LR, Holliday MJ, McCarthy EF, Nager GT. Fibrous dysplasia involving the skull base and temporal bone. *Archives of otolaryngology--head and neck surgery.* 2001;127(10):1239-47. Epub 2001/11/01.

[23] Maher CO, Friedman JA, Meyer FB, Lynch JJ, Unni K, Raffel C. Surgical treatment of fibrous dysplasia of the skull in children. *Pediatric neurosurgery.* 2002;37(2):87-92. Epub 2002/07/30.

[24] Fitzpatrick KA, Taljanovic MS, Speer DP, Graham AR, Jacobson JA, Barnes GR, et al. Imaging findings of fibrous dysplasia with histopathologic and intraoperative correlation. *AJR American journal of roentgenology.* 2004;182(6):1389-98. Epub 2004/05/20.

[25] Wyke BD. Primary hemangioma of the skull; a rare cranial tumor; review of the literature and report of a case, with special reference to the roentgenographic appearances. *The American journal of roentgenology and radium therapy.* 1949;61(1):302-16. Epub 1949/03/01.

[26] Khanam H, Lipper MH, Wolff CL, Lopes MB. Calvarial hemangiomas: report of two cases and review of the literature. *Surgical neurology.* 2001;55(1):63-7; discussion 7. Epub 2001/03/15.

[27] Sargent EN, Reilly EB, Posnikoff J. Primary hemangioma of the skull. Case report of an unusual tumor. *The American journal of roentgenology, radium therapy, and nuclear medicine.* 1965;95 (4):874-9. Epub 1965/12/01.

[28] Peterson DL, Murk SE, Story JL. Multifocal cavernous hemangioma of the skull: report of a case and review of the literature. *Neurosurgery.* 1992;30(5):778-81; discussion 82. Epub 1992/05/01.

[29] Ramamurthi B, Kalyanaraman S. Rationale for surgery in growing fractures of the skull. *Journal of neurosurgery.* 1970;32(4):427-30. Epub 1970/04/01.

[30] Muzumdar DP, Vengsarkar US, Bhatjiwale MG, Goel A. Diffuse calvarial meningioma: a case report. *Journal of postgraduate medicine.* 2001; 47(2):116-8. Epub 2002/02/08.

[31] Whicker JH, Devine KD, MacCarty CS. Diagnostic and therapeutic problems in extracranial meningiomas. *American journal of surgery.* 1973;126(4):452-7. Epub 1973/10/01.

[32] Lang FF, Macdonald OK, Fuller GN, DeMonte F. Primary extradural meningiomas: a report on nine cases and review of the literature from the era of computerized tomography scanning. *Journal of neurosurgery.* 2000;93(6):940-50. Epub 2000/12/16.

[33] Crawford TS, Kleinschmidt-DeMasters BK, Lillehei KO. Primary intraosseous meningioma. Case report. *Journal of neurosurgery.* 1995;83(5):912-5. Epub 1995/11/01.

[34] Pritchard PB, 3rd, Martinez RA, Hungerford GD, Powers JM, Perot PL, Jr. Dural plasmacytoma. *Neurosurgery*. 1983;12(5):576-9. Epub 1983/05/01.

[35] Bollar A, Allut AG, Prieto A, Gelabert M, Becerra E. Sinus pericranii: radiological and etiopathological considerations. Case report. *Journal of neurosurgery*. 1992;77(3):469-72. Epub 1992/09/01.

[36] Ruscalleda J, Feliciani M, Avila A, Castaner E, Guardia E, de Juan M. Neuroradiological features of intracranial and intraorbital meningeal haemangiopericytomas. *Neuroradiology*. 1994;36(6):440-5. Epub 1994/08/01.

In: Bone Tumors: Symptoms, Diagnosis and Treatment
Editor: Moncef Berhouma

ISBN: 978-1-62618-190-8
© 2013 Nova Science Publishers, Inc.

Chapter 9

SECONDARY BONE TUMORS IN PROSTATE CANCER: NEW TREATMENTS ON THE HORIZON

*Justin Sturge**

School of Biological, Biomedical & Environmental Sciences,
University of Hull, Hull, UK

ABSTRACT

Secondary bone tumors associated with the advancement of solid tumors of the prostate and other tissue sites result in the increased risk of intractable bone pain, pathological skeletal fracture and spinal-cord compression. In addition to increasing morbidity the occurrence of metastatic bone lesions results in a marked reduction in patient survival. Once lesions have established in the bone the disease is able to progress by homotypic and heterotypic cellular interactions between the invading tumor cells and bone-associated osteoblasts and osteoclasts.

The vicious cycle of bone matrix remodeling that ensues in lesions with an osteolytic phenotype is largely driven by increased osteoclast-mediated bone degradation - which leads to the subsequent loss of normal bone structure and compromised bone strength. In prostate cancer there is the additional complication of a predominantly osteosclerotic lesion phenotype - where osteoblasts become activated to overproduce a highly disorganized new bone matrix.

Advances have been made in the treatment of osteolytic bone lesions - for which the currently approved treatment is the delivery of intravenous bisphosphonates or subcutaneous inhibitors of receptor activator of nuclear factor κB ligand (RANKL). Current clinical trials are focused on blocking the activity of kinases (SRC and cABL) and enzymes (cathepsin K) involved in osteolytic lesion progression.

In contrast, few options exist for the treatment of osteosclerotic lesions – isolated lesions can be treated using palliative radiotherapy whereas multifocal lesions require systemic taxane-based chemotherapy. Pre-clinical and clinical studies have now started to address this shortfall in anti-osteosclerotic therapeutics and provide a significant focus of this chapter.

---

* E-mail: j.sturge@hull.ac.uk.

1. INTRODUCTION

This chapter expands upon a review focused on emerging therapeutic strategies for bone metastasis in prostate cancer [1]. The premise being that skeletal metastases occur in >80% of advanced prostate cancer cases and confer an increased level of morbidity, a 5-year survival rate of 25% and median survival time of approximately 40 months. Of the estimated one million deaths associated with bone metastasis in the USA, EU and Japan per annum, approximately 20% are attributed to cases of advanced prostate cancer [2]. In patients presenting with metastatic prostate cancer — and who are treatment naïve — the disease remains sensitive to androgen-deprivation therapy for an average of 18–24 months, at which point progression to castrate resistant prostate cancer (CRPC) and metastatic dissemination to visceral organs and bone is a frequent occurrence [3].

Secondary lesions in the bone impart some of the most distressing symptoms associated with metastatic prostate cancer. Estimates indicate that treatment of bone pain is required in 30% of cases of prostate cancer with associated bone metastasis [4]: with 22% requiring treatment for singular or multiple pathological skeletal fractures; 7% for spinal cord compression; and 3-4% for hemiparesis or paresis [4]. These clinical outcomes pose a significant challenge to the treating clinician — since in most cases a multidisciplinary approach will be required.

Despite the complexities involved in the management of bone metastasis a number of guidelines for treatment have been recommended [5]. Following diagnosis, therapeutic intervention will usually involve systemic chemotherapy, hormonal therapy and bisphosphonates. These options are mostly palliative with the primary intention being the reduction of pain [5]. Once the disease progresses and symptoms reoccur — or there is significant risk of skeletal fracture or spinal cord compression — the use of localized radiotherapy, in the case of solitary (single) bone lesions, or radiopharmaceuticals, for wide-spread (multiple) bone lesions, will be considered [5].

Taxane-based chemotherapy (docetaxel) in combination with a synthetic corticosteroid analogue (prednisone) became standard care following the outcome of the TAX327 phase III trial, reported in 2004 and followed up in 2008, in which patients with progressive metastatic CRPC (n = 1006) were randomized to receive docetaxel or mitoxantrone (both with prednisone) [6, 7].

The findings were a significant increase in overall survival of nearly 2 months ($P = 0.02$), improved quality of life, lower levels of cancer-induced bone pain, decreased serum levels of prostate specific antigen (PSA) and an objective (measurable) tumor response in the docetaxel group. Also reported in 2004, the SWOG 99-16 phase III trial ($n = 620$) — in which mitoxantrone in combination with prednisone was compared to docetaxel in combination with estramustine — a similar survival advantage in the group treated with docetaxel was observed [8]. However, the prognosis for patients with CRPC who start taxane-based chemotherapy for metastatic disease is relapse within their first year of treatment, for which the molecular basis is linked to fundamental changes in the bone microenvironment, which — in addition to genetic changes — can confer increased tumor cell survival, proliferation and drug efflux [9].

These multiple phenomena have led to the current strategy of implementing bone-targeted therapeutic intervention in the management of bone metastasis.

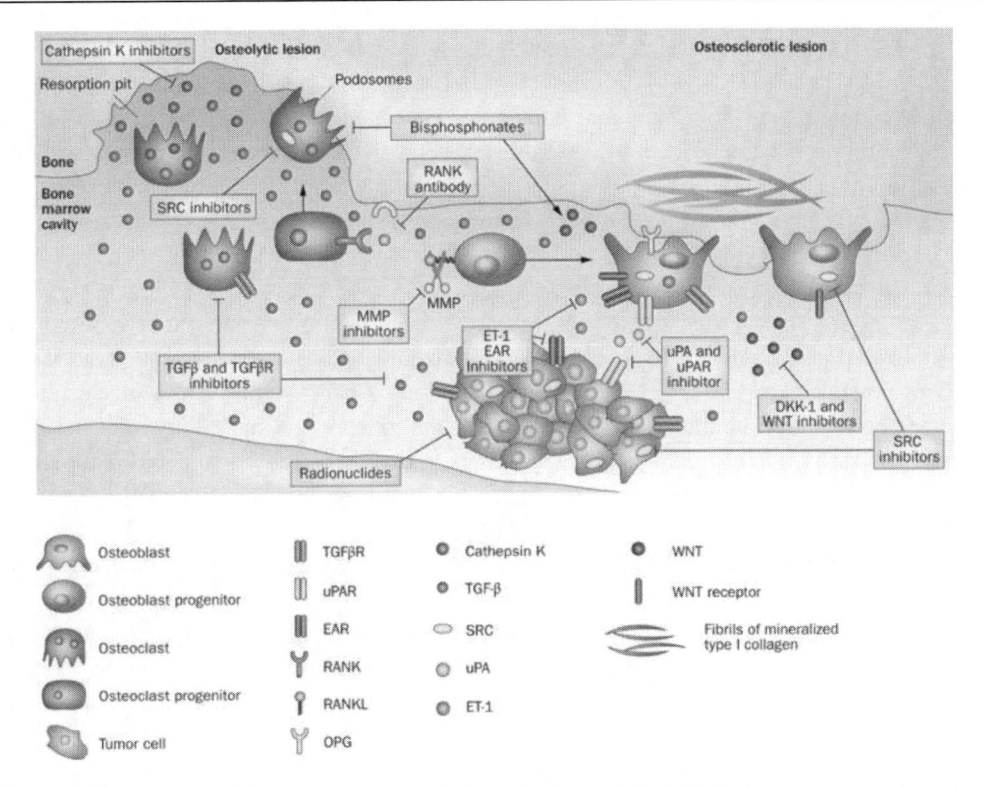

Figure 1. *Bone-targeted therapy in metastatic bone lesions*. Osteolytic lesions progress via vicious cycles of bone destruction and tumor growth. Osteoclastic factors secreted by tumor cells promote bone resorption by osteoclasts [2, 10, 11]. Subsequent osteolysis releases bone matrix factors, including TGF-β [12-17], which promotes the growth and survival of tumor cells. Tumor cells release matrix metalloproteases that can activate RANKL released by osteoblast precursors [18-20]. RANKL stimulates osteoclastogenesis by binding RANK on osteoclast precursors [21]; and its decoy receptor OPG (also released by osteoblast precursors) can protect against osteolysis [22]. Bone degradation is mediated by cathepsin K release in bone resorption pits [23-25], which form at the osteoclast-bone interface via the SRC-dependent and Rho GTPase-dependent assembly of podosomes [26, 27]. Osteosclerotic lesions progress via increased osteoblastogenesis and type I collagen production, deposition and mineralization. Osteoblastic factors like ET-1 [28-31], Wnts[32-36], TGF-β [12, 13] and uPA [37-42] drive poor quality woven bone formation in osteosclerotic lesions. Therapeutic approaches to target the osteolytic and osteosclerotic microenvironment of bone metastasis in prostate cancer include: bisphosphonates [43, 44]; radionuclides [45-51]; and targeted inhibition of RANKL [52-55], cathepsin K [56], SRC [57-59], EAR [60-67], TGFβ [68-73] and uPA [41, 42]. Collagen remodeling,which involves Endo180, is a proposed target [74, 75]. Abbreviations: DKK-1, dickopff-related protein-1 ET-1, endothelin-1; EAR, ET-1 receptor; OPG, osteoprotegerin; RANK, receptor activator of nuclear factor-κB; RANKL, RANK ligand; TGF-β, transforming growth factor-β; TGFβR, transforming growth factor-β receptor; uPA, urokinase-type plasminogen activator; uPAR, urokinase-type plasminogen activator receptor. Reproduced from Sturge, J. *et al.* (2011) Bone metastasis in prostate cancer: emerging therapeutic strategies *Nature Reviews in Clinical Oncology* 8 357-368 doi:10.1038/nrclinonc.2011.67 [1].

The complex pathology of bone lesions in metastatic CRPC, bone-targeted therapies currently under clinical evaluation and promising new therapeutic strategies and targets emerging in pre-clinical studies are the focus of the following sections in this chapter.

2. REMODELING OF BONE IN BONE METASTASIS

In healthy skeletal bone an equal balance of new bone matrix formation and old bone matrix resorption is achieved via the coordinated activity of bone-degrading osteoclasts and bone-forming osteoblasts [76]. To degrade bone the osteoclast must first create a resorption pit (Figure 1). The osteoclast does this by forming large arrays of multiple F-actin rich cell-matrix adhesion structures — called podosomes — that create a basolateral sealing-zone on the bone surface.

This allows the osteoclast to control bone degradation by the rapid assembly or disassembly of podosomes in response to the intracellular signaling cues generated via Rho GTPases [26] and Src kinases [27]. Once the resorption pit is formed proteases are secreted to facilitate the localized degradation of the underlying bone — the most important being the cysteine protease, cathepsin K, which is the only mammalian protease that can directly cleave the helical and non-helical type I collagen fibres that comprise mineralized bone [77].

The products of osteolysis, which include cleaved collagen fragments, can be cleared by internalization and transported to the acidic lysosomal compartment of the osteoclast [78]. Alternatively the products of osteolysis can be released into the bone microenvironment, for example — transforming growth factor-β-1 (TGF-β_1) — which, following its production by bone forming osteoblasts, is subsequently stored in its inactive latent form within the bone matrix. TGF-β_1 and other matricellular factors can be activated during osteolysis and stimulate the initiation of new bone formation by osteoblasts (Figure 1). Bone formation by osteoblasts involves the production of type I pro-collagen followed by its processing, modification and secretion by exocytosis [79]. Secreted type I pro-collagen is then processed and covalently cross-linked by lysyl oxidases to form aligned helical arrangements of multiple collagen fibrils and fibres. Once deposited and organized, this collagen-rich matrix (which also contains other matrix proteins) undergoes mineralization following exosomal release of bone alkaline phosphatase (ALPL, also known as BALP) from osteoblasts [80].

Osteoblasts can also act as direct modulators of the bone resorption process via the production of receptor activator of nuclear factor-kappa B ligand (RANKL) and its interaction with receptor activator of nuclear factor-kappa B (RANK) on pre-osteoclastic cells [21]. This heterotypic cell-cell interaction induces the fusion of pre-osteoclasts and the formation of mature multinucleated osteoclasts that are capable of bone resorption (Figure 1) [81]. Osteoblasts can also act as negative modulators of osteoclastogenesis and bone resorption via the secretion of the soluble decoy receptor for RANKL, osteoprotegerin (OPG), which has a protective effect against osteolytic bone metastasis [22].

During bone metastasis the normal balance that exists between bone resorption and formation is disrupted by the homotypic and heterotypic cell-cell interactions that occur between invading tumor cells, osteoblasts and osteoclasts (Figure 1). The dysregulation of bone resorption and formation is underpinned by the activation of a complex network of autocrine and paracrine signals that involve multiple soluble factors, signaling pathways and transcriptional regulators and drive continuous cycles of highly destructive bone remodeling [10, 11]. The majority of patients with secondary bone tumors — including those associated with prostate cancer — present with osteolytic lesions. Therefore the majority of treatment strategies in current use or under evaluation in bone metastasis have been designed to protect the bone matrix from the increased bone degrading activity of osteoclasts. The anti-osteolytic treatments under investigation for treatment of bone metastasis in prostate cancer are depicted in Figure 1 and are covered in *Sections 3.1-3.4.*

Of particular note, an additional complication that presents in more than 80% of prostate cancer patients with bone metastasis is the osteosclerotic lesion phenotype (also known as bony or bone-forming lesions) — or a combination of both osteolytic and osteosclerotic lesions — also referred to as mixed lesions [82, 83]. Osteosclerotic lesions are typified by bony deposits with multiple layers of poorly organized type I collagen fibrils that have a woven appearence and reduced mechanical strength [10]. The molecular mechanisms involved in this aberrant deposition of collagen fibrils by osteoblasts in osteosclerotic lesions have not been defined. Nevertheless, a number of osteogenic regulators are currently being considered as anti-osteosclerotic targets — these are depicted together with anti-osteolytic targets in Figure 1 — and are covered in *Sections 3.5-3.10.*

The severity of the bone matrix remodeling process initiated by metastatic prostate cancer is evident from the high serum levels of both bone-degradation and bone-formation markers when compared with those observed in patients with bone metastasis from other solid tumors [84, 85]. Interestingly the serum levels of the bone-degradation marker, amino-terminal propeptide of type I collagen (NTX), which is released following cathepsin K mediated osteolysis [86], was found to be a stronger predictor of disease progression and overall survival in CRPC patients with bone metastasis than the bone-formation marker, BALP, which suggests that osteolysis may be essential for osteosclerotic disease progression [84, 85]. Further studies that correlate bone lesion phenotypes with a wide range of available bone turnover markers may help to bring further clarity to the aetiology, mechanisms of progression and response to therapy of bone metastasis in prostate cancer — and may also help to direct new approaches for future treatment [87].

3. TREATMENT OF PROSTATE CANCER ASSOCIATED BONE METASTASIS

3.1. Bisphosponates

Treatment with intravenous or oral bisphosphonates has emerged as an effective measure for limiting osteolytic complications in prostate cancer patients [43, 44]. Bisphosphonates are chemically stable derivatives of inorganic pyrophosphate that inhibit calcification by binding to hydroxyapatite (also known as bone mineral) and then preventing its breakdown by osteoclasts [44].

Compared to first generation (etidronate, clodronate and tiludronate) second and third generation nitrogen-containing bisphosphonates (pamidronate, alendronate, risedronate, zoledronate) have the added effect of inhibiting mevalonate pathway enzymes, which directly suppresses osteoclast function. The second and third generation bisphosphonates also have direct effects on osteoblasts and tumor cells — they can block apoptosis and promote differentiation in osteoblasts and in tumor cells they can inhibit growth factor production, adhesion to bone matrix, invasion and promote apoptosis [88-91]. Some of these modes of action have been depicted in Figure 1.

Table 1. Clinical trials of bisphosphonates in metastatic and non-metastatic prostate cancer

Study and phase	Population	n	Treatment groups	End points	
				Primary	Secondary
NCT00039104 (II)	CRPC+MBD	50	ZA±rebimastat	DFS	TT
NCT00582556 (II)	PCa	45	ZA+GnRH analog (various doses)	BMD	BMM, PSA
NCT00151073 (II)	CRPC+MBD	34	ZA±docetaxel+estramustine	BMM	PSA, TT
NCT00181584 (II)	PCa−MBD	60	ZA vs placebo	BMD	BMM, TT
NCT00554918 (II) TRAPEZE	CRPC+MBD	300	Docetaxel+ZA vs docetaxel+Sr-89 vs docetaxel+ZA+Sr-89	TT	BMD, HCE, PPI profiling
ISRCTN66626762 (III) ZEUS	CRPC−MBD	1,300	ADT±ZA	MBD	BMD, BMM, OS, PSA, TT
NCT00058188 (III)	CRPC−MBD	70	Ca²⁺ gln+CCF±ZA	BMD	BALP, DFS, PSA, SRE
NCT00330759 (III)	AdCa−(PCa/BCa)+MBD; MM	745	ZA vs denosumab	SRE	TT, DS antibody titer
NCT00005073 (III)	PCa−MBD	500	ZA vs placebo	MBD, OS	QOL, SRE
NCT00329797 (III)	PCa−MBD	1,272	Ca²⁺ gln+CCF±ZA	SRE	BMD, QOL
NCT00869206 (III) CALGB-70604	(BCa/PCa)+MBD; MM	1,538	ZA (4 weeks vs 12 weeks)	SRE	BP; SRE rate; TT
NCT00079001 (III) SWOG-CALGB-90202	CRPC+MBD	680	ZA vs placebo	SRE	OS, PFS, TT
NCT00698308 (III)	CRPC+MBD	680	ZA vs placebo	SRE	OS, PFS, TT
NCT00193856 (III) RADAR	PCa−MBD	1,000	LHRH analog (6 months or 18 months)+SDR±ZA	DFS	BMD, OS, QOL, SRE, TT
NCT00268476 (II–III) STAMPEDE	CRPC±MBD	3,300	ADT±docetaxel+prednisone+ZA vs ADT+celecoxib±ZA	OS	HCE, PFS, QOL, SRE, TT
NCT01198457 (no phase indicated) BONA	BCa/PCa/MM+MBD	200	CA	ATT	BP, SRE
NCT00426777 (III)	PCa+MBD+BP	160	RA vs placebo	BMD	TT
NCT00216060 (III)	PCa+MBD	60	ADT±RA	SRE	BMM, PSA, OS, PFS, TR
NCT00082927 (III) RIB	PCa+MBD+BP	580	IA vs SDR	BP	QOL, OC activity
NCT00019695 (II)	PCa+MBD	72	Ketoconazole±AA	Pharmacokinetics	MMP activity

Abbreviations: AA, alendronic acid; AC, analgesic consumption; AdCa, advanced cancer; ADT, androgen-deprivation therapy; ATT, adherence to treatment; BALP, bone alkaline phosphatase; BCa, breast cancer; BMD, bone mineral density; BMM, bone metabolism markers; BP, bone pain; CA, clodronic acid; Ca²⁺gln, Ca²⁺ gluconate; CCF, cholecalciferol; CRPC, castration-resistant prostate cancer; DFS, disease-free survival; D, denosumab; GnRH, gonadotrophin releasing hormone; HCE, healthcare economics; IA, ibandronic acid; M, mitoxantrone; MBD, metastatic bone disease; MM, multiple myeloma; OC, osteoclast; OS, overall survival; P, prednisone; PCa, prostate cancer; PFS, progression-free survival; PPI, prognostic and predictive indicators; PSA, prostate specific antigen; QOL, quality of life; RA, risedronic acid; RP, radical prostatectomy; SDR, single dose radiotherapy; Sm-153, samarium-153; SRE, skeletal-related event; Sr-89, strontium-89; TR, tumor response; TT, tolerance and toxicity; Vit D, vitamin D; ZA, zoledronic acid.

Reproduced from Sturge, J. et al. (2011) Bone metastasis in prostate cancer: emerging therapeutic strategies Nature Reviews in Clinical Oncology 8 357-368 doi:10.1038/nrclinonc.2011.67 (1).

A review published in 2006 compiled ten randomized and controlled trials of bisphosphonate treatment of patients with CRPC and bone metastasis [92]. The meta-analysis carried out included seven studies of clodronate (Bonefos®, Bayer Schering Pharma AG, Wedding, Mitte, Berlin, Germany) (n = 911) and one study of each of the following compounds: pamidronate (Aredia®, Novartis International AG, Basel, Switzerland) (n = 350), etidronate (Didronel®, Warner Chilcott Company, LLC, Dublin, Ireland) (n = 51), and zoledronate (Zometa®, Novartis International AG, Basel, Switzerland) (n = 643). The overall response rate for bone pain was marginal and for reduced skeletal related events (SREs) reached significance (hazard ratio (HR) = 1.54; P = 0.07 and HR = 0.79; P = 0.05, respectively). The results of this review indicated no change in overall survival, disease-free progression, radiological response or serum PSA following bisphosphonate treatment.

However, follow-up data from two aligned Medical Research Council randomized trials (PR04 and PR05) revealed that clodronate increased overall survival in men with prostate cancer and bone metastasis (median follow-up of 11.5 years; $P = 0.032$) with a predicted 5-year survival of 21% in the placebo group and 30% in the treatment group [93]. By contrast, there was a negative trend in the overall survival of men with prostate cancer free of bone metastasis in the clodronate treatment group (median follow-up of 12 years; $P = 0.94$) with a predicted 5-year survival rate of 80% in the placebo group and 78% in the treatment group [93].

Intravenous infusion of 4 mg zoledronate every 3 to 4 weeks, in conjunction with standard therapy, prevents bone loss and SREs in cases of prostate cancer with bone metastasis [94, 95]. The effect of zoledronate on overall survival has been the focus of several phase II and III clinical studies in prostate cancer. The multicentre, multi-group and multi-stage MRC-STAMPEDE trial [96-99] is designed to involve more than 4,000 patients and provide definitive information about treatment options for men diagnosed with metastatic or high-risk non-metastatic prostate cancer. The first results compared hormonal therapy with celecoxib ($n = 291$) and hormonal therapy alone ($n = 584$) and confirmed that no benefit was provided by the addition of the non-steroidal anti-inflammatory drug [99]. Results for all other treatment arms in the MRC-STAMPEDE trial, including zoledronic acid with and without docetaxel are expected by 2017. The efficacy of several other bisphosphonates in prevention of bone pain, bone loss or SREs in men with prostate cancer and secondary bone metastasis are the focus of several studies. Risedronate (Actonel®, Warner Chilcott Company, LLC, Dublin, Ireland), which has previously been proven effective in the reversal of androgen-deprivation therapy associated bone loss [100-102], is the focus of two trials (SA-CMX-01 and HOG GU02-41). Alendronate (Fosamax®, Merck and Company Incorporated, Whitehouse Station, New Jersey, USA), which also protects against bone loss associated with androgen-deprivation therapy [103], is combined with ketoconazole for the treatment of stage IV prostate cancer in *NCT00019695*. CRUK report that the RIB trial found no difference between ibandronate (Boniva®, Roche Therapeutics Incorporated, Basel, Switzerland) and radiotherapy for the relief of bone pain, however these findings have not been published. Details of recent clinical trials of bisphosphonates in metastatic and non-metastatic prostate cancer are summarized in Table 1.

3.2. Cathepsin K Inhibition

The critical role of cysteine protease cathepsin K in osteoclast-mediated degradation of mineralized type I collagen during bone resorption [23, 77] made the inhibition of its activity an attractive anti-osteolytic strategy in the treatment of bone metastasis. The importance of cathepsin K in the pathology of osteolytic bone metastasis has been confirmed in preclinical studies: where bone marrow-derived cathepsin K has been shown to contribute to the progression of an osteolytic lesion phenotype in mouse models of metastatic prostate cancer [24] and intravenous cathepsin K inhibitors (Novartis International AG, Basel, Switzerland) have been shown to reduce skeletal tumor burden in a mouse model of osteolytic breast cancer by 60% ($P < 0.0001$) when administered alone or by 74% ($P < 0.0001$) when administered in combination with zoledronate [25]. The expression of cathepsin K during prostate cancer progression and on tumor cells localized in bone lesions [104] — together with the ability of transformed cells to assemble podosomes that promote degradation of the extracellular matrices and invasion [105-109] — also has implications for bone metastasis pathology and treatment. First, it suggests that invading tumor cells have the potential to directly contribute to the bone remodeling process in bone metastasis. Second, it suggests that cathepsin K inhibitors may limit bone degradation via the combined suppression of tumor cell and osteoclast mediated bone degradation.

Safety concerns regarding the toxic effects of the cathepsin K inhibitor, balicatib (AAE581, Novartis International AG, Basel, Switzerland) prevented its continued clinical evaluation. These adverse effects became apparent after phase II trials for the treatment of osteoporosis and osteoarthritis, in which the development of dermal morphea lesions was observed in some patients [110, 111]. This complication results from balicatib accumulation in lysosomes and the off-target inhibition of cathepsins in dermal fibroblasts.

The non-lysosomotropic cathepsin K inhibitor, odanacatib (MK-0822, Merck and Company Incorporated, Whitehouse Station, New Jersey, USA) has been evaluated in a phase II trial in breast cancer patients with bone metastasis ($n = 40$) [56]. The study reported that following 4 weeks of treatment odanacatib was as effective as zoledronate in reducing bone turnover measured using urinary NTX [56]. Despite these promising results, two phase III trials of odanacatib that were initiated in patients with breast and prostate cancer with bone metastasis were closed before their completion and no further evaluation is ongoing in the oncology setting. However, odanacatib remains under investigation in phase II/III trials for the treatment of osteoporosis.

3.3. RANKL-RANK Inhibition

Denosumab (XGEVA™, Amgen Incorporated, Thousand Oaks, California, USA) is a fully human RANKL monoclonal antibody that received FDA approval for sub-cutaneous administration in the treatment of osteoporosis. In November 2010 denosumab was also approved for the treatment of patients with bone metastasis derived from solid tumors following the completion of a randomized trial where its efficacy as an anti-osteolytic agent was compared with zoledronate in breast cancer patients with bone metastasis ($n = 2046$) [52].

The study reported a delay in the first on-study SRE by 18% ($P = 0.01$) and time to first and subsequent (multiple) on-study SREs by 23% ($P = 0.001$) in the denosumab treatment arm. Rates of renal toxicity with denosumab were 42% lower than in the zoledronate treatment arm [52].

An improved efficacy of denosumab over bisphosphonates was also reported in a phase II trial of patients with multiple tumor types (prostate cancer, 45%; breast cancer, 40%; other tumors, 15%) [53]. Further analysis of a subset of prostate cancer patients ($n = 50$) from this trial revealed the superiority of denosumab over bisphosphonate for normalization of bone turnover (<50 nM urinary NTX) — this was achieved in 69% of patients in the denosumab arm and only 19% of patients in the bisphosphonate arm of the trial [54, 55]. In addition, the first on-study SRE rate observed in this subset of patients was 8% and 17% respectively in the denosumab and bisphosphonate arms [54, 55].

In an Amgen phase III trial (*NCT000321620*) (Table 2), where 1904 patients with CRPC and bone metastasis were randomized to receive denosumab ($n = 950$) or zoledronic acid ($n = 951$) the median first on-study SRE was 20·7 months for denosumab compared to 17·1 months for zoledronic acid ($P = 0.008$) [112]. In a second Amgen phase III trial (*NCT00286091*) (Table 2), where 1432 patients were randomized to receive denosumab ($n = 716$) or placebo ($n = 716$), denosumab significantly increased bone-metastasis-free survival by a median of 4.2 months compared to placebo ($P = 0.028$) and significantly delayed time to first bone metastasis from 33.2 to 29.5 months ($P = 0.032$). The promising results of this trial provide strong evidence that targeting the bone microenvironment can delay bone metastasis in men with CRPC.

3.4. SRC Kinase Inhibition

The tyrosine kinase SRC promotes cell proliferation and survival [113] and has several pro-metastatic functions in prostate cancer cells, including the promotion of cell adhesion [114], migration [114] and invasion [115] and dissemination to distant organs [116]. Genetic ablation of *Src* results in osteopetrosis associated with a decrease in osteoclast mediated bone resorption and increased osteoblast differention and bone formation [117, 118]. In preclinical studies the dual SRC and BCR-ABL tyrosine kinase inhibitor, dasatinib (Sprycel®, Bristol-Myers Squibb, New York City, USA), has been shown to stimulate the bone forming activity of primary mouse osteoblasts, osteoblast cell lines and osteoblasts derived from human bone marrow [119, 120].

Dasatinib can also induce a concomitant decrease in RANKL production by osteoblasts leading to the inhibition of osteoclastogenesis. In a prostate cancer model of osteolytic bone metastasis, treatment with dasatinib alone was found to be sufficient to increase bone mineral density in the osteolytic lesions by 25% when compared with the control group ($P< 0.001$), whereas the combined treatment of dasatinib with docetaxel was more effective than dasatinib alone ($P = 0.01$) [57]. Dasatinib already has FDA approval for the treatment of imatinib-intolerant or resistant chronic myelogenous leukemia and Philadelphia chromosome-positive acute lymphoblastic leukaemia and is the focus as a potential treatment for different solid tumor types in phase I/II studies. Upon completion the phase III READY trial (*NCT00744497*) (Bristol-Myers Squibb) aims to report on the impact of docetaxel plus dasatinib compared to docetaxel plus placebo on the incidence of SREs — and overall survival — in CRPC patients with metastatic disease (Table 2).

Saracatinib (AZD0503, AstraZeneca plc, London, UK) — another SRC and BCR-ABL tyrosine kinase inhibitor that can limit RANKL-induced osteoclastogenesis and protect the bone architecture in the presence of prostate cancer cells [58] — is the focus of a phase II trial (*NCT00558272*) that aims to assess its effect on NTX levels and safety in the treatment of bone metastasis in prostate and breast cancer (Table 2).

A third SRC and BCR-ABL tyrosine kinase inhibitor, bosutinib (SKI-606, Pfizer Incorporated, New York City, USA) — which is being considered for the treatment of chronic myelogenous leukemia and breast pancreatic, colorectal and non small cell lung cancer — was recently reported to be effective in a preclinical model of prostate cancer bone metastasis, leading to the proposal for its future evaluation as a potential therapeutic in this clinical setting [59].

Table 2. Clinical trials of RANKL, SRC kinase and EAR inhibitors in metastatic and non-metastatic prostate cancer

Trial and phase	Population	n	Treatment groups	End points	
				Primary	Secondary
RANKL inhibition					
NCT00104650 (II)	ST+MBD	135	Bis vs denosumab (4 weeks or 12 weeks)	NTX	CTX, H, NTX, SRE
NCT00286091 (III)	CRPC–MBD	1,435	Denosumab vs placebo	PFS	–
NCT00321620 (III)	CRPC+MBD	1,904	Denosumab vs ZA	SRE	AnR, SRE, TT
SRC kinase inhibition					
NCT00792545 (I)	MBD	48	Dasatinib+BE	TT	–
NCT00558272 (II)	CRPC/BCa+MBD	132	ZA+Vit D+Ca^{2+} gln±SA	CTX	TT
NCT00744497 (III)	CRPC+MBD	1,500	Docetaxel±dasatinib	OS	BP, NTX, PSA, SRE, TT
Endothelin A receptor inhibition					
NCT00090363 (II)	CRPC+MBD	447	Zibotentan vs placebo	DFS	PSA, TTD, ORR, NBM
NCT00554229 (III)	CRPC+MBD	848	Zibotentan vs placebo	OS	BP, NBM, PFS, PSA, QOL, SRE, TTD
NCT00617669 (III) ENTHUSE M1C	CRPC+MBD	1,445	Docetaxel±zibotentan	OS	BP, PSA, QOL, SRE, TT
NCT00626548 (III) ENTHUSE MO	CRPC–MBD	1,500	Zibotentan vs placebo	PFS, OS	PSA, QOL, TT

Abbreviations: AnR, antibody response to treatment; BCa, breast cancer; BE, bevacizumab; Bis, bisphosphonate; BMD, bone mineral density; BP, bone pain; CAT, cataracts; CRPC, castration-resistant prostate cancer; CTX, C-telopeptide of collagen; DFS, disease-free survival; F, fractures; H, hypercalcemia; MBD, metastatic bone disease; MD, metastatic disease; NBM, number of bone metastases; NTX, N-telopeptide of collagen; ORR, objective response rate; OS, overall survival; PFS, progression-free survival; PSA, prostate-specific antigen; QOL, quality of life; RANKL, receptor activator of nuclear factor κB, SRE, skeletal-related event; ST, solid tumor; TT, tolerance and toxicity; TTD, time to death; ZA, zoledronate.

Reproduced and adapted from Sturge, J. et al. (2011) Bone metastasis in prostate cancer: emerging therapeutic strategies Nature Reviews in Clinical Oncology 8 357-368 doi:10.1038/nrclinonc.2011.67(1).

3.5. Endothelin-A-Receptor Inhibition

Endothelin-1 (ET1) is secreted by the epithelial cells of the normal prostate and can activate signaling pathways downstream of the G-protein coupled receptor, endothelin-1 receptor (ET-A, also known as EAR). The ET1-EARsignaling axis is linked to both the activation of osteoblasts and the formation of osteosclerotic bone lesions [28, 29] and preclinical studies have clearly demonstrated that EAR inhibition attenuates osteosclerotic lesion development [30, 31].

A phase II clinical study in prostate cancer reported a 34% reduction in time to disease progression ($P = 0.021$) [60], a 54% reduction in time to PSA progression ($P = 0.002$) [60], and improved quality of life ($P = 0.032$) in the group treated with the EAR inhibitor atrasentan (XINLAY™, Abbott Laboratories Ltd., Maidenhead, UK) [61]. A phase II study in CRPC ($n = 200$) reported that patients treated with placebo displayed continued increases in BALP and NTX, whereas these increases were either completely or partially blocked following treatment with atrasentan and this regression in BALP and NTX levels correlated with a measurable bone scan response [62]. However, the only relevant finding in a subsequent phase III study in CRPC ($n = 801$) was the suppression of BALP in the atrasentan treatment arm compared to the placebo arm ($P < 0.01$) [63]. A meta-analysis of these phase II and III data sets indicated that atrasentan treatment reduced time to disease progression by 14%, bone pain by 18%, PSA progression by 22% and BALP progression by 46% [64]. In a subsequent small phase II trial of atrasentan combined with zoledronate in CRPC ($n = 33$) there was no improvement in bone turnover markers in the treatment group versus atrasentan alone [65]. These fairly modest clinical outcomes and a correlation with increased adverse cardiovascular events [63], led to the rejection of its approval for the treatment of CRPC by the FDA. However, a review on anti-EAR targeted therapies in solid tumors published in 2010 gave an overall favorable opinion for this therapeutic approach [66].

Since the clinical assessment of atrasentan was ceased, focus has been turned to the evaluation of the alternate EAR inhibitor, zibotentan (ZD4054, AstraZeneca plc, London, UK). Daily administration of 15 mg and 10 mg of oral zibotentan to patients with CRPC ($n = 312$) resulted in respective survival advantages of 24% ($P = 0.103$) and 17% ($P = 0.254$) over placebo in a phase II study assessing its efficacy [67]. Modest effects on disease free progression were also observed in both treatment groups of the same study. The ENTHUSE M0 trial, which aimed to assess the efficacy of zibotentan in non-metastatic CRPC (Table 2), was closed early due to the detection of asymptomatic metastasis in 45% of the 2577 patients recruited to the study [121]. The ENTHUSE M1C trial (Table 2) ($n = 594$) median overall survival was 24.5 months in zibotentan-treated patients versus 22.5 months for placebo, but this did not reach statistical significance ($P = .240$). Statistically significant differences were also not found for any secondary endpoint, however, cardiac failure events were higher in the zibotentan group than placebo but were considered to be manageable and reversible [122].

3.5. Systemic Radionuclide Therapy

Radionuclides are systemically administered radiopharmaceuticals currently under investigation for the palliative treatment of severe pain in osteoscerotic bone metastasis. The effectiveness of these agents requires the specific targeting of tumor cells in metastatic bone lesions without affecting the adjacent bone marrow [123]. Some radionuclides have an intrinsic affinity with bone and following systemic administration rapidly accumulate in metastatic bone lesions. These include the particle β-emitter strontium-89 (Metastron™, GE Healthcare, Little Chalfont, Buckinghamshire, UK) and the α-emitter radium-223 (Alpharadin®, Algeta, Oslo, Norway). Other radionuclides are conjugated to bone-seeking ligands — such as phosphonates — to direct their selective delivery to bone lesions, for example the beta emitter samarium-153 is conjugated to ethylenediaminetetramethylene phosphonate (EDTMP) (Quadramet®, EUSA Pharma, Langhorne, PA, USA).

Radionuclides provide overall benefit in the palliation of painful bone metastases and their combined use with other systemic therapies is recommended [45]. In a clinical study strontium-89 increased the overall survival of patients with CRPC ($n = 103$) who had responded to doxorubicin (HR = 2.76; $P = 0.0014$) [46].

Likewise a phase I/II trial reported that samarium-153-EDTMP increased disease free survival with a trend towards increased overall survival in patients with CRPC with bone metastasis ($n = 52$) [47]. For radium-223, a meta-analysis of two phase I trials ($n = 37$) and three phase II trials ($n = 255$) calculated a 29% increase in overall survival ($P = 0.017$) and decreases in bone pain, bone markers and median time to PSA progression in the radium-223 treatment arm versus placebo [48].

Table 3. Clinical trials of radionuclides in metastatic prostate cancer

Trial and phase	Population	n	Treatment groups	End points	
				Primary	Secondary
Strontium-89					
NCT00081159 (II)	CRPC + MBD	80	ADT + doxorubicin + ZA ± Sr-89	DFS	BSR
NCT00554918 (II)	CRPC + MBD	300	Docetaxel + prednisone ± ZA ± Sr-89	TT	BMD, BP, HCE, PSA, OS, QOL, TTP
NCT00002503 (III)	CRPC + MBD	200	Sr-89 vs RT	TTP	HCE, OS, QOL, TT
NCT00024167 (III)	CRPC + MBD	480	ICT + doxorubicin ± Sr-89	OS	NBM
Samarium-153-EDTMP					
NCT00450619 (II)	CRPC + MBD	68	Sm-153 ± TRICOM	PFS	OS, PSA, TT
NCT00365105 (III)	ST + MBD	352	ZA + Vit D + Ca²⁺ ± Sr-89 or Sm-153	SRE	BP, OS, QOL, SRE
Radium-223					
NCT01106352 (I–II)	CRPC + MBD	60	Docetaxel ± Rad-223	TT	BP, BMM, PSA, TT
NCT00699751 ALSYMPCA (III)	CRPC + MBD	900	Rad-223 vs placebo	OS	BMM, PSA, QOL, TT, TTP

Abbreviations: ADT, androgen-deprivation therapy; BMD, bone mineral density; BMM, bone metabolic markers; BP, bone pain; BSR, bone scan response; CRPC, castration-resistant prostate cancer; DFS, disease-free survival; HCE, health care economic analysis; ICT, induction chemotherapy; MBD: metastatic bone disease; NBM, number of bone metastases; OS, overall survival; PSA, prostate-specific antigen; QOL, quality of life; Rad-223, radium 223; RT, radiotherapy, Sm-153, samarium-153 conjugated to ethylenediaminetetramethylene phosphonate; Sr-89, strontium-89; SRE, skeletal-related event; ST, solid tumor; TRICOM, triad of costimulatory molecules; TT, tolerance and toxicity; TTP, time to progression; ZA, zoledronate.

Reproduced from Sturge, J. et al. (2011) Bone metastasis in prostate cancer: emerging therapeutic strategies *Nature Reviews in Clinical Oncology* 8 357-368 doi:10.1038/nrclinonc.2011.67 (1).

The ALSYMPCA trial, an international, randomized, double-blind, placebo-controlled Phase III study of radium-223 chloride plus best standard of care compared with placebo plus best standard of care in men with symptomatic metastatic CRPC ($n = 922$) (Table 3) reported on its favorable efficacy and finished early with placebo controls being offered treatment with radium-223 [124, 125].

Treatment with radium-223 improved overall survival by 44 percent compared to placebo ($P = 0.00185$) with a median overall survival of 14.0 months for men treated with radium-223 and 11.2 months for men treated with placebo. The median time to first SRE was 13.6 months for men treated with radium-223 and 8.4 months for men treated with placebo and levels of BALP were normalized in 33 percent of men treated with radium-223 compared to 1 percent of men treated with placebo. Treatment with radium-223 improved time to PSA progression by 49 percent compared to placebo ($P = 0.00015$).

Radionuclide therapy in combination with other systemic therapies has shown favorable results. In particular, a number of phase I/II trials of samarium-153-EDTMP in combination with docetaxel reported good tolerance, a marked improvement in bone pain and a trend towards increased overall survival [49-51].

Data from phase I trials of samarium-153-EDTMP in combination with zoledronate reported that the bisphosphonate did not alter skeletal uptake of samarium-153-EDTMP [126, 127] and a case study has also suggested that their combined use may be effective [128]. In a further phase I trial samarium-153-lexidronam and docetaxel ($n = 13$) were reported to have favorable efficacy and toxicity in patients with metastatic CRPC [129].

3.6. WNT Signaling

A fundamental role for Wnt signaling in normal osteogenesis has been established in genetic models [32, 33]. Studies in human mesenchymal stem cells confirm the important role of different ligands from the Wnt family in osteogenesis [130]. Overexpression of WNT [131] or a deficiency in Wnt antagonists — noggin and dickkopf-related protein 1 (DKK1) [132, 133] — results in increased bone formation. The osteogenic effect of Wnt signaling has been linked to the promotion of osteosclerotic lesions [34, 35] and loss of endogenous noggin or DKK1 is correlated with osteosclerotic lesion formation [36] providing a basis for Wnt signaling as future target in osteosclerotic bone metastases in prostate cancer [134, 135].

3.7. TGF-β Signaling Axis

TGF-β_1 has a wide range of complex and often contradictory roles in bone homeostasis [12] and its dysregulation has extensive implications in human disease [136, 137]. A critical role for TGF-β_1 in normal bone homeostasis is to coordinate the temporal, spatial and quantitative coupling of new bone formation to sites where old bone degradation is occurring [13, 76]. This coupling is achieved following the release of active TGF-β_1 from the bone matrix during its degradation, which initiates the chemotactic recruitment of mesenchymal stem cells from the bone marrow to sites of osteolytic activity where they differentiate into osteoblasts that deposit new bone [13]. TGF-β_1 is also a key regulator of several other key stages in bone formation [12], including the proliferation of osteoblast progenitors and deposition of collagen type I [12]. It is also becoming clear that the TGF-β_1 signaling axis can also modulate osteoclastogenesis and bone resorption. This became evident following the targeted suppression of TGF-β-I/II receptors and their downstream signaling pathways in mouse models, which resulted in increased differentiation of osteoblasts, decreased differentiation of osteoclasts and the subsequent protection against skeletal fracture via enhanced bone formation and limited bone resorption [13-16]. Two critical findings have been that the TGF-β-signaling axis promotes the development of bone metastasis by regulating a gene expression signature [138] and by promoting tumor cell homing to bone [139]. Studies have also confirmed high levels of TGF-β_1 and subsequent downstream activation of the transcription factors SMAD-2 and -3 in osteolytic bone lesions and its targetability for limiting their progression [17].

The safety of a monoclonal antibody directed against all three isoforms of TGF-β — fresolimumab (GC1008) (Genzyme Oncology, Cambridge, Massachusetts, USA) — has been assessed in malignant melanoma, renal cell carcinoma, malignant pleural mesothelioma and focal segmental glomerulosclerosis and is under evaluation for safety in combination with radiation in a small cohort (n = 28) of metastatic breast cancer patients (*NCT01401062*). Several TGF-β-targeted therapies in development for the potential treatment of metastatic cancer include a second anti-TGF-β monoclonal antibody, 1D11 (Genzyme Oncology, Cambridge, Massachusetts, USA) [68, 69]. Also in the pipeline as therapeutic approaches are a TGFβRI kinase inhibitor, SD-208 (Tocris Bioscience, Ellisville, Missouri, USA) [72], soluble TGFβRII [70, 71] and inhibition of TGFβ-III receptor [73].

Its divergent roles in tumor cells and the bone microenvironment makes the TGF-β signalling axis a challenging target in bone metastasis. Blocking TGF-β is also considered problematic due to its role as a tumor suppressor in normal glandular epithelium and the ubiquitous expression of TGF-β receptors in most tissue types. However, since most preclinical data indicate that the TGF-β signaling axis promotes osteolytic bone lesions it is very likely that anti-TGF-β antibodies or TGF-β receptor inhibitors will undergo further evaluation in the metastatic cancer setting. Further evaluation in pre-clinical models of osteosclerotic bone lesions will inform on the outcome of targeting TGF-β in this context.

3.8. uPA-uPAR

Urokinase-type plasminogen activator (uPA) is a serine protease that binds to its cell surface receptor (uPAR) and promotes pericellular proteolysis and intracellular signaling, which can both coordinate multiple processes in cancer progression [140]. The clinical evaluation of uPA and uPAR in the serum of prostate cancer patients has revealed strong associations with multiple states of disease progression [141]. Serum levels of uPA and uPAR were significantly higher ($P < 0.044$) in patients with bone metastasis versus all other groups [141] and the detection of uPAR positive disseminated tumor cells in the bone marrow of patients with localized disease is associated with unfavorable Gleason score ($P = 0.004$), high-risk of cancer ($P = 0.005$) and decreased time to recurrence of increasing levels of PSA ($P = 0.01$) [142].

The finding that the amino-terminal fragment of uPA is mitogenic in osteoblasts [37, 38] and drives osteoblastic responses in three dimensional cocultures of prostate cancer cell and osteoblasts [39, 40] led to its consideration as a target in osteosclerotic bone metastasis. Subsequent preclinical studies have suggested that the regulation of the uPA-uPAR system can provide potential treatments for both osteosclerotic and osteolytic lesions. The former is evident from the finding that intracardiac injection of prostate cancer cells engineered to overexpress uPA in a rat model was associated with the formation of osteosclerotic lesions, increased serum BALP, osteogenesis and spinal cord compression [41]. The latter is evidenced by the development of a potential anti-osteolytic therapy based on overexpression of the amino-terminal fragment of uPA in bone marrow-derived mesenchymal stem cells and their targeted delivery to osteolytic lesions where they differentiate into osteoblasts and promote new bone formation [42].

MESUPRON® (WX-671) and WX-UK1 (Wilex AG, Munich, Germany) are the first uPA inhibitors to enter oncology trials. WX-UK1 has efficacy in preclinical models [143, 144] and both agents have been tested for safety in advanced malignancies (*NCT00499265* and*NCT0083525*) [145]. MESUPRON® has also been shown to have efficacy in breast cancer [146]. Given the role of uPA in osteosclerotic bone lesion pathology MESUPRON® and WX-UK1 could become future considerations for the treatment of CRPC and associated bone metastasis.

3.9. Endo180

Endocytic receptor 180 (Endo180, encoded by C-type mannose receptor 2, *MRC2*) is a uPA-uPAR associated protein [147] that is expressed on the surface of osteoblasts, interacts directly with the C-terminal region of type I collagen via its fibronectin type II domain [148] and localizes to sites of cell-matrix contact [149]. The ostoblastic effect of uPA and uPAR and their contribution to metastatic bone lesions with an osteosclerotic phenotype is discussed above in *Section 3.8*. In normal tissue Endo180 is localized to areas of active bone remodeling [150]. The genetic silencing and mutation of *Mrc2* is associated with skeletal defects [151, 152]. Although the precise biological function of Endo180 in adult bone has not been fully elucidated, its transcriptional regulation by the TGF-β_1-TGFβR1-SMAD-2 and -3 signaling axis [153, 154] suggests a direct link to turnover of the bone extracellular matrix. The contribution of TGF-β_1-TGFβR1-SMAD-2 and -3 signaling axis to metastatic bone lesion pathology was covered in *Section 3.7*.

In vitro and *in vivo* studies have demonstrated that Endo180 can bind exogenous collagen ligands at the plasma membrane and facilitate their rapid internalization into early endosomes, trafficking to lysosomes and subsequent degradation by cathepsins [155-158]. At the cellular and tissue level Endo180 is able to spatially localize to sites of osteoblast-like cell-matrix contact [149], expressed in areas of active bone remodeling [150, 159, 160], correlates with Gleason score [74] and is expressed on tumor cells with invasive potential in prostate cancer [74].

In recent work the functional implications of Endo180 expression in bone metastasis have been investigated using co-cultures of primary human osteoblasts and human prostate cancer cell lines [75]. It is important to note that primary cultures of human trabecular bone osteoblasts produce extracellular matrix enriched with the factors found in human bone [161] thereby providing a clinically relevant platform for modelling the tumor-bone stromal interface. When primary human osteoblasts are treated with osteogenic medium they display strong levels of alkaline phosphatase activity (a marker of osteoblast differentiation) and are able to deposit phosphate (a marker of bone matrix mineralization). Co-culture of primary human osteoblasts with human prostate cells (originating from different stages of prostatic disease) resulted in a significant reduction in their alkaline phosphatase activity in direct co-cultures with PC3 and DU145 cells or indirect co-culture with PC3 and DU145 conditioned medium [75].

The suppression of mineralized matrix production by osteoblasts that was induced by PC3 and DU145 cells, in both direct and indirect co-culture [75], was consistent with their osteolytic properties in mouse bone xenografts [162-164]. Endo180 positive PC3 and DU145 cell numbers were significantly increased after their co-culture with osteoblasts [75]. In contrast, the number of Endo180 positive osteoblasts was significantly decreased following their co-culture with PC3 and DU145 cells [75]. In accordance with these *in vitro* findings immunohistochemistry of metastatic bone lesion biopsies (Figure 2A) revealed high levels of Endo180 expression on cells within tumor foci (Figure 2B). Positive Endo180 staining was also observed on cells located in the stroma adjacent to small tumor foci (Figure 2C) but absent on cells located in stroma adjacent to large tumor foci (Figure 2D). These findings consolidate the high levels of Endo180 previously observed in prostate tumor cells localized in metastatic bone lesions [74]. The high expression of Endo180 in metastatic breast cancer cell foci [75] is consistent with the pattern of staining that has been reported for phospho-SMAD-2 (an indicator of TGFβ$_1$ activation) in osteolytic bone lesions [139]. Together with the lower levels of Endo180 staining in areas of the stroma near to the main tumor mass [75], these observations suggest that when tumor cells invade the bone they are able to disrupt TGFβ$_1$-dependent autocrine and paracrine signalling and reduce the stromal expression of Endo180. In line with this potential mechanism, PC3 and DU145 cells have been shown to reduce TGFβ$_1$ production in stromal fibroblasts [165].

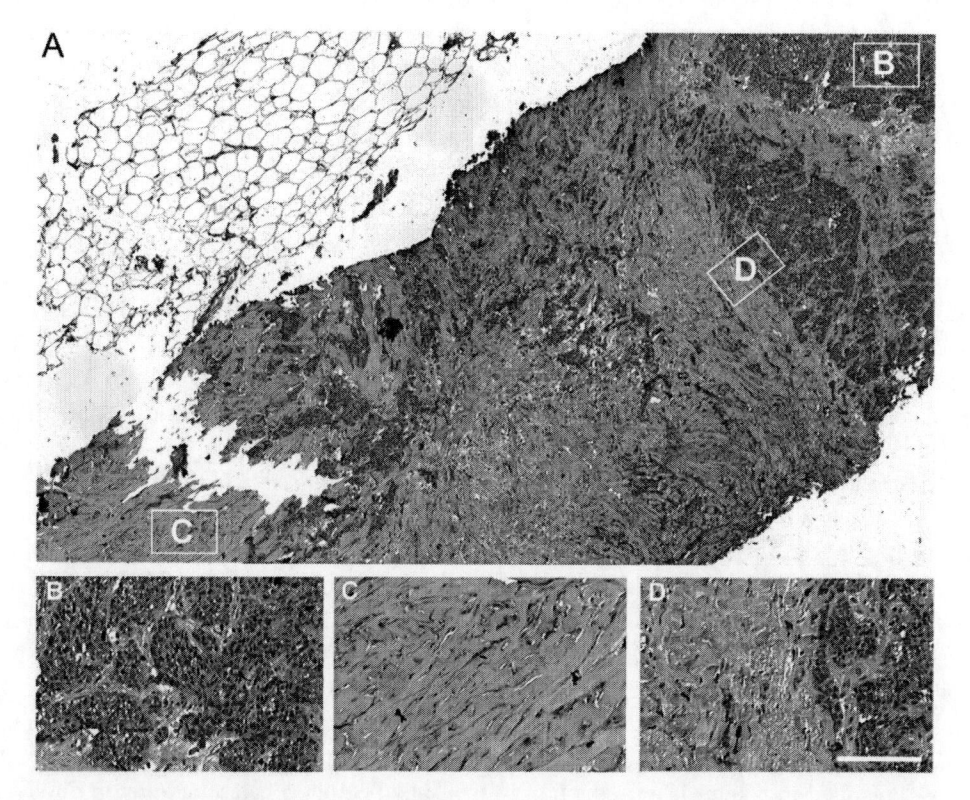

Figure 2. *Endo180 expression in a metastatic bone lesion.* (A) Low power image of a bone core biopsy including its associated fatty tissue core mounted to the left hand side. Fibro-collagenous tissue containing invasive tumor cells can be seen. The biopsy was taken to maximize tumor sample. Trabeculae and bone-lining osteoblasts were not present. Strong Endo180 staining can be observed in tumor cells (B) and stromal cells located near small tumor foci (C). Weak Endo180 staining can be observed in cells adjacent to the larger tumor foci (D). Data shown is representative of observations made from four patient biopsies. Scale bar = 100 μm. Reproduced from Caley et al., 2012 Journal of Pathology 226, 775-783 (Publisher: John Wiley and Sons, Incorporated) [75].

Moreover, as discussed below, TGFβ$_1$ *per se* was capable of reinstating normal levels of collagen type I deposition and Endo180 expression in primary human osteoblast and 'osteolytic' prostate cancer cell cocultures [75]. To investigate the effect of increased Endo180 expression on the ability of osteolytic prostate tumor cells to internalize collagen fragments PC3 cells were transfected with an Endo180 overexpression construct and internalization assays using fluorescently labelled gelatin were carried out [75]. Consistent with findings in a range of other cell types [154, 155, 157, 158] the increased expression of Endo180 was sufficient to facilitate OG-gelatin uptake by PC3 cells [75].

To investigate whether Endo180 is important during collagen deposition by osteoblasts we visualized and quantified type I collagen following the silencing of Endo180 in unstimulated osteoblasts and osteoblasts stimulated with osteogenic factors. The partial reduction in Endo180 expression (-60%) in osteoblasts following direct coculture with prostate cells could be mimicked in osteoblast monolayers using siRNA oligonucleotides to genetically silence Endo180. Intracellular type I collagen levels were increased in unstimulated osteoblasts following Endo180 silencing, which suggests that it does not participate in the internalization of native extracellular type I collagen produced by primary human osteoblasts. The negligible change in total type I collagen levels further indicates that Endo180 silencing confers a net decrease in extracellular type I collagen deposition and this was confirmed by the finding that type I collagen deposition by osteoblasts stimulated with osteogenic factors was significantly decreased following Endo180 silencing [75].

The fact that TGFβ$_1$ can induce Endo180 expression in osteoblasts and different tumor cell types [153, 154], including PC3 and DU145 cells [75], led us to investigate whether dysregulated TGFβ$_1$ paracrine signaling underlies the divergent regulation of Endo180 function in our coculture model. In accordance, decreased Endo180 expression in osteoblasts followed TGFβR1 inhibition, which directly correlated with reduced type I collagen fibril deposition [75]. Moreover, and as pointed out earlier in this section, the addition of exogenous TGFβ$_1$ restored osteoblastic Endo180 expression and reinstated normal levels of type I collagen deposition in osteoblast-PC3 and osteoblast-DU145 cell cocultures [75].

According to these results — and the results of immunohistochemical analysis of osteolytic bone lesions (Figure 2) — a potential model that emerges is that type I collagen deposition mediated by the TGF-β$_1$-TGFβR1-SMAD-2/3-Endo180 pathway is suppressed in osteoblasts and that — concomitantly — the Endo180-dependent internalization of collagen fragments by invading tumor cells is activated in osteolytic bone lesions. We have therefore proposed a heterotypic cellular mechanism in bone metastasis in which the TGFβ$_1$-TGFβ1R-Endo180-type I collagen deposition pathway becomes suppressed by competing TGFβ$_1$ paracrine and autocrine signaling loops that establish between adjacent tumor and stromal cells (Figure 3).

This phenomenon could involve: (a) sequestration of soluble TGFβ$_1$ by the tumor cell mass; (b) secretion of factors from tumor cells that can decrease TGFβ$_1$ production by adjacent stromal cells [165]; or (c) dysregulation of other soluble factors that can regulate Endo180 expression [166]. In conclusion, we propose the TGFβ-TGFβ1R-Endo180-dependent type I collagen deposition pathway as a future therapeutic target in bone metastasis and other conditions where aberrant collagen turnover is a major pathological feature. Following further work in the preclinical setting the Endo180-receptor may provide a future therapeutic opportunity where the use of a single agent with a dual mode of action in the tumor and bone compartments can be used to treat bone metastasis.

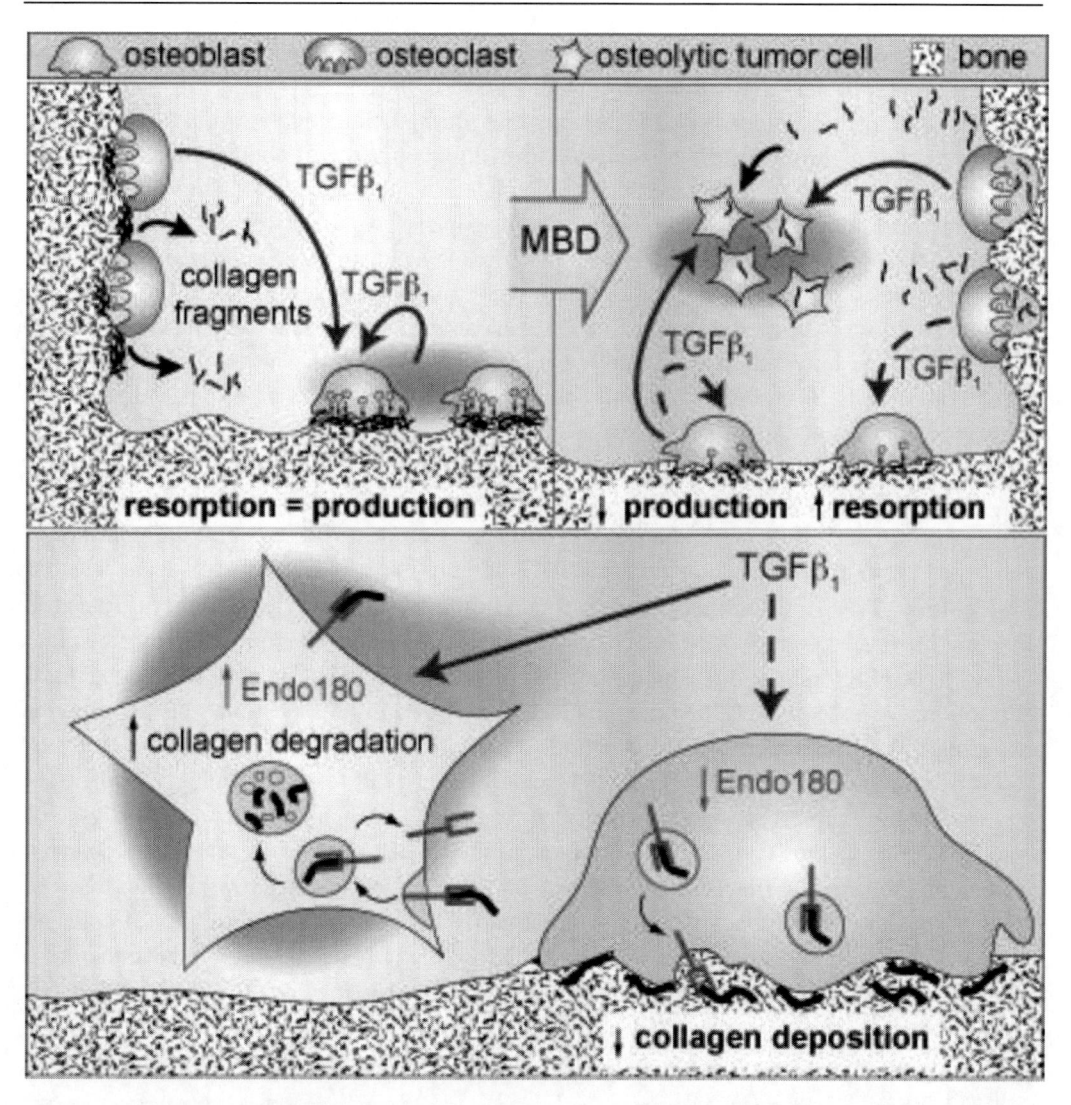

Figure 3. *Disruption of TGF-β₁-TGFβR1-Endo180 pathway at the tumor-bone stromal interface.* Upper left panel shows balanced bone-resorption/production in normal bone homeostasis, where bone-resorption releases cleaved collagen (black fragments) and matricellular factors, including transforming growth factor-beta (TGF-β₁) (blue cloud) [13]. TGF-β is an autocrine factor that maintains osteoblast differentiation and collagen deposition during bone formation [12]. Upper right panel shows metastatic bone disease (MBD) where invasive tumor cells promote osteoclastogenesis/bone-resorption and concomitantly suppress osteoblast differentiation, collagen deposition and new bone formation [2, 10, 11]. Lower panel shows dysregulated TGF-β₁ leading to increased Endo180 (red receptor) mediated internalization of collagen fragments into intracellular compartments (pink circles) and Endo180 suppression in osteoblasts leading to decreased collagen deposition (Lower Panel). Reproduced from Caley et al., 2012 Journal of Pathology 226, 775-783 (Publisher: John Wiley and Sons, Incorporated) [75].

3.10. Collagen Deposition

Bone metastasis in prostate cancer involves new bone deposits with multiple layers of poorly organized collagen fibrils [1, 10]. As discussed in *Section 3.9* the identification of Endo180 as an osteoblastic receptor that can promote collagen deposition [75] has led us to propose that a new avenue for bone-targeted therapy of osteosclerotic lesions is direct suppression of the collagen deposition pathway.

The initial stage of new bone formation by osteoblasts involves their orchestrated production and organization of osteoid matrix, which is comprised of approximately 90% type I collagen fibres [1, 10]. Type I pro-collagen formation by osteoblasts and other stromal cells is initiated in the rough endoplasmic reticulum where processing, modification and assembly of its constituent two alpha-1 chains and one alpha-2 chain into a triple helix is completed before trafficking to the Golgi apparatus for secretion by exocytosis [1]. Once outside the cell, pro-collagen undergoes processing and covalent cross-linking by lysyl oxidase to form the multiple collagen fibrils required for the assembly of each collagen fibre. The highly collagenous osteoid is then mineralized following exocytic deposition of alkaline phosphatase by osteoblasts [1].

The proposed target in this pathway, Endo180, is likely to play a role at the later stages of the pathway, either during pro-collagen exocytosis or the extracellular organization of collagen fibres. A better understanding about how Endo180 helps to direct type I collagen fibril deposition in normal bone and the aberrant molecular mechanisms that lead to inappropriate deposition of type I collagen fibrils in osteosclerotic bone lesions have potential application in addressing this unmet clinical need.

CONCLUSION

The conventional use of chemotherapy and radiotherapy to treat bone metastasis is mainly palliative. However, the use of adjuvant treatment with bisphosphonates or RANKL inhibitor can significantly reduce the progression of bone metastases and improve survival, which is a clear indication that bone-targeted therapies can provide a significant clinical benefit in patients with bone metastasis. The intense research that has rapidly evolved in this area of oncology indicates there will be new therapeutic options for the treatment of bone metastases from solid cancers over the coming decade.

The improved treatment of osteolytic and osteosclerotic bone lesions associated with prostate cancer will require the concomitant targeting of the critical molecular pathways in invading tumor cells, osteoclasts and osteoblasts that drive this complex bone remodeling process. This will involve therapeutic strategies where the tumor and bone compartments can be targeted together, either with a single agent that inhibits both compartments, or with appropriate combinations of anti-osteolytic and anti-osteosclerotic therapeutics.

At the same time it will also be important to identify those patients most likely to develop bone metastasis and those patients most likely to respond to therapy. This could be achieved by the validation of molecular signatures that can be used to better inform on effective treatment protocols for individual cases of bone metastasis [167].

KEY POINTS

1. The treatment of metastatic bone disease in men with prostate cancer is complicated by the occurrence of osteolytic (bone-degrading), osteosclerotic (bone-forming) and mixed osteolytic and osteosclerotic lesions; the aetiology of these contrasting phenotypes is unclear.
2. It is essential to study the complex interactions between tumor cells, osteoblasts and osteoclasts in the bone metastatic niche using clinically relevant models (such as primary human osteoblast and prostate cancer cell co-cultures) so that the mechanisms of osteolytic and osteoscleroticbone metastasis can be applied in the development of targeted treatments for both disease components.
3. Bisphosphonates are used as a palliative treatment to protect against the osteolytic effects of bone metastasis. To date, clodronate has been shown to improve the survival of prostate cancer patients with bone metastasis.
4. Denosumab, the inhibitor of RANKL has been approved for the treatment of bone metastasisthat originated from a solid tumor; however, its efficacy in bone metastasis associated with CRPC will not become clear until several clinical trials are completed.
5. EAR inhibition has limited efficacy for the treatment of bone metastasis associated with CRPC.
6. Systemic radionuclide therapy has good efficacy in the treatment of bone metastasis associated with CRPC.
7. Improved understanding of the molecular mechanisms of dysregulated type collagen I collagen deposition and degradation in bone metastasis will open up new avenues for therapeutic exploitation; this may involve targeting Endo180.

ACKNOWLEDGMENT

The author would like to thank Dr Ana-Violeta Fonseca for help in schematic design and Dr Matthew Caley for help with database searches.

DATABASES

The National Cancer Institute database for clinical trials (www.cancer.gov/clinicaltrials) and current controlled clinical trials database were used as reference tools.

REFERENCES

[1] Sturge J, Caley MP, Waxman J. Bone metastasis in prostate cancer: emerging therapeutic strategies. *Nat. Rev. Clin. Oncol.* 2011 8: 357-368.
[2] Mundy GR. Metastasis to bone: causes, consequences and therapeutic opportunities. *Nat. Rev. Cancer.* 2002 2: 584-593.

[3] Eisenberger MA, Walsh PC. Early androgen deprivation for prostate cancer? *N. Engl. J. Med.* 1999 341: 1837-1838.

[4] Smith MR, Brown, G.A., Saad, F. New opportunities in the management of prostate cancer-related bone complications. *Urologic Oncology: Seminars and Original Investigations.* 2009 27: S1-S20.

[5] Janjan N, Lutz ST, Bedwinek JM, Hartsell WF, Ng A, Pieters RS, Jr., et al. Therapeutic guidelines for the treatment of bone metastasis: a report from the American College of Radiology Appropriateness Criteria Expert Panel on Radiation Oncology. *J. Palliat. Med.* 2009 12: 417-426.

[6] Tannock IF, de Wit R, Berry WR, Horti J, Pluzanska A, Chi KN, et al. Docetaxel plus prednisone or mitoxantrone plus prednisone for advanced prostate cancer. *N. Engl. J. Med.* 2004 351:1502-1512.

[7] Berthold DR, Pond GR, Soban F, de Wit R, Eisenberger M, Tannock IF. Docetaxel plus prednisone or mitoxantrone plus prednisone for advanced prostate cancer: updated survival in the TAX 327 study. *J. Clin. Oncol.* 2008 26: 242-245.

[8] Petrylak DP, Tangen CM, Hussain MH, Lara PN, Jr., Jones JA, Taplin ME, et al. Docetaxel and estramustine compared with mitoxantrone and prednisone for advanced refractory prostate cancer. *N. Engl. J. Med.* 2004 351:1513-1520.

[9] Seruga B, Ocana A, Tannock IF. Drug resistance in metastatic castration-resistant prostate cancer. *Nat. Rev. Clin. Oncol.* 2011 8: 12-23.

[10] Clines GA, Guise TA. Molecular mechanisms and treatment of bone metastasis. *Expert Rev. Mol. Med.* 2008 10: e7.

[11] Rose AA, Siegel PM. Breast cancer-derived factors facilitate osteolytic bone metastasis. *Bull. Cancer.* 2006 93: 931-943.

[12] Janssens K, ten Dijke P, Janssens S, Van Hul W. Transforming growth factor-beta1 to the bone. *Endocr. Rev.* 2005 26: 743-774.

[13] Tang Y, Wu X, Lei W, Pang L, Wan C, Shi Z, et al. TGF-beta1-induced migration of bone mesenchymal stem cells couples bone resorption with formation. *Nat. Med.* 2009 15: 757-765.

[14] Mohammad KS, Chen CG, Balooch G, Stebbins E, McKenna CR, Davis H, et al. Pharmacologic inhibition of the TGF-beta type I receptor kinase has anabolic and anti-catabolic effects on bone. *PLoS. One.* 2009 e5275.

[15] Alliston T, Choy L, Ducy P, Karsenty G, Derynck R. TGF-beta-induced repression of CBFA1 by Smad3 decreases cbfa1 and osteocalcin expression and inhibits osteoblast differentiation. *EMBO J.* 2001 20: 2254-2272.

[16] Qiu T, Wu X, Zhang F, Clemens TL, Wan M, Cao X. TGF-beta type II receptor phosphorylates PTH receptor to integrate bone remodelling signalling. *Nat. Cell Biol.* 2010 12: 224-234.

[17] Korpal M, Yan J, Lu X, Xu S, Lerit DA, Kang Y. Imaging transforming growth factor-beta signaling dynamics and therapeutic response in breast cancer bone metastasis. *Nat. Med.* 2009 15: 960-966.

[18] Hikita A, Kadono Y, Chikuda H, Fukuda A, Wakeyama H, Yasuda H, et al. Identification of an alternatively spliced variant of Ca2+-promoted Ras inactivator as a possible regulator of RANKL shedding. *J. Biol. Chem.* 2005 280: 41700-41706.

[19] Hikita A, Yana I, Wakeyama H, Nakamura M, Kadono Y, Oshima Y, et al. Negative regulation of osteoclastogenesis by ectodomain shedding of receptor activator of NF-kappaB ligand. *J. Biol. Chem.* 2006 281: 36846-36855.

[20] Lynch CC, Hikosaka A, Acuff HB, Martin MD, Kawai N, Singh RK, et al. MMP-7 promotes prostate cancer-induced osteolysis via the solubilization of RANKL. *Cancer Cell.* 2005 7: 485-496.

[21] Lacey DL, Timms E, Tan HL, Kelley MJ, Dunstan CR, Burgess T, et al. Osteoprotegerin ligand is a cytokine that regulates osteoclast differentiation and activation. *Cell.* 1998 93:165-176.

[22] Honore P, Luger NM, Sabino MA, Schwei MJ, Rogers SD, Mach DB, et al. Osteoprotegerin blocks bone cancer-induced skeletal destruction, skeletal pain and pain-related neurochemical reorganization of the spinal cord. *Nat. Med.* 2000 6: 521-528.

[23] Saftig P, Hunziker E, Wehmeyer O, Jones S, Boyde A, Rommerskirch W, et al. Impaired osteoclastic bone resorption leads to osteopetrosis in cathepsin-K-deficient mice. *Proc. Natl. Acad. Sci. U S A.* 1998 95: 13453-13458.

[24] Podgorski I, Linebaugh BE, Koblinski JE, Rudy DL, Herroon MK, Olive MB, et al. Bone marrow-derived cathepsin K cleaves SPARC in bone metastasis. *Am. J. Pathol.* 2009 175: 1255-1269.

[25] Le Gall C, Bellahcene A, Bonnelye E, Gasser JA, Castronovo V, Green J, et al. A cathepsin K inhibitor reduces breast cancer induced osteolysis and skeletal tumor burden. *Cancer Res.* 2007 67: 9894-9902.

[26] Ory S, Brazier H, Pawlak G, Blangy A. Rho GTPases in osteoclasts: orchestrators of podosome arrangement. *Eur. J. Cell Biol.* 2008 87: 469-477.

[27] Heckel T, Czupalla C, Expirto Santo AI, Anitei M, Arantzazu Sanchez-Fernandez M, Mosch K, et al. Src-dependent repression of ARF6 is required to maintain podosome-rich sealing zones in bone-digesting osteoclasts. *Proc. Natl. Acad. Sci. U S A.* 2009 106: 1451-1456.

[28] Nelson JB, Hedican SP, George DJ, Reddi AH, Piantadosi S, Eisenberger MA, et al. Identification of endothelin-1 in the pathophysiology of metastatic adenocarcinoma of the prostate. *Nat. Med.* 1995 1: 944-949.

[29] Yin JJ, Mohammad KS, Kakonen SM, Harris S, Wu-Wong JR, Wessale JL, et al. A causal role for endothelin-1 in the pathogenesis of osteoblastic bone metastases. *Proc. Natl. Acad. Sci. U S A.* 2003 100: 10954-10959.

[30] Drake JM, Danke JR, Henry MD. Bone-specific growth inhibition of prostate cancer metastasis by atrasentan. *Cancer Biol. Ther.* 2010 9: 607-614.

[31] Guise TA, Yin JJ, Mohammad KS. Role of endothelin-1 in osteoblastic bone metastases. *Cancer.* 2003 97: 779-784.

[32] Day TF, Guo X, Garrett-Beal L, Yang Y. Wnt/beta-catenin signaling in mesenchymal progenitors controls osteoblast and chondrocyte differentiation during vertebrate skeletogenesis. *Dev. Cell.* 2005 8: 739-750.

[33] Hill TP, Spater D, Taketo MM, Birchmeier W, Hartmann C. Canonical Wnt/beta-catenin signaling prevents osteoblasts from differentiating into chondrocytes. *Dev. Cell.* 2005 8: 727-738.

[34] Hall CL, Bafico A, Dai J, Aaronson SA, Keller ET. Prostate cancer cells promote osteoblastic bone metastases through Wnts. *Cancer Res.* 2005 65: 7554-7560.

[35] Dai J, Hall CL, Escara-Wilke J, Mizokami A, Keller JM, Keller ET. Prostate cancer induces bone metastasis through Wnt-induced bone morphogenetic protein-dependent and independent mechanisms. *Cancer Res.* 2008 68: 5785-5794.

[36] Schwaninger R, Rentsch CA, Wetterwald A, van der Horst G, van Bezooijen RL, van der Pluijm G, et al. Lack of noggin expression by cancer cells is a determinant of the osteoblast response in bone metastases. *Am. J. Pathol.* 2007 170: 160-175.

[37] Rabbani SA, Desjardins J, Bell AW, Banville D, Mazar A, Henkin J, et al. An amino-terminal fragment of urokinase isolated from a prostate cancer cell line (PC-3) is mitogenic for osteoblast-like cells. *Biochem. Biophys. Res. Commun.* 1990 Dec 31;173(3):1058-64.

[38] Rabbani SA, Gladu J, Mazar AP, Henkin J, Goltzman D. Induction in human osteoblastic cells (SaOS2) of the early response genes fos, jun, and myc by the amino terminal fragment (ATF) of urokinase. *J. Cell Physiol.* 1997 172: 137-145.

[39] Koutsilieris M, Sourla A, Pelletier G, Doillon CJ. Three-dimensional type I collagen gel system for the study of osteoblastic metastases produced by metastatic prostate cancer. *J. Bone Miner. Res.* 1994 9: 1823-1832.

[40] Mitsiades C, Sourla A, Doillon C, Lembessis P, Koutsilieris M. Three-dimensional type I collagen co-culture systems for the study of cell-cell interactions and treatment response in bone metastases. *J. Musculoskelet. Neuronal. Interact.* 2000 1: 153-155.

[41] Achbarou A, Kaiser S, Tremblay G, Ste-Marie LG, Brodt P, Goltzman D, et al. Urokinase overproduction results in increased skeletal metastasis by prostate cancer cells in vivo. *Cancer Res.* 1994 54: 2372-2377.

[42] Fritz V, Noel D, Bouquet C, Opolon P, Voide R, Apparailly F, et al. Antitumoral activity and osteogenic potential of mesenchymal stem cells expressing the urokinase-type plasminogen antagonist amino-terminal fragment in a murine model of osteolytic tumor. *Stem Cells.* 2008 26: 2981-2990.

[43] Saad F, Sternberg CN. Multidisciplinary management of bone complications in prostate cancer and optimizing outcomes of bisphosphonate therapy. *Nat. Clin. Pract. Urol.* 2007 4: S3-13.

[44] Drake MT, Clarke BL, Khosla S. Bisphosphonates: mechanism of action and role in clinical practice. *Mayo. Clin. Proc.* 2008 83: 1032-1045.

[45] Bauman G, Charette M, Reid R, Sathya J. Radiopharmaceuticals for the palliation of painful bone metastasis - a systemic review. *Radiother. Oncol.* 2005 75: 258-270.

[46] Tu SM, Millikan RE, Mengistu B, Delpassand ES, Amato RJ, Pagliaro LC, et al. Bone-targeted therapy for advanced androgen-independent carcinoma of the prostate: a randomised phase II trial. *Lancet.* 2001 357: 336-341.

[47] Collins C, Eary JF, Donaldson G, Vernon C, Bush NE, Petersdorf S, et al. Samarium-153-EDTMP in bone metastases of hormone refractory prostate carcinoma: a phase I/II trial. *J. Nucl. Med.* 1993 34: 1839-1844.

[48] Nilsson S, Parker C, Haugen I, Lokna A, Aksnes A, Bolstad B, et al. Radium-223 chloride, a first-in-class alpha-pharmaceutical with a benign safety profile for patients with castration-resistant prostate cancer (CRPC) and bone metastases: Combined analysis of phase I and II clinical trials. *ASCO Meeting Abstracts.* 2010; 28 (15): 4678.

[49] Morris MJ, Pandit-Taskar N, Carrasquillo J, Divgi CR, Slovin S, Kelly WK, et al. Phase I study of samarium-153 lexidronam with docetaxel in castration-resistant metastatic prostate cancer. *J. Clin. Oncol.* 2009 27: 2436-2442.

[50] Fizazi K, Beuzeboc P, Lumbroso J, Haddad V, Massard C, Gross-Goupil M, et al. Phase II trial of consolidation docetaxel and samarium-153 in patients with bone metastases from castration-resistant prostate cancer. *J. Clin. Oncol.* 2009 27: 2429-2435.

[51] Tu SM, Mathew P, Wong FC, Jones D, Johnson MM, Logothetis CJ. Phase I study of concurrent weekly docetaxel and repeated samarium-153 lexidronam in patients with castration-resistant metastatic prostate cancer. *J. Clin. Oncol.* 2009 27: 3319-3324.

[52] Stopeck AT, Lipton A, Body JJ, Steger GG, Tonkin K, de Boer RH, et al. Denosumab Compared With Zoledronic Acid for the Treatment of Bone Metastases in Patients With Advanced Breast Cancer: A Randomized, Double-Blind Study. *J. Clin. Oncol.* 2010 28 5132-5139.

[53] Fizazi K, Lipton A, Mariette X, Body JJ, Rahim Y, Gralow JR, et al. Randomized phase II trial of denosumab in patients with bone metastases from prostate cancer, breast cancer, or other neoplasms after intravenous bisphosphonates. *J. Clin. Oncol.* 2009 27: 1564-1571.

[54] Fizazi K, Bosserman L, Gao G, Skacel T, Markus R. Denosumab treatment of prostate cancer with bone metastases and increased urine N-telopeptide levels after therapy with intravenous bisphosphonates: results of a randomized phase II trial. *J. Urol.* 2009 182: 509-515.

[55] Body JJ, Lipton A, Gralow J, Steger GG, Gao G, Yeh H, et al. Effects of denosumab in patients with bone metastases with and without previous bisphosphonate exposure. *J. Bone Miner. Res.* 2010 25: 440-446.

[56] Jensen AB, Wynne C, Ramirez G, He W, Song Y, Berd Y, et al. The cathepsin K inhibitor odanacatib suppresses bone resorption in women with breast cancer and established bone metastases: results of a 4-week, double-blind, randomized, controlled trial. *Clin. Breast Cancer.* 2010 10: 452-458.

[57] Koreckij T, Nguyen H, Brown LG, Yu EY, Vessella RL, Corey E. Dasatinib inhibits the growth of prostate cancer in bone and provides additional protection from osteolysis. *Br. J. Cancer.* 2009 101: 263-268.

[58] Yang JC, Bai L, Yap S, Gao AC, Kung HJ, Evans CP. Effect of the specific Src family kinase inhibitor saracatinib on osteolytic lesions using the PC-3 bone model. *Mol. Cancer Ther.* 2010 9: 1629-1637.

[59] Rabbani SA, Valentino ML, Arakelian A, Ali S, Boschelli F. SKI-606 (Bosutinib) blocks prostate cancer invasion, growth, and metastasis in vitro and in vivo through regulation of genes involved in cancer growth and skeletal metastasis. *Mol. Cancer Ther.* 2010 9: 1147-1157.

[60] Carducci MA, Padley RJ, Breul J, Vogelzang NJ, Zonnenberg BA, Daliani DD, et al. Effect of endothelin-A receptor blockade with atrasentan on tumor progression in men with hormone-refractory prostate cancer: a randomized, phase II, placebo-controlled trial. *J. Clin. Oncol.* 2003 21: 679-689.

[61] Cella D, Petrylak DP, Fishman M, Teigland C, Young J, Mulani P. Role of quality of life in men with metastatic hormone-refractory prostate cancer: how does atrasentan influence quality of life? *Eur. Urol.* 2006 49: 781-789.

[62] Nelson JB, Nabulsi AA, Vogelzang NJ, Breul J, Zonnenberg BA, Daliani DD, et al. Suppression of prostate cancer induced bone remodeling by the endothelin receptor A antagonist atrasentan. *J. Urol.* 2003 169: 1143-1149.

[63] Carducci MA, Saad F, Abrahamsson PA, Dearnaley DP, Schulman CC, North SA, et al. A phase 3 randomized controlled trial of the efficacy and safety of atrasentan in men with metastatic hormone-refractory prostate cancer. *Cancer.* 2007 110: 1959-1966.

[64] Vogelzang NJ, Nelson JB, Schulman CC, Dearnaley DP, Saad F, Sleep DJ, et al. Meta-analysis of clinical trials of atrasentan 10 mg in metastatic hormone-refractory prostate cancer. *J. Clin. Oncol.* 2005 23 (16): 4563.

[65] Michaelson MD, Kaufman DS, Kantoff P, Oh WK, Smith MR. Randomized phase II study of atrasentan alone or in combination with zoledronic acid in men with metastatic prostate cancer. *Cancer.* 2006 107: 530-535.

[66] Russo A, Bronte G, Rizzo S, Fanale D, Di Gaudio F, Gebbia N, et al. Anti-endothelin drugs in solid tumors. *Expert Opin. Emerg. Drugs.* 2010 15: 27-40.

[67] James ND, Caty A, Payne H, Borre M, Zonnenberg BA, Beuzeboc P, et al. Final safety and efficacy analysis of the specific endothelin A receptor antagonist zibotentan (ZD4054) in patients with metastatic castration-resistant prostate cancer and bone metastases who were pain-free or mildly symptomatic for pain: a double-blind, placebo-controlled, randomized Phase II trial. *BJU Int.* 2010 106: 966-973.

[68] Ganapathy V, Ge R, Grazioli A, Xie W, Banach-Petrosky W, Kang Y, et al. Targeting the Transforming Growth Factor-beta pathway inhibits human basal-like breast cancer metastasis. *Mol. Cancer.* 2010 9: 122.

[69] Nam JS, Terabe M, Mamura M, Kang MJ, Chae H, Stuelten C, et al. An anti-transforming growth factor beta antibody suppresses metastasis via cooperative effects on multiple cell compartments. *Cancer Res.* 2008 68: 3835-3843.

[70] Hu Z, Zhang Z, Guise T, Seth P. Systemic delivery of an oncolytic adenovirus expressing soluble transforming growth factor-beta receptor II-Fc fusion protein can inhibit breast cancer bone metastasis in a mouse model. *Hum. Gene. Ther.* 2010 21: 1623-1629.

[71] Hu Z, Robbins JS, Pister A, Zafar MB, Zhang ZW, Gupta J, et al. A modified hTERT promoter-directed oncolytic adenovirus replication with concurrent inhibition of TGFbeta signaling for breast cancer therapy. *Cancer Gene. Ther.* 2010 17: 235-243.

[72] Mohammad KS, Javelaud D, Fournier PG, Niewolna M, McKenna CR, Peng XH, et al. TGF-beta-RI kinase inhibitor SD-208 reduces the development and progression of melanoma bone metastases. *Cancer Res.* 71: 175-184.

[73] Criswell TL, Dumont N, Barnett JV, Arteaga CL. Knockdown of the transforming growth factor-beta type III receptor impairs motility and invasion of metastatic cancer cells. *Cancer Res.* 2008 68: 7304-7312.

[74] Kogianni G, Walker MM, Waxman J, Sturge J. Endo180 expression with cofunctional partners MT1-MMP and uPAR-uPA is correlated with prostate cancer progression. *Eur. J. Cancer.* 2009 45: 685-693.

[75] Caley MP, Kogianni G, Adamarek A, Gronau JH, Rodriguez-Teja M, Fonseca AV, et al. TGFbeta1-Endo180-dependent collagen deposition is dysregulated at the tumour-stromal interface in bone metastasis. *J. Pathol.* 2012 226: 775-783.

[76] Zaidi M. Skeletal remodeling in health and disease. *Nat. Med.* 2007 13: 791-801.

[77] Garnero P, Borel O, Byrjalsen I, Ferreras M, Drake FH, McQueney MS, et al. The collagenolytic activity of cathepsin K is unique among mammalian proteinases. *J. Biol. Chem.* 1998 273: 32347-32352.

[78] Coxon FP, Taylor A. Vesicular trafficking in osteoclasts. *Semin. Cell Dev. Biol.* 2008 19: 424-433.

[79] Leblond CP. Synthesis and secretion of collagen by cells of connective tissue, bone, and dentin. *Anat. Rec.* 1989 224: 123-138.

[80] Rohde M, Mayer H. Exocytotic process as a novel model for mineralization by osteoblasts in vitro and in vivo determined by electron microscopic analysis. *Calcif. Tissue Int.* 2007 80: 323-336.

[81] Boyle WJ, Simonet WS, Lacey DL. Osteoclast differentiation and activation. *Nature.* 2003 423: 337-342.

[82] Cereceda LE, Flechon A, Droz JP. Management of vertebral metastases in prostate cancer: a retrospective analysis in 119 patients. *Clin. Prostate Cancer.* 2003 2: 34-40.

[83] Cheville JC, Tindall D, Boelter C, Jenkins R, Lohse CM, Pankratz VS, et al. Metastatic prostate carcinoma to bone: clinical and pathologic features associated with cancer-specific survival. *Cancer.* 2002 95: 1028-1036.

[84] Brown JE, Cook RJ, Major P, Lipton A, Saad F, Smith M, et al. Bone turnover markers as predictors of skeletal complications in prostate cancer, lung cancer, and other solid tumors. *J. Natl. Cancer Inst.* 2005 97: 59-69.

[85] Coleman RE, Major P, Lipton A, Brown JE, Lee KA, Smith M, et al. Predictive value of bone resorption and formation markers in cancer patients with bone metastases receiving the bisphosphonate zoledronic acid. *J. Clin. Oncol.* 2005 23: 4925-4935.

[86] Atley LM, Mort JS, Lalumiere M, Eyre DR. Proteolysis of human bone collagen by cathepsin K: characterization of the cleavage sites generating by cross-linked N-telopeptide neoepitope. *Bone.* 2000 26: 241-247.

[87] Brown JE, Sim S. Evolving role of bone biomarkers in castration-resistant prostate cancer. *Neoplasia* 2010 12: 685-696.

[88] Bellido T, Plotkin LI. Novel actions of bisphosphonates in bone: Preservation of osteoblast and osteocyte viability. *Bone.* 2010 49: 50-55.

[89] Roelofs AJ, Thompson K, Gordon S, Rogers MJ. Molecular mechanisms of action of bisphosphonates: current status. *Clin. Cancer Res.* 2006 20: 6222s-6230s.

[90] Roelofs AJ, Thompson K, Ebetino FH, Rogers MJ, Coxon FP. Bisphosphonates: molecular mechanisms of action and effects on bone cells, monocytes and macrophages. *Curr. Pharm. Des.* 2010 16: 2950-2960.

[91] Corey E, Brown LG, Quinn JE, Poot M, Roudier MP, Higano CS, et al. Zoledronic acid exhibits inhibitory effects on osteoblastic and osteolytic metastases of prostate cancer. *Clin. Cancer Res.* 2003 9: 295-306.

[92] Berry S, Waldron T, Winquist E, Lukka H. The use of bisphosphonates in men with hormone-refractory prostate cancer: a systematic review of randomized trials. *Can. J. Urol.* 2006 13: 3180-3188.

[93] Dearnaley DP, Mason MD, Parmar MK, Sanders K, Sydes MR. Adjuvant therapy with oral sodium clodronate in locally advanced and metastatic prostate cancer: long-term overall survival results from the MRC PR04 and PR05 randomised controlled trials. *Lancet Oncol.* 2009 10: 872-876.

[94] Saad F, Gleason DM, Murray R, Tchekmedyian S, Venner P, Lacombe L, et al. Long-term efficacy of zoledronic acid for the prevention of skeletal complications in patients with metastatic hormone-refractory prostate cancer. *J. Natl. Cancer Inst.* 2004 96: 879-882.

[95] Saad F, Gleason DM, Murray R, Tchekmedyian S, Venner P, Lacombe L, et al. A randomized, placebo-controlled trial of zoledronic acid in patients with hormone-refractory metastatic prostate carcinoma. *J. Natl. Cancer Inst.* 2002 94: 1458-1468.

[96] Sydes MR, Parmar MK, James ND, Clarke NW, Dearnaley DP, Mason MD, et al. Issues in applying multi-arm multi-stage methodology to a clinical trial in prostate cancer: the MRC STAMPEDE trial. *Trials.* 2009 10: 39.

[97] James ND, Sydes MR, Clarke NW, Mason MD, Dearnaley DP, Anderson J, et al. STAMPEDE: Systemic Therapy for Advancing or Metastatic Prostate Cancer - a multi-arm multi-stage randomised controlled trial. *Clin. Oncol.* (R Coll Radiol). 2008 20: 577-581.

[98] James ND, Sydes MR, Clarke NW, Mason MD, Dearnaley DP, Anderson J, et al. Systemic therapy for advancing or metastatic prostate cancer (STAMPEDE): a multi-arm, multistage randomized controlled trial. *BJU Int.* 2009 103: 464-469.

[99] James ND, Sydes MR, Mason MD, Clarke NW, Anderson J, Dearnaley DP, et al. Celecoxib plus hormone therapy versus hormone therapy alone for hormone-sensitive prostate cancer: first results from the STAMPEDE multiarm, multistage, randomised controlled trial. *Lancet Oncol.* 2012 13: 549-558.

[100] Ishizaka K, Machida T, Kobayashi S, Kanbe N, Kitahara S, Yoshida K. Preventive effect of risedronate on bone loss in men receiving androgen-deprivation therapy for prostate cancer. *Int. J. Urol.* 2007 14: 1071-1075.

[101] Izumi K, Mizokami A, Sugimoto K, Narimoto K, Miwa S, Maeda Y, et al. Risedronate recovers bone loss in patients with prostate cancer undergoing androgen-deprivation therapy. *Urology.* 2009 73: 1342-1346.

[102] Taxel P, Dowsett R, Richter L, Fall P, Klepinger A, Albertsen P. Risedronate prevents early bone loss and increased bone turnover in the first 6 months of luteinizing hormone-releasing hormone-agonist therapy for prostate cancer. *BJU Int.* 2010 106: 1473-1476.

[103] Greenspan SL, Nelson JB, Trump DL, Wagner JM, Miller ME, Perera S, et al. Skeletal health after continuation, withdrawal, or delay of alendronate in men with prostate cancer undergoing androgen-deprivation therapy. *J. Clin. Oncol.* 2008 26: 4426-4434.

[104] Brubaker KD, Vessella RL, True LD, Thomas R, Corey E. Cathepsin K mRNA and protein expression in prostate cancer progression. *J. Bone Miner. Res.* 2003 18: 222-230.

[105] Seals DF, Azucena EF, Jr., Pass I, Tesfay L, Gordon R, Woodrow M, et al. The adaptor protein Tks5/Fish is required for podosome formation and function, and for the protease-driven invasion of cancer cells. *Cancer Cell.* 2005 7: 155-165.

[106] Berdeaux RL, Diaz B, Kim L, Martin GS. Active Rho is localized to podosomes induced by oncogenic Src and is required for their assembly and function. *J. Cell Biol.* 2004 166: 317-323.

[107] Schramp M, Ying O, Kim TY, Martin GS. ERK5 promotes Src-induced podosome formation by limiting Rho activation. *J. Cell Biol.* 2008 181: 1195-1210.

[108] Mandal S, Johnson KR, Wheelock MJ. TGF-beta induces formation of F-actin cores and matrix degradation in human breast cancer cells via distinct signaling pathways. *Exp. Cell Res.* 2008 314: 3478-3493.

[109] Tu C, Ortega-Cava CF, Chen G, Fernandes ND, Cavallo-Medved D, Sloane BF, et al. Lysosomal cathepsin B participates in the podosome-mediated extracellular matrix

degradation and invasion via secreted lysosomes in v-Src fibroblasts. *Cancer Res.* 2008 68:
9147-9156.

[110] Peroni A, Zini A, Braga V, Colato C, Adami S, Girolomoni G. Drug-induced morphea: report of a case induced by halicatib and review of the literature. *J. Am. Acad. Dermatol.* 2008 59: 125-129.

[111] Bromme D, Lecaille F. Cathepsin K inhibitors for osteoporosis and potential off-target effects. *Expert Opin. Investig. Drugs.* 2009 18: 585-600.

[112] Fizazi K, Carducci M, Smith M, Damiao R, Brown J, Karsh L, et al. Denosumab versus zoledronic acid for treatment of bone metastases in men with castration-resistant prostate cancer: a randomised, double-blind study. *Lancet.* 2011 377: 813-822.

[113] Migliaccio A, Castoria G, Di Domenico M, de Falco A, Bilancio A, Lombardi M, et al. Steroid-induced androgen receptor-oestradiol receptor beta-Src complex triggers prostate cancer cell proliferation. *EMBO J.* 2000 19: 5406-5417.

[114] Slack JK, Adams RB, Rovin JD, Bissonette EA, Stoker CE, Parsons JT. Alterations in the focal adhesion kinase/Src signal transduction pathway correlate with increased migratory capacity of prostate carcinoma cells. *Oncogene.* 2001 20: 1152-1163.

[115] Asim M, Siddiqui IA, Hafeez BB, Baniahmad A, Mukhtar H. Src kinase potentiates androgen receptor transactivation function and invasion of androgen-independent prostate cancer C4-2 cells. *Oncogene.* 2008 27: 3596-3604.

[116] Xia W, Unger P, Miller L, Nelson J, Gelman IH. The Src-suppressed C kinase substrate, SSeCKS, is a potential metastasis inhibitor in prostate cancer. *Cancer Res.* 2001 61: 5644-5651.

[117] Marzia M, Sims NA, Voit S, Migliaccio S, Taranta A, Bernardini S, et al. Decreased c-Src expression enhances osteoblast differentiation and bone formation. *J. Cell Biol.* 2000 151: 311-320.

[118] Soriano P, Montgomery C, Geske R, Bradley A. Targeted disruption of the c-src proto-oncogene leads to osteopetrosis in mice. *Cell.* 1991 64: 693-702.

[119] Lee YC, Huang CF, Murshed M, Chu K, Araujo JC, Ye X, et al. Src family kinase/abl inhibitor dasatinib suppresses proliferation and enhances differentiation of osteoblasts. *Oncogene.* 2010 29: 3196-3207.

[120] Id Boufker H, Lagneaux L, Najar M, Piccart M, Ghanem G, Body JJ, et al. The Src inhibitor dasatinib accelerates the differentiation of human bone marrow-derived mesenchymal stromal cells into osteoblasts. *BMC Cancer.* 2010 10: 298.

[121] Yu EY, Miller K, Nelson J, Gleave M, Fizazi K, Moul JW, et al. Detection of previously unidentified metastatic disease as a leading cause of screening failure in a phase III trial of zibotentan versus placebo in patients with nonmetastatic, castration resistant prostate cancer. *J. Urol.* 2012 188:103-109.

[122] Nelson JB, Fizazi K, Miller K, Higano C, Moul JW, Akaza H, et al. Phase 3, randomized, placebo-controlled study of zibotentan (ZD4054) in patients with castration-resistant prostate cancer metastatic to bone. *Cancer.* 2012 118: 5709-5718.

[123] Jansen DR, Krijger GC, Kolar ZI, Zonnenberg BA, Zeevaart JR. Targeted Radiotherapy of Bone Malignancies. *Curr. Drug Discov. Technol.* 2010 7: 233-246.

[124] Radium-223 plus chemo shows clear OS benefit. *Oncology (Williston Park).* 2011 25: 1232-1234.

[125] Vengalil S, O'Sullivan J M, Parker CC. Use of radionuclides in metastatic prostate cancer: pain relief and beyond. *Current Opinion in Supportive and Palliative Care.* 2012 6: 310-315.

[126] Lam MG, Dahmane A, Stevens WH, van Rijk PP, de Klerk JM, Zonnenberg BA. Combined use of zoledronic acid and 153Sm-EDTMP in hormone-refractory prostate cancer patients with bone metastases. *Eur. J. Nucl. Med. Mol. Imaging.* 2008 35: 756-765.

[127] Waldert M, Klatte T, Remzi M, Sinzinger H, Kratzik C. Is (153)Samarium-ethylene-diamine-tetramethyl-phosphonate (EDTMP) bone uptake influenced by bisphosphonates in patients with castration-resistant prostate cancer? *World J. Urol.* 2012 30: 233-237.

[128] Lam MG, de Klerk JM, Zonnenberg BA. Treatment of painful bone metastases in hormone-refractory prostate cancer with zoledronic acid and samarium-153-ethylenediaminetetramethylphosphonic acid combined. *J. Palliat. Med.* 2009 12: 649-651.

[129] Lin J, Sinibaldi VJ, Carducci MA, Denmeade S, Song D, Deweese T, et al. Phase I trial with a combination of docetaxel and (153)Sm-lexidronam in patients with castration-resistant metastatic prostate cancer. *Urol. Oncol.* 2011 29: 670-675.

[130] Liu G, Vijayakumar S, Grumolato L, Arroyave R, Qiao H, Akiri G, et al. Canonical Wnts function as potent regulators of osteogenesis by human mesenchymal stem cells. *J. Cell Biol.* 2009 185: 67-75.

[131] Bennett CN, Ouyang H, Ma YL, Zeng Q, Gerin I, Sousa KM, et al. Wnt10b increases postnatal bone formation by enhancing osteoblast differentiation. *J. Bone Miner. Res.* 2007 22: 1924-1932.

[132] Morvan F, Boulukos K, Clement-Lacroix P, Roman Roman S, Suc-Royer I, Vayssiere B, et al. Deletion of a single allele of the Dkk1 gene leads to an increase in bone formation and bone mass. *J. Bone Miner. Res.* 2006 21: 934-945.

[133] ten Dijke P, Krause C, de Gorter DJ, Lowik CW, van Bezooijen RL. Osteocyte-derived sclerostin inhibits bone formation: its role in bone morphogenetic protein and Wnt signaling. *J. Bone Joint Surg. Am.* 2008 90 (Suppl 1): 31-35.

[134] Rentsch CA, Cecchini MG, Thalmann GN. Loss of inhibition over master pathways of bone mass regulation results in osteosclerotic bone metastases in prostate cancer. *Swiss Med. Wkly.* 2009 139: 220-225.

[135] Hall CL, Keller ET. The role of Wnts in bone metastases. *Cancer Metastasis Rev.* 2006 25: 551-558.

[136] Blobe GC, Schiemann WP, Lodish HF. Role of transforming growth factor beta in human disease. *N. Engl. J. Med.* 2000 342: 1350-1358.

[137] Gordon KJ, Blobe GC. Role of transforming growth factor-beta superfamily signaling pathways in human disease. *Biochim. Biophys. Acta.* 2008 1782: 197-228.

[138] Kang Y, Siegel PM, Shu W, Drobnjak M, Kakonen SM, Cordon-Cardo C, et al. A multigenic program mediating breast cancer metastasis to bone. *Cancer Cell.* 2003 3: 537-549.

[139] Kang Y, He W, Tulley S, Gupta GP, Serganova I, Chen CR, et al. Breast cancer bone metastasis mediated by the Smad tumor suppressor pathway. *Proc. Natl. Acad. Sci. U S A.* 2005 102: 13909-13914.

[140] Smith HW, Marshall CJ. Regulation of cell signalling by uPAR. *Nat. Rev. Mol. Cell Biol.* 2010 11: 23-36.

[141] Shariat SF, Roehrborn CG, McConnell JD, Park S, Alam N, Wheeler TM, et al. Association of the circulating levels of the urokinase system of plasminogen activation with the presence of prostate cancer and invasion, progression, and metastasis. *J. Clin. Oncol.* 2007 25: 349-355.

[142] Thomas C, Wiesner C, Melchior SW, Schmidt F, Gillitzer R, Thuroff JW, et al. Urokinase-plasminogen-activator receptor expression in disseminated tumour cells in the bone marrow and peripheral blood of patients with clinically localized prostate cancer. *BJU Int.* 2009 104: 29-34.

[143] Zengel P, Ramp D, Mack B, Zahler S, Berghaus A, Muehlenweg B, et al. Multimodal therapy for synergic inhibition of tumour cell invasion and tumour-induced angiogenesis. *BMC Cancer.* 2010 10: 92.

[144] Setyono-Han B, Sturzebecher J, Schmalix WA, Muehlenweg B, Sieuwerts AM, Timmermans M, et al. Suppression of rat breast cancer metastasis and reduction of primary tumour growth by the small synthetic urokinase inhibitor WX-UK1. *Thromb Haemost.* 2005 93: 779-786.

[145] Meyer JE, Brocks C, Graefe H, Mala C, Thans N, Burgle M, et al. The Oral Serine Protease Inhibitor WX-671 - First Experience in Patients with Advanced Head and Neck Carcinoma. *Breast Care (Basel).* 2008 3 (s2): 20-24.

[146] Schmitt M, Harbeck N, Brunner N, Janicke F, Meisner C, Muhlenweg B, et al. Cancer therapy trials employing level-of-evidence-1 disease forecast cancer biomarkers uPA and its inhibitor PAI-1. *Expert Review of Molecular Diagnostics.* 2011 11: 617-634.

[147] Sturge J, Wienke D, East L, Jones GE, Isacke CM. GPI-anchored uPAR requires Endo180 for rapid directional sensing during chemotaxis. *J. Cell Biol.* 2003 162: 789-794.

[148] Thomas EK, Nakamura M, Wienke D, Isacke CM, Pozzi A, Liang P. Endo180 binds to the C-terminal region of type I collagen. *J. Biol. Chem.* 2005 280: 22596-22605.

[149] Sturge J, Wienke D, Isacke CM. Endosomes generate localized Rho-ROCK-MLC2-based contractile signals via Endo180 to promote adhesion disassembly. *J. Cell Biol.* 2006 175: 337-347.

[150] Wu K, Yuan J, Lasky LA. Characterization of a novel member of the macrophage mannose receptor type C lectin family. *J. Biol. Chem.* 1996 271: 21323-21330.

[151] Fasquelle C, Sartelet A, Li W, Dive M, Tamma N, Michaux C, et al. Balancing selection of a frame-shift mutation in the MRC2 gene accounts for the outbreak of the Crooked Tail Syndrome in Belgian Blue Cattle. *PLoS Genet.* 2009 5: e1000666.

[152] Wagenaar-Miller RA, Engelholm LH, Gavard J, Yamada SS, Gutkind JS, Behrendt N, et al. Complementary roles of intracellular and pericellular collagen degradation pathways in vivo. *Mol. Cell Biol.* 2007 27: 6309-6322.

[153] Huijbers IJ, Iravani M, Popov S, Robertson D, Al-Sarraj S, Jones C, et al. A role for fibrillar collagen deposition and the collagen internalization receptor Endo180 in glioma invasion. *PLoS One.* 2010 5: e9808.

[154] Wienke D, Davies GC, Johnson DA, Sturge J, Lambros MB, Savage K, et al. The collagen receptor Endo180 (CD280) is expressed on basal-like breast tumor cells and promotes tumor growth in vivo. *Cancer Res.* 2007 67: 10230-10240.

[155] East L, McCarthy A, Wienke D, Sturge J, Ashworth A, Isacke CM. A targeted deletion in the endocytic receptor gene Endo180 results in a defect in collagen uptake. *EMBO Rep.* 2003 4: 710-716.

[156] Engelholm LH, List K, Netzel-Arnett S, Cukierman E, Mitola DJ, Aaronson H, et al. uPARAP/Endo180 is essential for cellular uptake of collagen and promotes fibroblast collagen adhesion. *J. Cell Biol.* 2003 160: 1009-1015.

[157] Wienke D, MacFadyen JR, Isacke CM. Identification and characterization of the endocytic transmembrane glycoprotein Endo180 as a novel collagen receptor. *Mol. Biol. Cell.* 2003 14: 3592-3604.

[158] Madsen DH, Ingvarsen S, Jurgensen HJ, Melander MC, Kjoller L, Moyer A, et al. The non-phagocytic route of collagen uptake: adistinct degradation pathway. *J. Biol. Chem.* 2011 286: 26996-27010.

[159] Howard MJ, Chambers MG, Mason RM, Isacke CM. Distribution of Endo180 receptor and ligand in developing articular cartilage. *Osteoarthritis Cartilage.* 2004 12: 74-82.

[160] Engelholm LH, Nielsen BS, Netzel-Arnett S, Solberg H, Chen XD, Lopez Garcia JM, et al. The urokinase plasminogen activator receptor-associated protein/endo180 is coexpressed with its interaction partners urokinase plasminogen activator receptor and matrix metalloprotease-13 during osteogenesis. *Lab. Invest.* 2001 81: 1403-1414.

[161] Reichert JC, Quent VM, Burke LJ, Stansfield SH, Clements JA, Hutmacher DW. Mineralized human primary osteoblast matrices as a model system to analyse interactions of prostate cancer cells with the bone microenvironment. *Biomaterials.* 2010 31: 7928-7936.

[162] Nemeth JA, Harb JF, Barroso U, Jr., He Z, Grignon DJ, Cher ML. Severe combined immunodeficient-hu model of human prostate cancer metastasis to human bone. *Cancer Res.* 1999 59: 1987-1993.

[163] Akech J, Wixted JJ, Bedard K, van der Deen M, Hussain S, Guise TA, et al. Runx2 association with progression of prostate cancer in patients: mechanisms mediating bone osteolysis and osteoblastic metastatic lesions. *Oncogene.* 2009 29: 811-821.

[164] Lee Y, Schwarz E, Davies M, Jo M, Gates J, Wu J, et al. Differences in the cytokine profiles associated with prostate cancer cell induced osteoblastic and osteolytic lesions in bone. *J. Orthopaed. Res.* 2003 21: 62-72.

[165] Coulson-Thomas VJ, Gesteira TF, Coulson-Thomas YM, Vicente CM, Tersariol ILS, Nader HB, et al. Fibroblast and prostate tumor cell cross-talk: Fibroblast differentiation, TGF-[beta], and extracellular matrix down-regulation. *Experimental Cell Research.* 2010 316: 3207-3226.

[166] Ye Q, Xing Q, Ren Y, Harmsen MC, Bank RA. Endo180 and MT1-MMP are involved in the phagocytosis of collagen scaffolds by macrophages and is regulated by interferon-gamma. *European Cells and Materials.* 2010 20: 197-209.

[167] Wang G, Haile S, Comuzzi B, Tien AH, Wang J, Yong TM, et al. Osteoblast-derived factors induce an expression signature that identifies prostate cancer metastasis and hormonal progression. *Cancer Res.* 2009 69 (8): 3433-3442.

In: Bone Tumors: Symptoms, Diagnosis and Treatment   ISBN: 978-1-62618-190-8
Editor: Moncef Berhouma   © 2013 Nova Science Publishers, Inc.

Chapter 10

SKULL-BASE METASTASES: CLINICAL FEATURES AND MANAGEMENT STRATEGIES

Julie Dubourg[1] and Mahmoud Messerer[2]

[1]Research and Education Unit of Medicine, Claude Bernard University Lyon 1, France
[2]Department of Clinical Neurosciences, Department of Neurosurgery,
Centre Hospitalier Universitaire Vaudois, Lausanne, Switzerland

ABSTRACT

Skull base metastasis (SBM) is a malignant bone tumor originating from distant malignancies occurring in approximately 4% of oncologic patients. The most frequent primary malignancies sources of dissemination are breast, lung, prostate cancers and lymphomas. The common pathophysiologic mechanism of dissemination is a haematogenous spreading from a systemic primary tumor resulting from the access of tumor emboli to the skull base (SB) through anastomotic vessels at the neural foramina or via Batson's venous plexus. Spreading can also arise from regional neoplasms or along perineural spaces. Skull base metastases may involve cranial nerves and craniobasal vascular structures but are frequently asymptomatic for prolonged periods until their growth induces pain and/or neurological deficit. Therefore SBM represent common findings in autopsy studies contrasting with very rare clinical reports. Symptoms are various but most of them can be gathered in five main syndromes with localizing value: orbital (anterior SB), jugular foramen (posterior SB), middle-fossa or gasserian ganglion (lateral middle SB), parasellar or cavernous sinus (medial middle SB), and occipital condyle (posterior SB) syndromes. Systematic imaging during the oncological assessment allows an earlier diagnosis. Computed Tomography – Scan with high resolution and bone windowing permits the detection of lytic bone lesions but the best diagnostic tool to detect SBM remains magnetic resonance imaging using T2 and T1-weighted sequences before and after injection of intravenous gadolinium. Survival of patients depends on the nature and dissemination of primary malignancy but also of characteristics of SBM itself. To our knowledge, there are no guidelines for the management of SBM. Based on limited available literature data, the first line strategy is radiotherapy that provides an excellent relief of pain and can offer symptoms regression. Others options include radiosurgery, chemotherapy or hormonal therapy, and surgery.

In this chapter, we highlight clinical and radiological features, and, summarize available evidence on current management strategies of SBM.

INTRODUCTION

The skull base (Figure 1) is formed of the ethmoid, sphenoid, occipital, paired frontal and paired parietal bones. It can be divided into 3 regions: the anterior, middle and posterior skull base.

The skull base is a common site of metastases and was first reported by Paget in 1889. Most of these metastases are clinically silent and are diagnosed incidentally on routine imaging for cancer staging or for another cause. SBM can also be diagnosed by typical symptoms described in five main clinical syndromes determined by the anatomic location of the metastases. SBM represent an important management challenge because of its rarity, deep location and proximity to critical neurovascular structures.

EPIDEMIOLOGY

The incidence of SBM is approximately 4% [1-3].

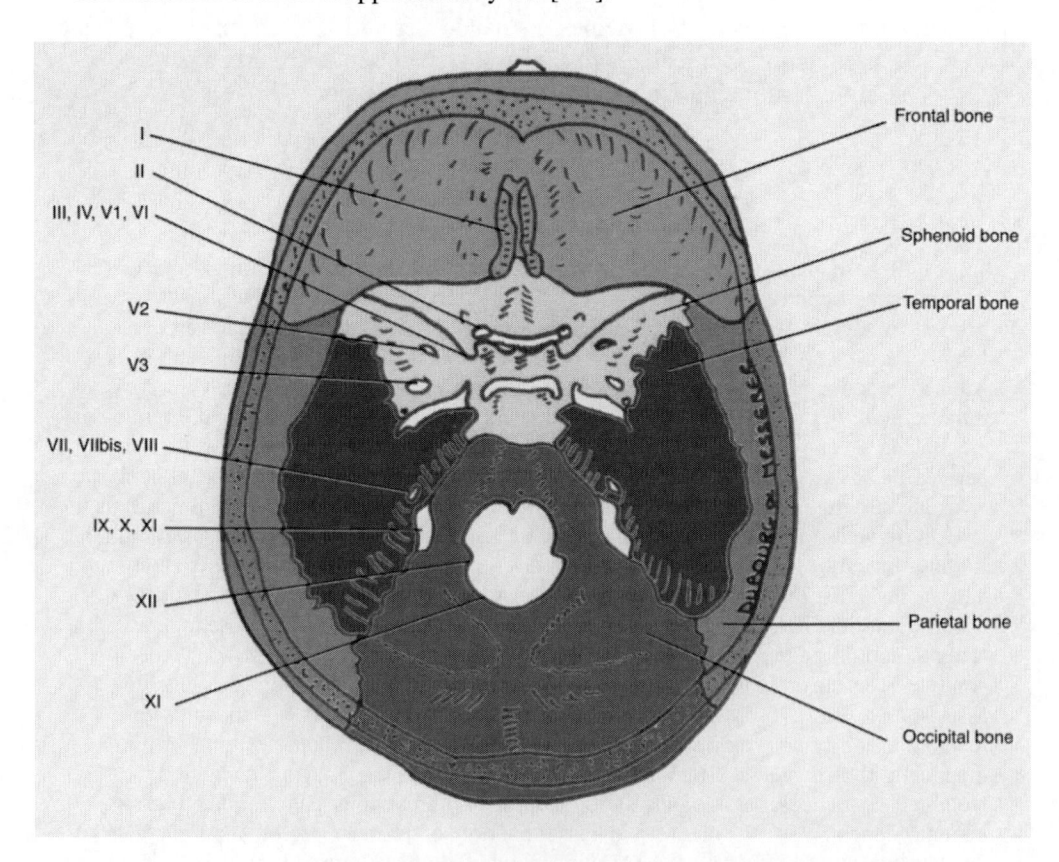

Figure 1. Illustration of skull base with its bony constitution and cranial nerves foramina.

The most common primary tumours engendering SBM are: breast (40%), lung (14%) and prostate (12%); knowing that breast cancer is the first cause of SBM in women whereas prostate cancer is the first cause in men [3]. Others potential primary cancer are: neuroblastoma, lymphoma, thyroid, renal, colorectal and melanoma.

Classically, at the stage of diagnosis of SBM, the primary localization is known however, sometimes, the diagnosis of SBM can be the first sign of cancer in 28% of cases [3] thus can be the revelation mode of the primary cancer [3].

PHYSIOPATHOLOGY

The most likely mechanism responsible for skull base metastases formation is a direct hematogeneous spread from a distant primary tumor [1]. Another mechanism is a retrograde spreading through the Batson's valveless venous plexus connecting, through the epidural and dural veins, the skull with pelvic structures [4]. Local invasion by cancer arising from adjacent structures (nasopharynx, external ear, salivary glands, paranasal sinuses) is also possible.

CLINICAL PRESENTATION

SBM are frequently asymptomatic and are discovered on a systematic imaging realized for staging primary cancer or for another brain check-up. When symptomatic, there are various potential symptoms depending on the location of the lesion.

Most of them can be gathered in five main syndromes with localizing value: orbital (anterior SB), jugular foramen (posterior SB), middle-fossa or Gasserian ganglion (lateral middle SB), parasellar or cavernous sinus (medial middle SB), and occipital condyle (posterior SB) syndromes. Clinical presentation of these syndromes is summarized in Table 1.

The jugular foramen syndrome occurs in around 3.5 % to 21 % of SBM [1, 3] and results from a metastatic involvement of the jugular foramen region in the posterior skull base.

The main structures of this region are represented by cranial nerves (IX, X, XI, XII), jugular vein and transverse sinus (Figure 2).

Clinical presentation depends on the metastatic involvement of the jugular foramen structures and is characterized by unilateral occipital or postauricular pain associated with hoarseness and dysphagia [5].

Others symptoms may be: glossopharyngeal neuralgia with syncope [1], Horner's syndrome, Collet-Sicard syndrome and others [6]. Clinical examination reveals cranial nerves palsy with amyotrophy, affecting: palate, vocal cord, sternocleidomastoid and upper part of the trapezius palsies. Papilledema may be noticed when there is jugular vein compression.

The occipital condyle syndrome occurs approximately in 21% of SBM [1] and results from a metastatic involvement of occipital condyle region that contains the cranial nerve XII (Figure 2).

Clinical presentation is typically a progressive and severe occipital pain associated with neck pain. At examination, there are an ipsilateral atrophy and paresis of the tongue due to the XII cranial nerve palsy, tenderness and a neck stiffness exacerbated by movements.

Table 1.

SYNDROME	LOCATION	ANATOMY	SYMPTOMS	EXAMINATION
JUGULAR FORAMEN	Posterior Skull Base	Cranial nerves (IX, X, XI, XII), jugular vein, transverse sinus	Occipital pain, dysphagia, hoarseness	Cranial nerve palsies, papilledema
OCCIPITAL CONDYLE	Posterior Skull Base	Cranial nerve XII	Occipital pain	Cranial nerve palsy (XII)
MIDDLE FOSSA (GASSERIAN GANGLION)	Middle Skull Base	Cranial nerves (III, IV, V, VI, VII)	Frontal pain, facial paresthesias, facial weakness	Sensory loss (V2, V3), Cranial nerve palsies (III, IV, VI, VII)
PARASELLAR (CAVERNOUS SINUS)	Middle Skull base	Cranial nerves (III, IV, V1, VI)	Frontal supraorbital headache, diplopia	Cranial nerves palsies (III, IV, VI), periorbital swelling
ORBITAL	Anterior Skull Base	Extraocular muscles, Cranial nerves (III, IV, V_1, VI)	Frontal headache, diploplia, blurred vision, decreased visual acuity	Ophtalmoplegia, proptosis, periorbital swelling and tenderness

This XII nerve palsy may be the only sign [7]. Others potential symptoms are dysarthria and dysphagia.

The middle fossa or Gasserian ganglion syndrome occurs in 6% to 35 % of SBM [1, 3] results from a metastatic involvement of the middle fossa region including the Gasserian ganglion and cranial nerves (III, IV, V, VI, VII) (Figure 2).

It is characterized by a progressively pain in the frontal region (cheek, jaw, forehead) associated with facial paresthesias, numbness in lower face and cheek region. Symptoms may also mick an idiopathic trigeminal neuralgia due to the involvement of cranial nerve V. Others symptoms can be: headaches, diplopia. At examination, physicians classically discovered a sensory loss in V2 and V3 cranial nerves territory and rarely in VI division territory. To be noted that this sensory loss may be a difficult diagnosis and may be required an electromyography. Others cranial nerve palsied can be noted: VII (facial weakness), VI (abducens), III, IV …

The parasellar or cavernous sinus syndrome occurs in 16% to 29 % of SBM [1, 3] and results from a metastatic involvement of the cavernous sinus region in the middle skull base. This region contains cranial nerves (III, IV, V1, VI) (Figure 2).

Typically, patients present with an unilateral progressive supraorbital headache associated with diplopia.

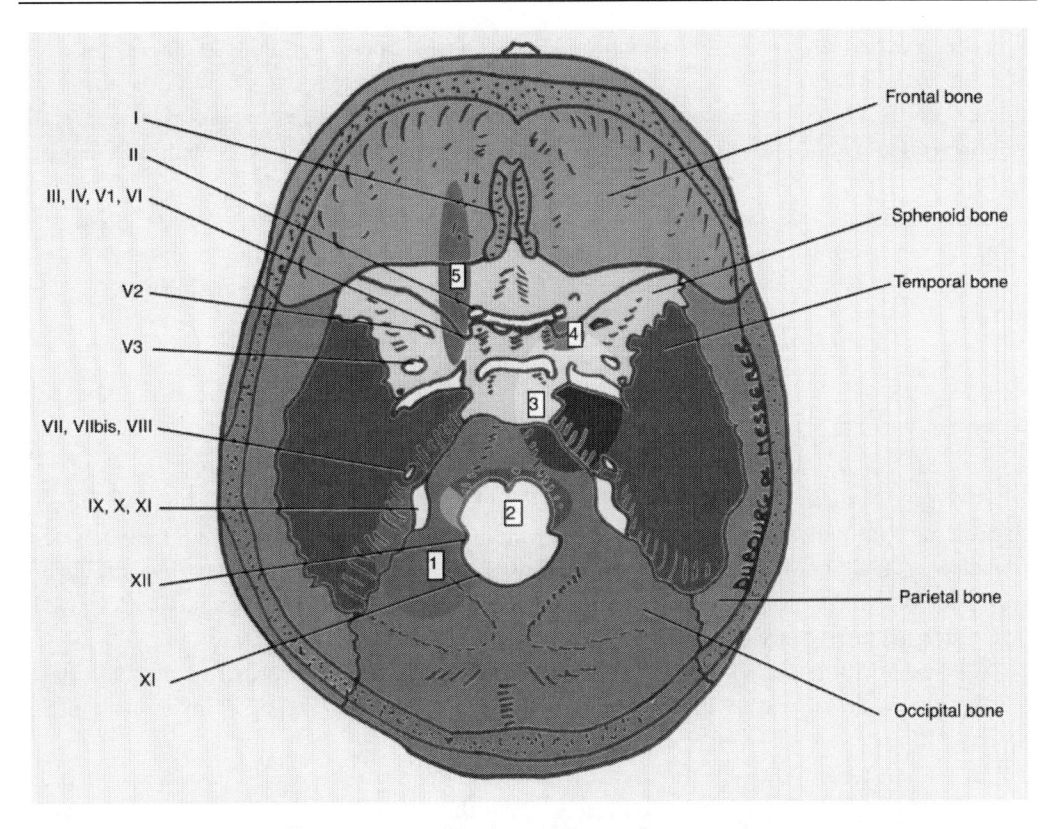

Figure 2. Main potential localization for SBM: 1: Jugular foramen region; 2: Occipital condyle region; 3: Middle fossa (or Gasserian ganglion region 4: Parasellar (or cavernous sinus) region; 5: Ocular region.

Others potential symptoms are: dysestesia in V1 division territory, facial numbness. At examination, there are nerve palsies (III, IV, VI) without proptosis, periorbital swelling, rarely opthalmoplegia.

The orbital syndrome occurs in 7% to 11.9% of SBM [1,8], is rarely isolated [9] and results of the metastatic involvement of the bony structure and adjacent structures in the anterior skull base. The main structures of the orbital region are extraocular muscles and cranial nerves (III,IV,V_1 and VI)(Figure 2).

The most common primary tumour at the origin of this metastases localization are: prostate carcinoma (56%), lymphoma (23%), and breast carcinoma (15%) [3].

Clinical presentation depends on the involvement of orbital region structures and is often characterized by persistent frontal headache associated with diploplia and/or numbness of the frontal region [1]. Others symptoms may be: blurred vision, decreased visual acuity. At clinical examination, patients usually presented with ophtalmoplegia, proptosis and, sometimes, sensory loss in the region of the ophthalmic segment of the trigeminal nerve [10]. The lesion may also be palpable during orbit examination.

Additional syndromes can be caused by other SBM locations, including the sellar syndrome, the temporal bone syndrome and symptoms due to the invasion of the nose and paranasal sinuses.

The *sellar syndrome* is often asymptomatic or cause diabetes insipidus in case of invasion of posterior pituitary. Sometimes, it also induces anterior hypopituitarism and/or visual loss. When there is a tumor extension in the cavernous sinus, these symptoms are associated with the parasellar syndrome. It is therefore possible to group these two syndrome entities together.

The temporal bone syndrome is characterized by a dysfunction of the Eustachian tube inducing serous otitis media. Symptoms are otalgia, periauricular swelling and cranial nerve palsy (VII). *The invasion of the nose and paranasal sinuses* often causes periorbital swelling and epistaxis.

IMAGING

The gold standard for the diagnostic of SBM is neuroimaging. The objectives are to characterize the lesion (vascularity, bone involvement location, invasion of adjacent structures: soft tissue, meninges) and Plain X rays may demonstrate bone erosion but have a very poor diagnostic accuracy. Computed Tomography (CT) scan and Magnetic Resonance (MR) imaging are more accurate to diagnose and to delineate such lesions.

CT scans with bone windows is able to detect lytic lesions or sclerosis of the skull base. In CT scans with soft tissue windows and contrast enhancement, it may delineate enhancing lesions within the bones.

In some patients, the diagnosis can be uncertain either because there is an atypical clinical and/or radiological feature or because the primary cancer is unknown.

PET scan is also useful in atypical lesion and as a systemic screening exam.

MANAGEMENT

First line treatment is obviously the symptomatic treatment including analgesic and steroids. This treatment may be the only treatment in case of palliative care when the prognosis of the cancer is very poor and the discovery of SBM is a late event in the course of the disease. However, sometimes the survival rate may be more important and in these cases, more aggressive treatments should be performed such as surgery, radiotherapy and/or chemotherapy.

Surgical therapy is not the first line of aggressive treatment but it can provide a good palliation. It is most often considered in patients with a single metastasis in an accessible location (sellar and parasellar regions) or in case of resistant to radiation primary cancer. Surgery may also be envisaged when patients present with a rapid neurological deterioration or chronic intractable pain and may potentially improve the quality of life of patients. Tumor debulking may also offer a good alternative thanks to decompression of vital structures such as optic nerve and chiasm. Finally surgery may also be the way to diagnose the primary cancer by achieving histopathological diagnosis. The main complications of surgery are cerebrospinal fluid leakage and infection.

Chemotherapy, immunotherapy and hormonal therapy are most often use in combination with radiotherapy because these therapies are generally ineffective when used as the only treatment modality.

Radiotherapy has emerged as the gold standard treatment of SBM. Some cancer diseases are particularly sensitive to radiotherapy and/or chemotherapy: breast, prostate and small cell lung cancer. However, others are relatively resistant: melanoma, sarcoma, renal cell carcinoma. The most frequently used is standard, fractionated, external beam radiotherapy [3]. This treatment modality seems to markedly improve the symptomatology of patients with partial or complete improvement of cranial nerve deficits in the majority of cases [1, 11]. However, the efficacy of radiotherapy decline with the delay in the management [12]. Stereotactic radiosurgery is a new treatment modality allowing delivering a very high dose of radiation to a small target while avoiding damage due to the surrounding healthy structures. These last decades, radiosurgery including Gamma-Knife and Linear accelatot-based techniques [13, 14] has been used to primary treat SBM or to treat its recurrence or residue. Tumor control rates vary from 65 % to 90 % [13, 15, 16]. The main limitation of this treatment modality is related to the size of the lesion. Complications reported are cranial neuropathy, trismus and cerebrospinal fluid leakage, which occur in 6 % to 12 % of cases [13-15].

CONCLUSION

Skull base metastases are rare but extremely severe indicating an active cancer disease. SBM is a disease where aggressive treatment is decided on a multidisciplinary debate. Surgery is often included in a palliative management but can provide an important improvement of quality of life. Radiotherapy remains the gold standard. Physicians should be familiar with the five main classical clinical presentations in order to early diagnose these lesions. Indeed the later the lesion is diagnose the poorest is the rate of improvement of extremely disabling symptoms.

REFERENCES

[1] Greenberg HS, Deck MD, Vikram B, Chu FC, Posner JB. Metastasis to the base of the skull: clinical findings in 43 patients. *Neurology.* 1981;31(5):530-7. Epub 1981/05/01.

[2] Stark AM, Eichmann T, Mehdorn HM. Skull metastases: clinical features, differential diagnosis, and review of the literature. *Surgical neurology.* 2003;60(3):219-25; discussion 25-6. Epub 2003/08/19.

[3] Laigle-Donadey F, Taillibert S, Martin-Duverneuil N, Hildebrand J, Delattre JY. Skull-base metastases. *Journal of neuro-oncology.* 2005; 75 (1): 63-9. Epub 2005/10/11.

[4] Castaldo JE, Bernat JL, Meier FA, Schned AR. Intracranial metastases due to prostatic carcinoma. *Cancer.* 1983; 52 (9):1739-47. Epub 1983/11/01.

[5] Dichiro G, Fisher RL, Nelson KB. The Jugular Foramen. *Journal of neurosurgery.* 1964; 21:447-60. Epub 1964/06/01.

[6]   Svien HJ, Baker HL, Rivers MH. Jugular Foramen Syndrome And Allied Syndromes. *Neurology*. 1963;13:797-809. Epub 1963/09/01.

[7]   Pavithran K, Doval DC, Hukku S, Jena A. Isolated hypoglossal nerve palsy due to skull base metastasis from breast cancer. *Australasian radiology*. 2001; 45 (4):534-5. Epub 2002/03/21.

[8]   Font RL, Ferry AP. Carcinoma metastatic to the eye and orbit III. A clinicopathologic study of 28 cases metastatic to the orbit. *Cancer*. 1976;38(3):1326-35. Epub 1976/09/01.

[9]   Boldt HC, Nerad JA. Orbital metastases from prostate carcinoma. *Archives of ophthalmology*. 1988;106(10):1403-8. Epub 1988/10/01.

[10]   Long MA, Husband JE. Features of unusual metastases from prostate cancer. *The British journal of radiology*. 1999;72(862):933-41. Epub 2000/02/16.

[11]   McDermott RS, Anderson PR, Greenberg RE, Milestone BN, Hudes GR. Cranial nerve deficits in patients with metastatic prostate carcinoma: clinical features and treatment outcomes. *Cancer*. 2004; 101 (7): 1639-43. Epub 2004/10/07.

[12]   Vikram B, Chu FC. Radiation therapy for metastases to the base of the skull. *Radiology*. 1979;130(2):465-8. Epub 1979/02/01.

[13]   Miller RC, Foote RL, Coffey RJ, Gorman DA, Earle JD, Schomberg PJ, et al. The role of stereotactic radiosurgery in the treatment of malignant skull base tumors. *International journal of radiation oncology, biology, physics*. 1997; 39 (5):977-81. Epub 1997/12/10.

[14]   Cmelak AJ, Cox RS, Adler JR, Fee WE, Jr., Goffinet DR. Radiosurgery for skull base malignancies and nasopharyngeal carcinoma. *International journal of radiation oncology, biology, physics*. 1997; 37 (5): 997-1003. Epub 1997/03/15.

[15]   Iwai Y, Yamanaka K. Gamma Knife radiosurgery for skull base metastasis and invasion. *Stereotactic and functional neurosurgery*. 1999; 72 Suppl 1:81-7. Epub 2000/02/22.

[16]   Kocher M, Voges J, Staar S, Treuer H, Sturm V, Mueller RP. Linear accelerator radiosurgery for recurrent malignant tumors of the skull base. *American journal of clinical oncology*. 1998; 21 (1): 18-22. Epub 1998/03/14.

ISBN: 978-1-62618-190-8
© 2013 Nova Science Publishers, Inc.

Chapter 11

PAINFUL BONEY METASTASES

Howard S. Smith *

Pain Management, Albany Medical College, Department of Anesthesiology,
Albany, NY, US

ABSTRACT

Carcinoma from breast, lung, and prostate cancers account for about 80% of secondary metastatic bone disease. Bone metastases may cause devastating clinical complications associated with dramatic reductions in quality of life, mobility, and independence as well as excruciating refractory pain. Treatments for painful osseous metastases may not only diminish pain, but may also improve quality of life and independence/mobility, and reduce skeletal morbidity, potential pathologic fractures, spinal cord compression, and other "skeletal-related events." Treatment strategies for painful osseous metastases include systemic analgesics, intrathecal analgesics, glucocorticoids, radiation (external beam radiation, radiopharmaceuticals), ablative techniques (radiofrequency ablation (RFA) and cryoablation), bisphosphonates, chemotherapeutic agents, inhibitors of RANK-RANKL interaction (e.g., denosumab), hormonal therapies, interventional techniques (e.g., kyphoplasty), and surgical approaches. Although the precise mechanisms underlying the development of bone metastases remain uncertain, there appears to be important bi-directional interactions between the tumor and the bone microenvironment. A greater understanding of the pathophysiology of painful osseous metastases may lead to improved and more selective targeted analgesic therapy. Additionally, potential future therapeutic approaches may lead to optimal outcomes with maximal pain relief and minimal adverse effects.

INTRODUCTION

World health experts estimated that in 2008 there were over12 million new cases of cancer diagnosed and 7.6 million deaths from cancer [1]. It has been reported that up to 75–

---

* Phone: 518-262-4461. Fax: 518-262-4462. E-mail: smithh@mail.amc.edu.

90% of patients with metastatic or advanced stage cancer will experience significant cancer-induced pain [2-5].

Approximately half or more of patients diagnosed with cancer may experience bone pain [6]. Bone is the third most common site of metastatic disease. Breast, lung, and prostate cancers are collectively responsible for about 80 percent of secondary metastatic bone disease [7]. Other common types of cancer, such as thyroid, lung, and renal cell carcinomas, also display significant osteotropism. Carinomas are more likely to metastasize to bone than sarcomas. The axial skeleton is seeded more than the appendicular skeleton, particularly due to the persistence of red bone marrow in the former. The ribs, pelvis and spine are generally involved early with distal bone involvement being infrequent. Batson's vertebral venous plexus permits malignant cells to enter the vertebral circulation without first passing through the lungs. Malignant cell survival with the development of spinal metastases may occur is common due to the sluggish blood flow in this plexus. In general, when a tumor grows in bone it may become more of a challenge to achieve a "cure" status, and it may cause devastating clinical complications, such as intractable severe pain, pathological fractures, spinal cord and nerve compression, hypercalcemia, and bone marrow aplasia, collectively referred as "skeletal-related events" (SRE) [7]. Not all patients with bone metastases have pain, but about 83% of patients with osseous metastases complain of pain at some point with wide variation in pattern and severity [8,9].

CIBP often results in hospice or hospital admission and is associated with reduced quality of life, increased psychological distress and decreased physical and social functioning [10-12]. With higher levels of disability, advanced illness and pain, comes an increased incidence of depression and anxiety [13].

CIBP does not exist as a single entity, but instead may be considered as a combination of background pain and breakthrough pain. Breakthrough pain (BTP) has been defined as 'a transitory exacerbation of pain experienced by the patient who has relatively stable and adequately controlled baseline pain' [14]. Breakthrough pain can be divided into spontaneous pain at rest and incident pain (either volitional or non-volitional) [15,16]. Breakthrough pain was present in 75% of cases of CIBP [9]. Patients with breakthrough pain had greater interference on aspects of life (mood, relationships, sleep, activity, walking ability, work, enjoyment of life) than those with no breakthrough pain (P <0.01). Almost half of breakthrough pain episodes were rapid in onset (<5 min) and short in duration (<15 min).

Forty-four per cent of patients with breakthrough pain had pain that was unpredictable [9]. These clinical characteristics make the successful treatment of CIBP challenging. This has been supported by other studies that have shown that up to 45% of patients with CIBP report poor pain control [17,18].

Payne and Janjan recommend specialized interdisciplinary cancer center bone metastasis clinics for patients with painful osseous metastases, if available. Payne and Janjan have published an algorithm for assessment and management of these patients [19,20].

Treatment strategies have employed various therapies for the treatment of painful osseous metastases including: bisphosphonates [21], chemotherapeutic agents---mitoxantrone (a chemotherapeutic agent that inhibits DNA synthesis) [22], hormonal therapy, interventional, and surgical approaches [23]. Additional agents may include systemic analgesics, steroids, radiation, (external beam radiation, radiopharmaceuticals), and ablation (radiofrequency ablation (RFA) and cryoablation), and intrathecal analgesics.

Metastatic bone disease is classified as osteolytic (e.g. breast) and osteblastic (e.g. prostate); however, usually lesions lie within a spectrum of these two entities (Figure 1).

As denoted by their names, osteolytic metastases, which are considerably more common, are characterized by significant bone disruption due to augmented osteoclastic activity; on the contrary, osteoblastic metastases are characterized by overproduction of osseous tissue by activated osteoblasts [24].

PATHOPHYSIOLOGY OF BONE METASTASES

In order for bone metastases to develop, cancer cells first have to metastasize to the bone marrow which is mainly composed of hematopoietic stem cells (HSCs) residing in two different biological structures known as osteoblastic and vascular niches [25].

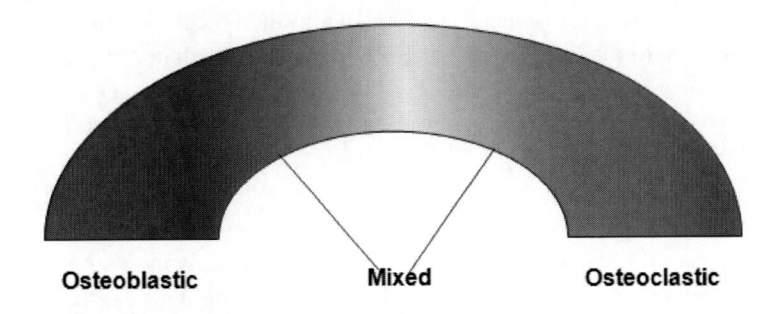

Osteoblastic   **Mixed**   **Osteoclastic**

Figure 1. The Spectrum of Metastatic Bone Disease.

Ommunications between osteoblasts as well as other tumor stromal cells and HSCs are mainly driven *via* chemoattractive factors such as the stromal-derived factor 1 (SDF-1) on stromal cells and its receptor CXCR4 on HSCs [26]. Communication between the tumor cells and bone marrow hematopoietic stem cells is vitally important in for the development of osseous metastases. A significant role in the interaction between cancer and bone is played by stromal-d factor 1 (SDF-1, also known as CXCL12) binding to CXCR4 with resultant CXCR4 signaling. The attachment/adherence of osteoclasts to bone/collagen is in large part due to $\alpha_v\beta_3$. This is facilitated by cathepsin K exposing the RGD sequence from collagen to $\alpha_v\beta_3$. Osteoclast activation appears to contribute to osteolytic lesions/erosions and pain. C-Src kinase activity is increased in response to integrin binding as well as RANKL/RANK interaction, and increased c-Src is involved in promoting osteoclast function/activation. The development of bone metastases is a multi-step process which includes the following sequence of events: (1.) tumor growth, detachment of cancer cells, and invasion of the tissue stroma; (2.) neoangiogenesis; (3.) escape from the tissue by intravasation; (4.) survival in the circulation; (5.) chemoattraction and arrest (docking and locking) in the bone marrow endothelial vessel wall; (6.) extravasation; and (7.) establishment of the metastatic microenvironment (osteoblastic metastasis) via the cross-talk between the cancer and bone cells [27-30].

PATHOPHYSIOLOGY OF BONE RESORPTION

Bone metastases may lead to pain via stimulation of nociceptors by algesic mediators (e.g., cytokines [Geis et al. demonstrated that evoked pain behavior and spinal glia activation is at least in part dependent on tumor necrosis factor receptor 1 and 2 in a mouse model of bone cancer [31].], prostaglandins, bradykinin, serotonin, substance P). Involvement or invasion, stretching, or compression of pain-sensitive structures such as nerves, vasculature, and periosteum and microfractures of various joint structures may also lead to pain. Pain from osseous metastic lesions may also occur from mechanical instability of "weakened bone" or high intra-osseous pressures (>50 mm Hg) [32]. Although numerous contributing factors lead to the pain of osseous metastases, a significant portion of the pain seems to be related to osteoclastic bone resorption. Osteoclasts solubilize the mineral (e.g., hydroxyapatite) and degrade the organic matrix (e.g., type 1 collagen) with cysteine-proteinases. The bone resorption occurs in an acidic microenvironment produced by proton secretion via vacuolar H^+ATPases in osteoclastic membranes. The first step in the process of bone resorption is that the osteoclast adheres to the bone surface. This adherence is mediated by specific membrane receptors. Podosomes are osteoclastic processes that become the primary attachment sites to bone. The podosomes are made up of integrins and cytoskeletal proteins: actin microfilaments surrounded by vinculin and talin [33].

The predominant attachment site is the vitronectin receptors (e.g. $\alpha v \beta_3$ integrin), which recognizes the RGD (Arg-Gly-Asp) amino acide sequence in various bone matrix proteins (osteopontin, vitronectin, bone sialoprotein) [33]. Integrin activation appears to result in Pyk2-dependent recruitment of c-Src to the plasma membrane and lead to c-Src activation and association with Pyk2 and subsequent c-Src-dependent phosphorylation of the nonreceptor isoform of tyrosine phosphatase epsilon (cyt-PTPe) at its C-terminal residue Y638, supports osteoclast adhesion and activation as well as proper structure, stability, and dynamics of podosomes [34]. A highly convoluted membrane area termed the *ruffled border* and *sealing zone* appears in the osteoclast during bone resorption. The accumulation of podosomes at the bone surface occurs first with ligand binding to the vitronectin receptor [33]. Subsequently, a tight sealing zone is formed where osteoclastic acid and proteases reorganize elements to form a "double circle" of vinculin and talin around a core of F-actin [33].

In order to effectively "digest" inorganic bone matrix components (e.g. hydroxyapatite) at least two major factors are needed: a) acid (e.g. HCl) and b) energy (e.g. ATP). The osteoclats generate H+ and Cl^- utilizing carbonic anhydrase II (CAII) that catalyzes conversion of carbon dioxide [CO2] and water [H2O] into carbonic acid [H2CO3], which in turn dissociates into hydrogen ion [H+] and bicarbonate [$HCO3^-$] [35, 36].

The $HCO3^-$ ions are then exchanged for Cl^- through the basolaterally located Anion Exchanger 2 (AE2) [37,38], providing the Cl^- ions required for acidification [HCl] occurring in the resorption lacuna (Figure 2).

Inside the sealing zone, bone resorption is induced by active secretion of protons to the bone surface through a specialized vacuolar type ATPase (V-ATPase) requiring ATP, containing the a3 subunit [39-42] and passive transport of chloride through the chloride channel [ClC-7], also to the bone surface [43-47] (Figure 2). Hydrochloric acid lowers the pH to approximately 4.5, leading to dissolution of the inorganic matrix of bone [48].

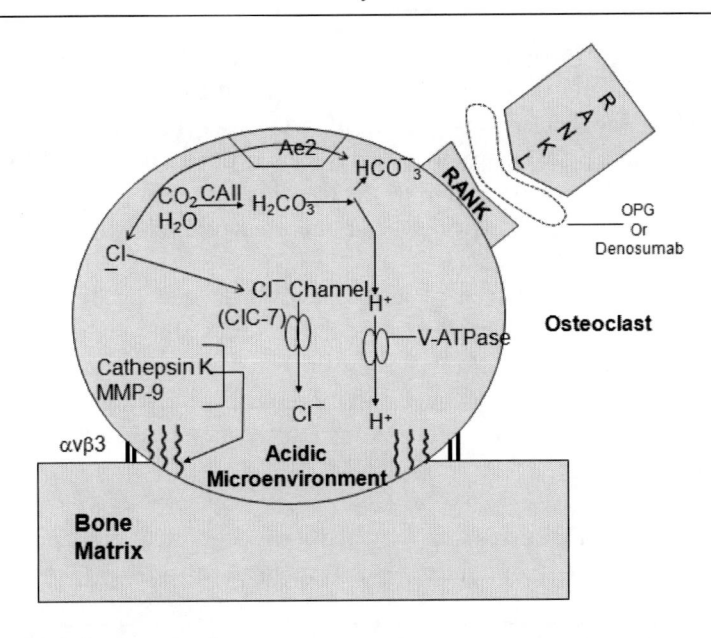

Figure 2. Osteoclastic bone resorption.

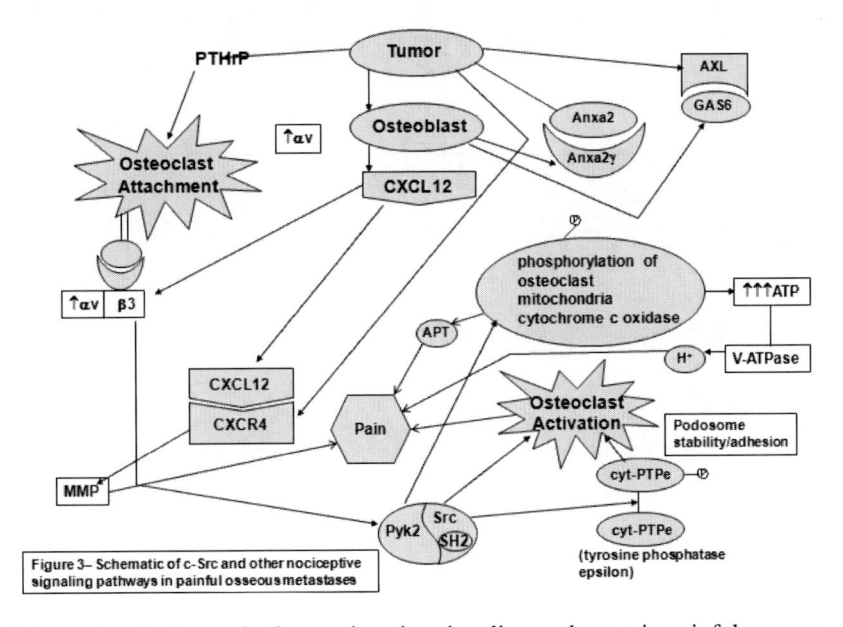

Figure 3. Schematic of c-Src and other nociceptive signaling pathways in painful osseous metastases.

Thus, involvement of vacuolar H^+-ATPase and carbonic anhydrase are crucial to "digesting" bone with subsequent creation of osteolytic lesions. c-Src may contribute to bone resorption, in part by: a.) preventing the inhibitory effects of calcitonin on osteoclast function and facilitating osteoclast activation, b.) enhancing the normal organization of the osteoclast actin cytoskeleton and contributing to the formation of the "ruffled border" [after c-Src is recruited to the plasma membrane, c.) facilitating podosome activities by promoting a shift from stable focal adhesions with actin stress fibers to more dynamic podosome assemblies, d.) by phosphorylating cytochrome c oxidase within the mitochondria, thereby increasing cytochrome c oxidase activity, and subsequently contributing to the generation of high levels of ATP required for bone resorbing actions of osteoclasts [49-51] (Figure 3). The ATP produced by c-Src-induced cytochrome c oxidase activity may be utilized by V-ATPase to provide energy for the proton pump to secrete hydrogen ions by the bone surface. Furthermore, the ATP generated may also contribute to nociception via binding to purinergic receptors (P2X2/3 and P2X3).

Cleavage of the type I collagen fibers is mainly mediated by the cysteine proteinase cathepsin K, which is active at low pH [52-55], and performs almost complete removal of the type I collagen fibers [56]. The MMPs are also involved in the degradation of the organic matrix of the bones; however, their precise role is remains uncertain (Figure 2). Targeting major processes involved in painful osseous metastases may lead to novel potential future therapeutic agents (Table 1).

Table 1. Major Processes that may be therapeutic targets for palliation of painful osseous metastases

Target	Process	Potential Therapy
CXCR4	Communication (between tumor and hematopoetic stem cell)	CXCR4 Antagonists
$\alpha v \beta 3$	Attachment (between osteoclast [$\alpha v \beta 3$] and bone/collagen {RGD]	$\alpha v \beta 3$ antagonists
Cathepsin K (exposes RGD)		Cathepsin K Inhibitors
RANKL-RANK interaction	Osteoclast Activation	Denosumab
Prenylation of Src		Bisphosphonates
Src		Src Inhibitors
Src	Src →ATP binding to: P2Y1R, P2X3R, P2X2/3R Energy ⇓ Nociception	Src Inhibitors
Vacuolar H⁺-ATPase	Bone Resorption - Acidic Microenvironment (proton secretion) - dissolution of Inorganic Matrix	Inhibitor of vacuolar H⁺-ATPase [V-ATPase] (e.g. bafilomycin A1) – subunit $\alpha 3$
Carbonic Anhydrase		Carbonic Anhydrase Inhibitors
CIC-7 (Chloride Channel)		Inhibitors of CIC-7 (Chloride Channel)
Ae2 (Anion Exchanger)		Inhibitors of Ae2 (anion exchanger)
Cathepsin K	Bone Resorption Proteolysis – removal of collagen fibers	Inhibitors of Cathepsin K
MMP-9		Inhibitors of MMP-9

NONPHARMACOLOGIC APPROACHES TO THE MANAGEMENT OF POM

Treatment strategies for painful osseous metastases include multiple nonpharmacologic approaches. These may include: physical medicine approaches, tai chi, yoga, stretching modalities, heat, cold, galvanic ultrasound, behavioral medicine approaches, cognitive behavioral therapy, mediation, hypnosis, relaxation techniques, guided imagery, and acupuncture. Bradt and colleagues performed a systematic review indicating that music interventions may have beneficial effects on anxiety, pain, mood, and QOL in people with cancer [57]. Jane and colleagues conducted a randomized clinical trial was to compare the efficacy of message therapy (MT) to a social attention control condition on pain intensity, mood status, muscle relaxation, and sleep quality in a sample (n=72) of Taiwanese cancer patients with bone metastases [58]. MT was shown to have beneficial within- or between-subjects effects on pain, mood, muscle relaxation, and sleep quality.

PHARMACOLOGIC APPROACHES TO THE MANAGEMENT OF POM

The "standard" or "traditional" pharmacologic approach to the treatment or palliation of painful osseous metastases follows the World Health Organization (WHO) analgesic stepladder guidelines approach to pain relief [59,60].

An international WHO Expert Committee on cancer pain, chaired by Dr. Kathleen Foley of Memorial Sloan-Kettering Cancer Center, was convened in 1982, and in 1986 the WHO monograph *Cancer Pain Relief was published* [61]. By 1993 it has been translated into 22 languages [61]. The WHO guidelines have been prospectively and cross-culturally validated and shown to work well clinically [61].

Zech et al. published the largest prospective trial of WHO guidelines to date and achieved favorable pain control in 76% of 2118 cancer patients who were treated over a 10-year interval [62].

Analgesic agents which may play a role in the WHO guidelines approach include: non-opioid analgesics [acetaminophen, traditional or nonselective nonsteroidal anti-inflammatory drugs (NSAIDs), cyclooxygenase-2 inhibitors], adjuvants [antidepressants, anticonvulsants, muscle relaxants, alpha-2 adrenergic agonists, n-methyl-d-aspartate (NMDA) receptor antagonists], and opioids/opioid-like analgesic agents.

ANTI-INFLAMMATORY AGENTS

NSAIDs appear to be particularly useful in patients with bone pain or pain related to inflammatory conditions and less useful in patients with neuropathic pain [63]. However, although clinicians regard anti-inflammatory agents as important drugs for the treatment of CIBP, this has largely been based on experience rather than a strong evidence base; and the use of traditional [nonselective (NS)] NSAIDs in CIBP has been questioned due to the lack of robust, clinical evidence [64]. Three randomized trials of NSAIDs in cancer pain did not separate out bone metastases, and six non-randomized trials mention bone metastases but did not record incident pain [65-72].

Eisenberg and colleagues performed a meta-analysis of the published randomized controlled trials to assess the efficacy and safety of nonsteroidal antiinflammatory drugs (NSAIDs) in the treatment of cancer pain by meta-analyses of the published randomized control trials (RCTs) [73]. Twenty-five studies met inclusion criteria for analysis. Of these, 13 tested a single-dose effect, nine multiple-dose effects, and three both single- and multiple-dose effects of 16 different NSAIDs in a total of 1,545 patients [73]. Better pain relief was obtained from NSAIDs than placebo in three scores (summed pain intensity difference [SPID], peal pain relief [PPAR], and total pain relief [TOPAR]) based on five or six studies, and in another score peak pain intensity difference [PPID] based on eight studies. Single doses of placebo produced a 15% to 36% rate of analgesia, whereas NSAIDs resulted roughly twice as much analgesia (31% to 60%).

All differences between NSAIDs and placebo comparisons were statistically significant [73]. Pain was related to bone metastases in seven studies. Four studies enrolled patients with either malignant bone pain, non-bone malignant pain, or both, but results were not reported separately for bone-related and non-bone-related pain in any study. Three studies [74-76] examined the analgesic efficacy of NSAIDs specifically for malignant bone pain, but not for other types of malignant pain. Analgesic efficacy data were extractable from only two of these studies, but were not combinable because one was a single-dose trial [76] and the other a multiple-dose trial [74]. The single-dose with ketoprofen study crossover reported a mean NSAID-induced PPID of 40% to 55% and SPID of 34% to 45%. The NSAID PPID in the multiple-dose study with naproxen 275 mg versus 550 mg was 23% to 33% [73].

McNicol and colleagues performed a Cochrane review and evaluated forty-two trials involving 3084 patients were included. Clinical heterogeneity of study methods and outcomes precluded meta-analyses and only supported a qualitative systematic review [77]. Sixteen studies lasted 1 week or longer and 11 evaluated a single doses [77,78].

They concluded that based upon limited data, NSAIDs appear to be more effective than placebo for cancer pain (7 out of 8 papers); clear evidence to support superior safety or efficacy of one NSAID over another is lacking; and trials of combinations of an NSAID with an opioid have disclosed either no difference (4 out of 14 papers), a statistically insignificant trend towards superiority (1 out of 14 papers), or at most a slight but statistically significant advantage (9 out of 14 papers), compared with either single entity. The short duration of studies undermines generalization of their findings on efficacy and safety of NSAIDs for cancer pain [77].

Cyclooxygenase (COX)-2 inhibitors may in theory be of greater therapeutic potential in well selected patients due to their anti-tumor/antiangiogenic properties [79,80]; especially in patients at high risk of gastrointestinal complications and those at risk of bleeding. Studies have shown in the sarcoma model of bone cancer pain that chronic inhibition of COX-2 activity with selective COX-2 inhibitors resulted in significant attenuation of bone cancer pain behaviors [both spontaneous and movement-evoked pain] as well as many of the neurochemical changes suggestive of both peripheral and central sensitization [81].

Microsomal prostaglandin E synthase-1 (mPGES-1) acts on COX-2 derived endoperoxide PGH_2 to catalyze its isomerization PGE_2. Thus, mPGES-1 inhibition may represent a therapeutic target to treating painful osseous metastases [82]. Lumiracoxib (Cyclooxygenase- 189; Prexige ®), is a highly selective COX-2 inhibitor which is not approved in the United States, Canada, Australia, England, and in some other countries due to hepatic related adverse events. Compared with diclofenac, lumiracoxib has substantially reduced affinity for COX-1, being 300-fold less potent.

The pKa of lumiracoxib is 4.3 and thus, lumiracoxib is predicted to be more effective in a low pH environment; which may potentially be beneficial for pain relief in sites of metastatic bone lesions, where the local environment is acidic in nature.

STEROIDS

Corticosteroids are commonly used for bone-related pain management which includes dexamethasone, methylprednisolone, and prednisone. Dexamethasone is often preferred orally because of its relatively high anti-inflammatory potency and low mineralcorticoid potency; therefore, dexamethasone has a lower risk of causing salt and water retention compared to equipotent doses of other corticosteroids. The mechanism of action of corticosteroid-induced analgesia is uncertain but may be related to decreasing tumor-related edema or inhibition of prostaglandin and leukotriene synthesis.

To date, only one study specifically addressed corticosteroid use for cancer-related bone pain. This study was a 14-day, randomized, double-blind, placebo-controlled, crossover study comparing 32 mg of oral methylprednisolone (MP) (16 mg twice daily) with placebo for symptoms in terminally ill cancer patients. After the initial 14 days, patients were continued on MP for a treatment period of 20 days.

Pain intensity was significantly lower after MP compared with baseline or placebo in the crossover phase; 68% of patients responded that their pain control was better with MP compared to placebo by the end of the treatment phase. Furthermore, the findings of this study suggest that MP exerts its action rapidly, and the chances of obtaining better responses after 5 days of treatment are poor [83].

ANTIEPILEPTIC DRUGS

Animal models of cancer pain have demonstrated that peripheral nerve destruction can take place in both skin [84] and bone [85]. Additionally, sensitization of unmyelinated primary afferent fibers and damage to small and medium sized sensory neurons may occur. Metastatic tumor cells and/or tumor stromal cells in bone appear to lead to sensory nerve injury as evidenced by changes that include: sprouting of sensory fibers into bone [86], increased expression of activating transcription factor-3 (ATF-3) in the nucleus of sensory neurons that innervate bone, as well as up-regulation of galanin and glial fibrillary acidic protein (GFAP) with hypertrophy of satellite cells surrounding ipsilateral dorsal roof ganglion (DRG) sensory neuron cell bodies and ipsilateral DRG macrophage infiltration [87].

Gabapentin and pregabalin are voltage-gated calcium channel blockers believed to exert their effects at the alpha-2-delta-1 subunit. It has been demonstrated in animal studies, that gabapentin reverses dorsal horn changes associated with POM resulting in relief of spontaneous and movement-related pain [88]. In a sarcoma model chronic treatment with gabapentin did not affect tumor growth, tumor-induced bone destruction or tumor –induced neurochemical reorganization in sensory neurons or spinal cord, but did attenuate both ongoing and movement-evoked bone cancer-related pain behaviors [85]. These changes suggest that there is likely a neuropathic component which exists in conjunction with nociceptive and inflammatory components in painful osseous metastases. Stimulated by favorable effects of gabapentin in animal models demonstrated modulation of continuous and stimulus-related bone pain [88,89] and by the observation that gabapentin is reported to be useful for the treatment of neuropathic cancer pain [90], and as a synergistic adjuvant to opioid analgesics; Caraceni and colleagues published an anecdotal report describing their treatment of six consecutive patients with incident pain caused by bone metastases with gabapentin not completely controlled by opioid medication [91].

The addition of gabapentin was associated with significant clinical improvement of pain at rest and incident pain exacerbated by movement, which was sustained for up to 3 months [91]. Clinical trials have been underway for assessing the effects of pregabalin on attenuating chronic bone pain related to metastases [92]. As far as therapeutic agents in the class of "anticonvulsants", it is conceivable that topiramate may be an antiepileptic drug which is particularly well-suited for the treatment of painful osseous metastases, since in addition to its multiple mechanisms of action, it also possesses actions as a carbonic anhydrase inhibitor. Topiramate is a calcium channel blocker, sodium channel blocker, glutamic acid inhibitor; GABA facilitator and may affect the NMDA receptor complex. Adequate hydration is recommended due to the potential formulation of calcium phosphate renal stones.

OPIOIDS

One of the major classes of agents for the pharmacologic management of POM is that of opioid analgesics. Preclinical research suggests that there may be varying efficacy for different opioids [93], however, clinically there does not appear to be any opioid that is better than any other opioid for the treatment of painful osseous metastases. Although some opioids may provide more analgesia than other opioids for a specific individual patient, currently, "trial and error" is the only way to determine this.

Opioids are considered an effective therapy for background pain in CIBP. However, their usefulness in breakthrough pain is less clear. It appears to be vitally important to match the characteristics of the opioid utilized to treat BTP; to the type of BTP experienced. Immediate release oral morphine has, at best, an onset of action of about 30 min [94]. This means that in patients with rapid-onset, short duration breakthrough pain, immediate release morphine will probably be ineffective. Furthermore, titration of opioids to doses that control episodes of breakthrough pain may result in unacceptable opioid side-effects [95]. Newer, rapid-onset opioids have been developed with the aim of mirroring the temporal features of breakthrough pain.

The author suggests a "triple opioid therapy (TOT) approach" to using opioid analgesics to treat painful osseous metastases. A triple opioid therapy approach utilizes three different opioid formulations (a controlled release opioid, an immediate release opioid, and a rapid onset opioid [ROO]). Enteral or transdermal extended release (ER) or controlled release (CR) opioids are employed for "maintenance" therapy to control the baseline or background constant pain.

The patient receiving TOT then evaluates breakthrough pain (BTP) episodes; a.) if a BTP episode seems relatively predictable and gradually intensifies over a half-hour or more [Gradual Onset Breakthrough Pain (GOBTP)] then it may be treated early with an immediate release (IR) opioid formulation, however, b.) if a BTP episode is unpredictable and/or the intensity suddenly increases rapidly [Rapid Onset Breakthrough Pain (ROBTP)], then it should be treated with a rapid-onset opioid (Figure 4).

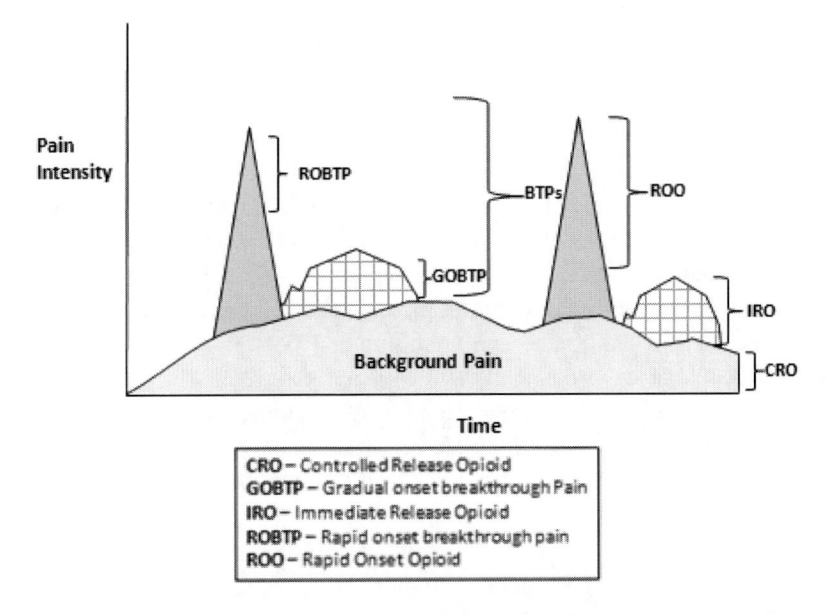

Figure 4. Two different types of breakthrough pain (BTPs) and their "matching" opioid treatment.

Rapid-onset opioids FDA approved in the United States include: oral transmucosal fentanyl citrate (OTFC) [Atiq®], fentanyl buccal tablet (FBT) [Fentora®], fentanyl buccal soluble film (FBSF) [Onsolis®], sublingual fentanyl (SLF) [Abstral®], and fentanyl pectin nasal spray (FPNS) [Lazanda®]. Potential future rapid-onset opioids may include: intranasal fentanyl spray (INFS) [Instanyl®] and fentanyl dry powder intrapulmonary inhaler [TAIFUN®].

BISPHOSPHONATES

Early-generation bisphosphonates (i.e., clodronate and etidronate) lack nitrogen and adhere to bone, where they are metabolized by osteoclasts. Metabolic products include cytotoxic ATP analogs that interfere with mitochondrial membrane potential and lead to osteoclast apoptosis [96,97]. Later generation, nitrogen-containing bisphosphonates (i.e., pamidronate, ibandronate and zoledronate) inhibit osteoclasts by a different mechanism. They are internalized – but not metabolized – by osteoclasts, where they subsequently inhibit an enzyme called farnesyl pyrophosphate (FPP) synthase. FPP synthase is required for producing intermediates (e.g. isoprenoid lipids) necessary for post-translational modification (prenylation) of several small GTPases, including Ras, Rho and Rac. These small GTPases are required for proper cellular vesicle transport, without which osteoclasts cannot form the tight sealing zones or ruffled borders at the bone surface that are required for resorption [96,97]. Additionally, nitrogen-contain bisphosphonates may lead to the accumulation of ispentyl pyrophosphate (IPP) which may be conjugated with adenosine monophosphate (AMP) to form an endogenous ATP analog triphosphoric acid 1-adenosin-5'-ylster 3-(3-methylbut 3-enyl) ester [ApppI] which may inhibit mitochondrial adenine nucleotide translocase (ANT) and cause osteoclast apoptosis [98]. In the United States bisphosphonates not used for osteoporosis include Zoledronic acid (indicated for a range of solid tumors, with osseous metastases--- breast, prostate, non-small cell lung, renal, and others), Pamidronate (included for breast cancer and multiple myeloma), ibandronate (indicated for breast cancer), and Clodronate (not approved in U.S.).

Multiple studies have demonstrated the efficacy of bisphosphonates in reducing skeletal complications and pain from bone metastases [99-102]. Intravenous zoledronic acid has demonstrated the broadest clinical activity [103]. Zoledronate (zoledronic acid) is the most potent of the nitrogen containing bisphosphonates, displaying superior efficacy in inhibiting FPP synthase activity, reducing bone resorption and relieving pain when compared with other bisphosphonates, such as clodronate and pamidronate [97, 104-107]. Zoledronic acid is the only bisphosphonate that has statistically shown significant reductions in skeletal morbidity, including bone pain, in patients with metastatic prostate cancer [108]. Fulfaro and colleagues demonstrated a relationship between a decrease in bone pain in 75% of patients and modification of C-telopeptide levels was identified in bone metastases from prostate cancer treated with zoledronic acid [109].

Zoledronate, in particular, has been reported to have direct antitumor properties in preclinical studies. It is capable of inducing tumor cell apoptosis [110], inhibiting cancer cell invasion [111] and limiting metastatic outgrowth in visceral tissues at extremely high doses [107]. Zoledronate treatment has been associated with a decline in circulating levels of the potent pro-angiogenic molecule, VEGF, in cancer patients [112]. Zoledronate -mediated reductions in VEGF levels were associated with increased time to a skeletal-related event, increased time to the progression of bone disease and longer time to the worsening of performance status [113]. Zoledronic acid distributes and bonds to osseous tissues and has a triphasic post-infusion decline process with a terminal half-life of 146 hours. Prior to therapy initiation of zoledronate, a dental evaluation and subsequent follow-up are needed in efforts to monitor for the occurrence and risk of osteonecrosis of the jaw.

Zoledronic acid can cause flu-like symptoms that are manageable with standard treatment. Renal monitoring is recommended due to association with iatrogenic renal function deterioration. Use of zoledronic acid should be avoided in patients with a Clcr of $\leq$ 30 ml/min and caution should be utilized when using coledronate in patients with other nephrotoxic agents. Dose reductions should be followed according to the package information sheet for patients with renal dysfunction.

HORMONAL APPROACHES TO THE MANAGEMENT OF POM

Only certain types of cancers (e.g. breast cancer, prostate cancer) may respond in some fashion to hormonal therapy. Intuitively, it would seem that any hormonal therapy which achieves antineoplastic results may also possess antinociceptive qualities under certain circumstances. An example of a cancer type which may respond to hormonal therapy is prostate cancer. Androgen deprivation therapy (ADT) is achievable with surgical castration (bilateral orchiectomy), or medical castration which may include agents such as: synthetic gonadotropin releasing hormone (GrRH) agonists (e.g. leuprolide, buserelin, goserelin, histrelin, [triptorelin-in phase II trials is a 60 month formulation triptorelin embonate that is under development]), cytochrome P450 enzyme 17A1 (CYP17A1) inhibitors [inhibition of androgen synthesis] (e.g. nonselective CYP17A1 inhibitors) ketoconazole, [aromatase inhibitors] aminoglutethimide], selective CYP17A1 inhibitors [abiraterone acetate – in phase III clinical trials, TOK-001 and TAK-700 in phase I/II trials], androgen receptor antagonists (e.g. bicalutamide, nilutamide, flutamide, and [MDV 31000 – in phase III clinical trials, BMS-641988 in phase I clinical trials]), inhibitors of 5α-reduction [which converts testosterone to the more potent dihydrotestosterone (DHT)] (e.g. finasteride, dustasterude).

Androgen-deprivation therapy (ADT) has become a vital component of treatment for certain types of cancer (e.g. advanced prostate cancer). Gonadotropin-releasing hormone (GnRH) agonists override the normal pulsatile control of the pituitary by providing continuous stimulation with resultant down regulation of pituitary GnRH receptors with consequent reduction of luteninizing hotrmone (LH) and follicle-stimulation hormone (FSH) production and testosterone suppression. However, before this occurs, there tends to be a transient increase in LH, FSH and testosterone. GnRH antagonists (e.g. degarelix and abarelic) bind directly to pituitary GnRH receptors blocking the effects of GnRH on the pituitary with immediate suppression of LH, FSH, and testosterone.

RADIOTHERAPY

External beam RT for osseous metastases may lead to improved analgesia, elimination or reduction of analgesic usage, functional improvement, such as increased ambulation, and reduction in the risk of fracture in weight-bearing bones. Large multiinstitutional randomized trials conducted by the Radiation Therapy Oncology Group have demonstrated that 80% of patients receiving RT for osseous metastases will experience complete to partial pain relief, typically within 10-14 days of the initiation therapy [114]. A correlation was also found between the incidence of pain relief and the site of bone metastases, in that a lower response was shown in limb localizations [115]. Dennis and colleagues found that patients suffering from painful bone metastases with an estimated survival of 3 months should still be considered for palliative radiotherapy [116].

Approximately 80% of patients may be successfully treated with sequential whole-skeleton radiation, in which 6-8 Gy is administered as a single fraction to either the upper and lower part of the body, followed by a second dose of 6-8 Gy, given 4-6 weeks later, to the remainder of the body [117]. Most prospective randomized trials evaluating differences in the outcomes have shown that single fraction regimens (mostly 8 Gy) are at least equal in analgesic efficacy to the various fractionated regimens [118]. These results have been confirmed in three meta- analyses [119-121]. Wu et al. [119] included eight randomized trials (3,260 patients) in a meta-analysis, comparing 1×8 Gy single fraction radiotherapy with various multi-fraction regimens and found that all multi-fraction regimens were essentially equal to single fraction therapy.

Similar results have been observed in the meta-analysis of Sze et al. [120], which included 3,621 patients from 12 randomized trials. The complete response rates were 34% (508/1,476) after single-fraction radiotherapy and 32% (475/1,473) after multi fraction radiotherapy (Odds ratio [OR] 1.10; 95% CI 0.94-1.30, P>0.05).

Overall response rates were 60% (1,080/1,814) and 59% (1,060/1,807), respectively (OR 1.03; 95% CI 0.90-1.19; P<0.05) [120, 122]. Chow and colleagues included 5,000 patients from 16 randomized trials in their meta-analysis [121].

The overall response rates (intention-to-treat analysis) were 58% (1,468/2,513) after single-fraction radiotherapy (mostly 1×8 Gy) and 59% (1,466/2,487) after multi-fraction radiotherapy (mostly 5×4 Gy or 10×3 Gy) (OR 0.99; 95% CI 0.95–1,03; P = 0.60) [121,122].

Nomiya and colleagues analyzed the time course of pain relief by radiotherapy for cancer pain [123]. Complete pain relief was obtained in 45/91 (49%) cases, and partial (> or =50%) pain relief was obtained in 83/91 (91%) cases. The mean time to obtain 50% pain relief was 13 days. The mean time to obtain complete pain relief (n=45) was 24 days [123].

Huisman and colleagues performed a systematic review in which 10 of 707 articles were selected for inclusion and seven entered a meta-analysis [124]. Overall, the study quality was mediocre. Of the 2,694 patients initially treated for metastatic bone pain, 527 (20%) patients underwent reirradiation. Overall, a pain response after reirradiation was achieved in 58% of patients (pooled overall response rate 0.58, 95% confidence interval = 0.49-0.67) [124].Reirradiation of painful bone metastases was found to be effective in terms of pain relief for a small majority of patients; approximately 40% of patients do not benefit from reirradiation [124].

Table 2. Treatment Guidelines

Complete history and physical (with thorough neurological exam)
Review bone scan; check for increased uptake (hot spots) at painful areas
Complete blood counts
Perform renal studies (minimal BUN/creatinine)
Acquire informed consent
Hydrate patient
Double-check that patient is suitable candidate for therapy
Complete blood counts every other week after injection for three months or recovery to baseline counts (generally, the usual hematological response is a 20-30 percent decrease in platelet count with a nadir in about five to six weeks and recovery by 12 weeks)
Maintain a close patient follow-up post injection
Change an aspirin products (including traditional NSAIDs) to COX-two selective inhibitors (e.g., celecoxib, refecoxib)
Have the patient keep a diary post injection with daily entries including evening temperature, 0-10 pain score (NRS-11), and side effects nausea, etc.)

RADIOPHARMACEUTICALS

Radiopharmaceuticals provide several advantages over conventional external beam radiotherapy: 1) they can be administered intravenously, 2) they can treat multiple, diffuse sites with mild bone marrow depression, and 3) they cause fewer adverse side-effects such as nausea, vomiting, diarrhea, and tissue damage [23].

Radiopharmaceuticals are relatively easy to administer but should be performed by clinicians appropriately trained in nuclear medicine. Although the preparation and steps for each patient surrounding radiopharmaceutical administration is different and should be individualized; certain common treatment guidelines exist (Table 2).

Absolute contraindications for using radiopharmaceuticals include pregnancy and patient refusal. Relative contraindications require careful consideration of risks versus potential benefits within the context of the patients' wishes (Table 3) [23]. Multiple radiopharmaceuticals exist which may provide analgesia from painful osseous metastases, some agents have appropriate energies to be imaged as well (Table 4).

Table 3. Contraindication for treatment of painful osseous metastases with radiopharmaceuticals

White blood cell count < 2.500
Platelet count < 60,000 (stable)
Recent rapid fall in platelet count (even if over 60,000)
Disseminated intravascular coagulopathy
Myelosupression chemotherapy within one month
Hemibody radiotherapy within two months
Extensive soft-tissue metastases
Pregnancy
Patient refusal
Inability of patient to follow radiation safety precautions
Impending spinal cord compression or pathological fracture
Estimated survival time < 2 months
Karnofsky performance < 50
Significant renal insufficiancy

Table 4. Characteristics of Radiopharmaceutical for the Treatment of POM

Radiopharmaceutical	Half-life (days)	Beta Energy MeV (Max)	Gamma Energy KeV	Usual Dose
Phosphorous- 32 phosphate	14.3	1.7	0	5-10 mCi
Strontium - 89 chloride	50.5	1.5	Essentially none	4 mCi
Samarium – 153 lexidroam	1.9	0.8	103	1 mCi/kg
Rhenium – 186 Hydroxyethylidene diphosphate*	3.8	101	137	35 mCi

* Not approved in U.S.

Figuls and colleagues updated a Cochrane Review to determine efficacy and safety of radioisotopes in patients with painful bone metastases. Their update includes 15 studies (1146 analyzed participants): four (325 participants) already included and 11 new (821 participants). They found a small benefit of radioisotopes for complete relief (risk ratio (RR) 2.10, 95% CI 1.32 to 3.35; Number needed to treat to benefit (NNT) = 5) and complete/partial relief (RR 1.72, 95% CI 1.13 to 2.63; NNT = 4) in the short and medium term (eight studies, 499 participants). Leucocytopenia and thrombocytopenia are secondary effects significantly associated with the administration of radioisotopes (RR 5.03; 95% CI 1.35 to 18.70; Number needed to treat to harm (NNH) = 13). Pain flares were not higher in the radioisotopes group (RR 0.74; 95% CI 0.27 to 2.06) [125].

Strontium-89 Chloride

Strontium is a divalent cation, like calcium, and is incorporated into hydroxyapatite in the bone after intravenous injection and is a bone specific radiosotope. Sr-89-chloride (Metastron; GE Healthcare Global, Bucks, UK) was the first FDA-approved radiopharmaceutical for bone pain palliation [126].

Pain relief usually begins within two weeks of treatment, with maximum benefit by six weeks, and lasts between four and 15 months [127,128]. Mild thrombocytopenia or leukopenia may occur in up to 80 percent of patients [127,128]. Platelets decline about 15-30 percent below pretreatment levels and usually completely recover in two to three months, enabling repeat treatment at that time [127,128]. Occasionally, recovery of platelet count to baseline may take about six month [127,128]. In addition, 15- 20 percent reductions in WBCs have also been recorded following 89Sr administration [127]. A transient flushing sensation immediately after rapid 89Sr injection has been noted and is self limited. Bone pain may transiently increase in some patients ($\leq$ 20% reported).

A recent systematic review of the available literature published by Finlay et al. showed a percentage of complete responders to Sr-89 ranging from 8% to 77%, with a mean value of 32%, and no responders ranging from 14% to 52% (mean, 25%). In general, 44% of patients had some degree of response to Sr-89 treatment, giving a mean overall response of 76%) [129].

Samarium-153 Lexidronam

Samarium-153 lexidronam (153Sm- EDTMP) was originally described by William Goeckler PhD in 1984, and it was approved by the Federal Drug Administration (FDA) on March 28, 1987 for relief of pain in patients with osteoblastic bone metastases [130,131]. 153Sm-EDTMP is a stable complex of radioactive samarium-153 and ethylene diamine tetramethylene phosphonic acid (EDTMP) [132-135]. Sartor and colleagues reported the safety and efficacy of repeated doses of Sm-153 in patients with metastatic bone pain [136]. Significant decreases in pain scores (P < 0.002) were observed at week 4 after each of the first 3 doses and maintained at week 8 after the first 2 doses (P < 0.003) but not after the third dose. Decreases in pain scores were observed in 70%, 63%, and 80% of patients, respectively, at week 4 after the first 3 administrations.

INTERVENTIONAL APPROACHES TO THE MANAGEMENT OF POM

Ablation

Patients Selection for Ablation

Patients may be offered focal ablative therapy (radiofrequency ablation [RFA] [137] or cryoablation) for painful metastases when 3 factors are present. First, a patient reports moderate or severe pain, typically ≥ 4 of 10 for worst pain in a 24-hour period. Second, a patient's local pain is limited to 1 or 2 sites and the patient's pain is associated with a corresponding abnormality evident with cross-sectional imaging. Third, treatment of the patient's painful metastatic lesion must be amenable to the use of ablative devices. Lesions that amenable to ablative therapy are typically osteolytic or mixed osteolytic/osteoblastic in nature or otherwise composed of soft tissue [138]. Exclusion of patients from focal ablative therapy usually occurs when one or more of the following situations are present. First, if a successful treatment requires the treatment of a portion of the lesion located within 1 cm of the spinal cord, major motor nerve, brain, artery of Adamkiewicz, bowel, or bladder [138]. Di Staso et al. suggest that radiofrequency ablation (RFA) followed by radiotherapy (RT) (RFA-RT) is safe and more effective than RT alone [139]. While cryoblation may effectively treat intact or sclerotic bone, RFA energy is poorly delivered into sclerotic or otherwise intact bone [140]. Cryoablation may have several other unique advantages over RFA for treatment of pain due to metastatic disease. Importantly, the zone of ablation is readily monitored with intermittent CT or MR imaging. The ice ball that is generated appears as a low attenuation region with a well-defined margin with CT and with various pulse sequences with MR imaging [138]. Cryoablation also allows the simultaneous use of multiple cryoprobes, which allows complete ablation of large lesions (up to approximately 8-cm diameter) in a single session. This approach avoids leaving residual neoplasm between the separate cryoprobes that is possible between sequential single overlapping ablations [138,141]. Furthermore, cryoblation may treat larger lesions than RFA, since the site of the ice ball generated is generally larger than the tip of the radiofrequency probe.

VERTEBRAL AUGMENTATION PROCEDURES

The incidence of spinal metastases and vertebral compression fractures continues to rise, with associated axial pain, progressive radiculomyelopathy, and mechanical instability. Vertebral augmentation procedures such as percutaneous vertebroplasty and percutaneous kyphoplasty can provide relief in patients with pathologic vertebral body compression fractures that do not cause neurological deficits but severely compromise quality of life largely because of intractable pain, but also due to loss of independence, mobility, and function often with resulting isolation/loneliness [142].

Vertebroplasty

Percutaneous vertebroplasty, first described in 1987, is a radiologically guided procedure in which percutaneous injection of polymethylmethacrylate, a surgical bone cement, is injected into a vertebra under imaging guidance [143]. Lee and colleagues reported on 19 percutaneous vertebroplasty procedures performed mainly in breast, prostate, lung and renal cancers [144]. Of these 19 cases, 10 patients (53%) were treated for solitary lesions, 3 (16%) were injected at two levels and the remaining 6 cases (31%) underwent cement injection at three levels. The majority of individuals (84%) reported short- and long-term symptomatic improvements [144]. Saliou et al. evaluated a total of 74 vertebrae in 51 patients, (22 women and 29 men) with a mean age of 62.5 years with malignant fractures of the spine with epidural involvements [145]. They concluded that percutaneous vertebroplasty provided effective analgesia in patients experiencing pain related to malignant spinal tumors with epidural extension, and was associated with a relatively low complication rate [145].

Kyphoplasty

Kyphoplasty has evolved from vertebroplasty and aims to offer the benefit of analgesia in vertebral fractures in combination with restoration of vertebral body height. A balloon-like device is inflated, which restores vertebral body height and creates a cavity into which cement is then injected [146].

Qian and colleagues performed a retrospective review of clinical outcome data for 48 patients with multiple spinal metastases treated with kyphoplasty [147]. Outcome data (vertebral body height variation, degree of kyphosis, visual analog scale score for pain, Oswestry Disability Index score, the Short Form-36 [SF-36] questionnaire score for function) were collected preoperatively, postoperatively, and at 1 month, 6 months, 1 year, and 2 years after treatment. The mean visual analog scale score decreased significantly from presurgery to postsurgery (7.4 ± 2.1 to 3.8 ± 1.6; $p < 0.001$), as did the Oswestry Disability Index score (71.5 ± 16.7 to 32.4 ± 9.6; $p < 0.001$). The SF-36 scores for bodily pain, physical function, vitality, and social functioning all also showed significant improvement ($p < 0.05$). Qian et al. concluded that kyphoplasty appears to be an effective, minimally invasive procedure for the stabilization of pathological vertebral fractures caused by metastatic disease, even in levels with vertebral wall deficiency [147].

INTRATHECAL THERAPIES FOR POM

The use of intrathecal analgesics is an important treatment consideration for many patients with chronic cancer pain [148]. Intrathecal analgesia has emerged as a key therapeutic option for pain relief for patients who have failed other treatment avenues as well as patients with adequate analgesia on high dose enteral or parenteral therapy but with unacceptable side effects [149].

Smith and colleagues performed a multicenter randomized, prospective trial evaluating intrathecal drug delivery for 202 cancer patients [150]. Specific outcomes from the Smith et al. study were that opioid-induced toxicities such as fatigue, sedation, and cognitive slowing were improved compared with patients receiving comprehensive medication management. Pain scores were also improved with respect to baseline and compared with the scores in patients receiving comprehensive medication management, with nearly 2/3 of IDDS patients, having scores in the target range of less than 4/10. The number of intrathecal drug choices are limited and should be guided by consensus guidelines [151]. First-line intrathecal analgesics include morphine, sulfate, hydromorphone and ziconotide [151], however, there are other alternative agents as well (Figure 5) [148,149,151]. Appropriate selection of patients with intractable cancer pain for chronic intrathecal analgesia therapy is paramount [152] and clear communication of the rationale for infusion is very important, as is regular education about infusion management [153].

POTENTIAL FUTURE APPROACHES TO THE MANAGEMENT OF POM

Inhibitors of the RANK–RANKL System

The RANK–RANKL system plays a fundamental role in the maturation and function of osteoclasts and thus in the development and progression of bone metastasis.

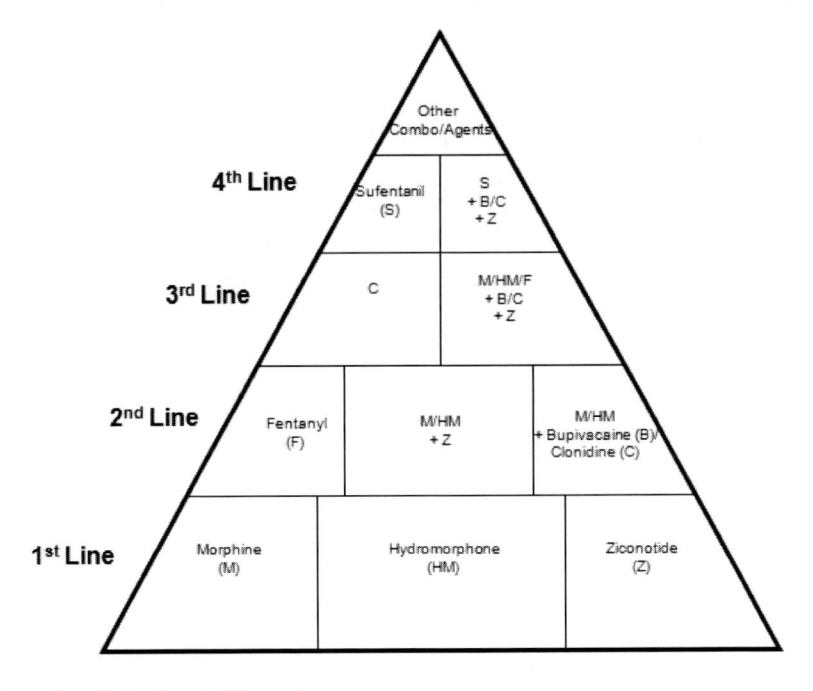

Figure 5. Intrathecal Analgesic Therapies.

Therefore, inhibition of this system has been evaluated as therapeutic target for the treatment of osteolytic diseases, including bone metastasis [24].

It appears that some of the pain from metastatic bone lesions may be secondary to the effects of osteoclastic activity, so that "shutting down" osteoclastic activity is paramount to incorporate in analgesic treatments. Osteoclast bone-resorbing activity is dependent on the binding of the (TNF family molecule osteoprotegerin ligand (OPGL) [154], which is expressed on activated T cells and osteoblasts, to a receptor termed receptor activator of nuclear factor kB (NF-kB), abbreviated RANK [154]. RANK is expressed on osteoclast precursors and mature osteoclasts [155]. Any treatment that impedes the OPGL-RANK interaction will impair RANK activation and therefore impair osteoclastic activity and bone resorption. Osteoprotegerin (OPG) is a soluble tumor necrosis factor receptor molecule that is secreted and binds to the RANK activating site of OPGL, acting as a "dummy" or "decoy" receptor and preventing OPGL from binding to and activating the osteoclast RANK receptor [154,156, 157] (Figure 2).

Amgen created a recombinant Fc-OPG (AMGN-0007) to treat multiple myeloma and bone metastatic breast cancer. Results from the Phase I trial were encouraging, in that Fc-OPG was well tolerated and its inhibitory effects on bone resorption were similar to the bisphosphonate, pamidronate [158]. However, due to the superior efficacy of their newer agent, denosumab (AMG-162) – a fully human monoclonal antibody that specifically neutralizes RANKL – thereby inhibiting bone resorption, and concerns regarding deleterious OPG-mediated protection from TRAIL mediated apoptosis in cancer cells, Amgen ceased further clinical development of AMGN-0007 [159].

Charles S. Cleeland, PhD, University of Texas M. D. Cancer Center, Houston, Texas, and colleagues elsewhere examined differences between patient-reported pain interference with daily functioning using data from a phase 3 trial that compared denosumab with zoledronic acid in women with advanced breast cancer and bone metastases; and their findings in December 2010 presented at the 33rd annual San Antonio Breast Cancer Symposium (SABCS) [160].

In the trial, patients completed the 11-point Brief Pain Inventory-Short Form (BPI-SF) to assess pain interference with general activity, walking, work, mood enjoyment of life, relations with others and sleep, and to assess pain severity. The analysis included 1,018 patients treated with denosumab and 1,011 patients treated with zoledronic acid. Results showed that time to improvement in pain interference with activity (PIWA) tended to occur more rapidly with denosumab than with zoledronic acid (a median of 70 vs 86 days; P =.09). Also, time to worsening PIWA tended to tended to be longer with denosumab than with zoledronic acid (median of 394 vs 310 days; P =.13). In women with no pain or only mild pain at enrollment, denosumab showed a trend for shorter time to improvement in PIWA and a longer time to worsening PIWA. Also, a shift in analgesic use from no or low analgesics to strong opioids occurred in fewer patients treated with denosumab.

PURINERGIC MODULATORS

Purinergic modulators appear to have the capacity to affect nociceptive processes. Kaan et al. utilized a rat model of bone cancer with MRMT-1 carcinoma cells and demonstrated that pain-related behaviors were increased and phosphorylation of ERK 1/2 (p-ERK 1/2) protein expression levels were increased in the spinal dorsal horn and DRG of the CIBP group relative to the sham group [161]. Using AF-353, an orally administered potent and selective P2X3 and P2X2/3 receptor antagonist, Kaan and colleagues demonstrated attenuation of bone cancer pain-related behaviors, reduced bone cancer-induced dorsal horn neuronal hyperexcitability in vivo, and reduced carcinoma cells-induced extracellular signal-regulated kinase activation (p-ERK 1/2) in dorsal root ganglion neurons [161].

Additionally, Chen et al. published that P2Y1R mRNA and phosphorylated ERK1/2 (p-ERK1/2) protein expression levels were increased in the spinal dorsal horn and DRG of the CIBP group relative to the sham group [162]. Intrathecal injection of the P2Y1R antagonist MRS2179 decreased P2Y1R mRNA and p-ERK1/2 protein expression in the spinal dorsal horn and DRG (P< 0.01), as well as pain-related behavior including tactile allodynia, spontaneous pain, and ambulatory-evoked pain [162]. These results provide supportingevidence that the inhibition of P2Y1R-mediated ERK1/2 phosphorylation in the spinal dorsal horn and DRG can attenuate nociception transmission [162].

Additionally, it is conceivable that potential future therapeutic agents may include cannabinoid receptor modulators [163], nerve growth factor modulators [164], inhibitors of cathepsin K, Src inhibitors, inhibitors of MMP-9 αVβ3 antagonists, CXCR4 antagonists, endothelin-A receptor antagonists (e.g. atrasentan [165]), and tyrosine kinase inhibitors (e.g. cabozantinib [XL184]).

CONCLUSION

Metastatic disease to the bone has been a crippling devastating complication of various cancers, leaving patients bedridden or wheelchair-bound and victims of suffering with unbearable pain. Knowledge surrounding the pathophysiology of painful osseous metastases is rapidly changing. Treatment approaches continue to be introduced into practice as they are approved. The advent of intravenous bisphosphonates has not only given clinicians another agent to reduce pain but also to reduce and/or postpone the risk of "skeletal-related events". RANK-L inhibition with denosumab represents a new therapeutic approach to also prevent or delay "skeletal-related events" as well as reduce pain. A greater understanding of the pathophysiology of painful osseous metastases may lead to improved analgesia with minimal adverse effects by utilizing tailor-made selective targeted therapy. It is hoped that potential future therapeutic agents for the treatment of painful osseous metastases may revolutionize current pharmacologic approaches and lead to improved patient outcomes with better quality of life.

ACKNOWLEDGMENT

The author would like to thank Pya Seidner for her enormous assistance in the preparation of this manuscript.

REFERENCES

[1]   P. Boyle, and B. Levin, World cancer report 2008. International Agency for Research on Cancer, Lyon: France, (2008).

[2]   Berruti, L. Dogliotti, R. Bitossi, G. Fasolis, G. Gorzegno, M. Bellina, M. Torta, F. Porpiglia, D. Fontana, and A. Angeli, *J. Urol.* 164, 1248 (2000).

[3]   T. Meuser, C. Pietruck, L. Radbruch, P. Stute, K. A. Lehmann, and S. Ground, *Pain.* 93, 247 (2001).

[4]   M. H. van den Beuken-van Everdingen, J. M. de Rijke, A. G. Kessels, H. C. Schouten, J. van Kleef, and M. Patijn, *Ann. Oncol.* 18, 1437 (2007).

[5]   M. H. van den Beuken-van Everdingen, J. M. de Rijke, A. G. Kessels, H. C. Schouten, J. van Kleef M. and Patijn, *Pain.* 132, 312 (2007).

[6]   M. Farhanghi, R. A. Holmes, W. A. Volkert, K. W. Logan, and A. Singh, *J. Nucl. Med.* 33, 1451 (1992).

[7]   R. E. Coleman and R. D. Rubens, *Br. J. Cancer.* 55, 61 (1987).

[8]   Delaney, S. M. Fleetwood-Walker, L. A. Colvin, and M. Fallon, *Br. J. Anaesth.*; 101, 87 (2008).

[9]   J. Laird, J. Walley, G. D. Murray, E. Clausen, L. A. Colvin, and M. T. Fallon, *Support Care Cancer.* 19, 1393 (2011).

[10]   R. E. Coleman, *Cancer.* 80, 1588 (1997).

[11]   H. Neville-Webbe, and R. E. Coleman, *Palliat. Med.* 17, 539 (2003).

[12]   T. Rustøen, T. Moum, G. Padilla, S. Paul, and C. Miakowski, *J. Pain Symptom. Manage.* 30, 234 (2005).

[13]   S. Mercadante, *Pain.* 69, 1 (1997).

[14]   R. K. Portenoy, K. Forbes, D. Lussier, and G. Hanks, *Oxford textbook of palliative medicine*, Oxford University Press, Oxford (2004).

[15]   L. Colvin, and M. Fallon, *Eur. J. Cancer.* 44, 1083 (2008).

[16]   S. Mercadante, and E. Arcuri, *Cancer Treat. Rev.* 24, 425 (1998).

[17]   R. de Wit, F. van Dam, S. Loonstra, L. Zandbelt, A. van Buuren, K. van der Heijden, G. Leenhouts, and H. Huijer Abu-Saad, *Pain.* 91, 339 (2001).

[18]   T. Meuser, C. Pietruck, L. Radbruch, P. Stute, K. A. Lehmann, and S. Grond, *Pain.* 93, 247 (2001).

[19]   R. Payne, and N. Janjan, Progress in Pain Research and Management. Vol 12. IASP Press, Seattle (1998).

[20]   N. A. Janjan, R. Payne, T. Gillis, D. Podoloff, H. I. Libshitz, R. Lenzi, R. Theriault, C. Martin, and A. Yasko. *J. Pain Symptom. Manage*; 16, 171 (1998).

[21]   F. Fulfaro, A. Casuccio, C. Ticozzi, and C. Ripamonti, *Pain.* 78, 157 (1998).

[22]   F. Tannock, D. Osoba, M. R. Stockler, D. S. Ernst, A. J. Neville, M. J. Moore, G. R. Armitage, J. J. Wilson, P. M. Venner, C. M. Coppin, and K. C. Murphy, *J. Clin. Oncol.* 14, 1756 (1996).

[23]   H. Smith, A. Navani, and S. M. Fishman, *Am. J. Hosp. Palliat. Care.* 21, 303 (2004).

[24]   D. J. Papachristou, E. K. Basdra, and A. G. Papavassiliou, *Med. Res. Rev.* 32, 611 (2012).

[25]   D. Santini, S. Galluzzo, A. Zoccoli, F. Pantano, M. E. Fratto, B. Vincenzi, L. Lombardi, C. Gucciardino, N. Silvestris, E. Riva, S. Rizzo, A. Russo, E. Maiello, G. Colucci, and G. Tonini G, *Cancer Treat. Rev.* 36, S6 (2010).

[26]   Y. Jung, J. Wang, A. Schneider, Y. X. Sun, A. J. Koh-Paige, N. I. Osman, L. K. McCauley, and R. S. Taichman RS, *Bone.* 38, 497 (2006).

[27]   M. Koutsilieris, *Anticancer Research.* 13, 443 (1993).

[28]   M. Koutsilieris, *Critical Reviews in Oncology/Hematology.* 18, 51 (1995).

[29] C. R. Pound, A. W. Partin, M. A. Eisenberger, D. W. Chan, J. D. Pearson, and P. C. Walsh, *JAMA* 281, 1591 (1999).

[30] P. Msaouel, N. Pissimissis, A. Halapas, and M. Koutsilieris, *Best. Pract. Res. Clin. Endocrinol. Metab.* 22, 341 (2008).

[31] C. Geis, M. Graulich, A. Wissmann, T. Hagenacker, J. Thomale, C. Sommer, and M. Schäfers, *Neuroscience.* 169, 463 (2010).

[32] H. S. Smith, *Drugs for Pain*. Hanley and Belfus, Philadelphia (2003).

[33] C. S. B. Galasko, *Clin. Orthop.* 169, 20 (1982).

[34] S. Granot-Attas, C. Luxenburg, E. Finkelshtein, and A. Elson, *Mol. Biol. Cell.* 20, 4324 (2009).

[35] W. S. Sly, D. Hewett-Emmett, M. P. Whyte, Y. S. Yu, and R. E. Tashian, *Proc. Natl. Acad. Sci. USA.* 80, 2752 (1983).

[36] J. Tolar, S. L. Teitelbaum, and P. J. Orchard, *N. Engl. J. Med.* 351, 2839 (2004).

[37] K. Josephsen, J. Praetorius, S. Frische, L. R. Gawanis, T-H. Kowon, P. Agre, S. Nielsen, and O. Fejerskov, *PNAS* 106, 1638 (2009).

[38] Teti, H. C. Blair, S. L. Teitelbaum, A. J. Kahn, C. Koziol, J. Konsek, A. Zambonin-Zallone, and P. H. Schlesinger, *J. Clin. Invest.* 83, 227 (1989).

[39] Frattini, P. J. Orchard, C. Sobacchi, S. Giliani, M. Abinun, J. P. Mattsson, D. J. Keeling, A. K. Andersson, P. Wallbrandt, L. Zecca, L. D. Notarangelo, P. Vezzoni, and A. Villa, *Nat. Genet.* 25, 343 (2000).

[40] U. Kornak, A. Schulz, W. Friedrich, S. Uhlhaas, B. Kremens, T. Voit, C. Hasan, U. Bode, T. J. Jentsch, and C. Kubisch, *Hum. Mol. Genet.* 9, 2059 (2000).

[41] Y. P. Li, W. Chen, Y. Liang, E. Li, and P. Stashenko, *Nat. Genet.* 23, 447 (1999).

[42] J. C. Scimeca, A. Franchi, C. Trojani, H. Parrinello, J. Grosgeorge, C. Robert, O. Jaillon, C. Poirier, P. Gaudray, and G. F. Carle, *Bone.* 26, 207 (2000).

[43] H. C. Blair, S. L. Teitelbaum, R. Ghiselli, S. Gluck, *Science.* 245, 855 (1989).

[44] H. C. Blair, S. L. Teitelbaum, H. L. Tan, C. M. Koziol, and P. H. Schlesinger, *Am. J. Physiol.* 260, C1315 (1991).

[45] K. Henriksen, J. Gram, S. Schaller, B. H. Dahl, M. H. Dziegiel, J. Bollerslev, and M. A. Karsdal, *Am. J. Pathol.* 164, 1537 (2004).

[46] M. A. Karsdal, K. Henriksen, M. G. Sørensen, J. Gram, S. Schaller, M. H. Dziegiel, A. M. Heegaard, P. Christophersen, T. J. Martin, C. Christiansen, and J. Bollerslev, *Am. J. Pathol.* 166, 467 (2005).

[47] U. Kornak, D. Kasper, M. R. Bosl, E. Kaiser, M. Schweizer, A. Schulz, W. Friedrich, G. Delling, and T. J. Jemtsch, *Cell.* 104, 205 (2001).

[48] R. Baron, L. Neff, D. Louvard, and P. J. Courtoy, *J. Cell Biol.* 101, 2210 (1985).

[49] T. Miyazaki, l. Neff, S. Tanaka, W. C. Horne, and R. Baron, *J. Cell Biol.* 160, 709 (2003).

[50] T. Miyazaki, A. Sanjay, L. Neff, S. Tanaka, W. C. Horne, and R. Baron, *J. Biol. Chem.* 279, 17660 (2004).

[51] Miyazaki T, Tanaka S, Sanjay A, Baron R. The role of c-Src kinase in the regulation of osteoclast function. *Mod. Rheumatol.* 2006; 16:68-74.

[52] M. J. Bossard, T. A. Tomaszek, S. K. Thompson, B. Y. Amegadzie, C. R. Hanning, C. Jones, J. T. Kurdyla, D. E. McNulty, F. H. Drake, M. Gowen, and M. A. Levy, *J. Biol. Chem.* 271, 12517 (1996).

[53] M. Gowen, F. Lazner, R. Dodds, R. Kapadia, J. Field, M. Tavaria, I. Bertoncello, F. Drake, S. Zavarselk, I. Tellis, P. Hertzop, C. Debouck, and I. Kola, *J. Bone Miner. Res.* 14, 1654 (1999).

[54] Y. Nishi, L. Atley, D. E. Eyre, J. G. Edelson, A. Superti-Furga, T. Yasuda, R. J. Desnick, and B. D. Gelb, *J. Bone Miner. Res.* 14, 1902 (1999).

[55] P. Saftig, E. Hunziker, O. Wehmeyer, S. Jones, A. Boyde, W. Rommerskirch, J. D. Moritz, P. Schu, and K. von Figura, *Proc. Natl. Acad. Sci. USA.* 95, 13453 (1998).

[56] V. Everts, J. M. Delaissé, W. Korper, D. C. Jansen, W. Tigchelaar-Gutter, P. Saftig, and W. Beertsen, *J. Bone Miner. Res.* 17, 77 (2002).

[57] J. Bradt, C. Dileo, D. Grocke, and L. Mahill, *Cochrane Database Syst. Rev.* Aug 10;(8):CD006911 (2001).

[58] S. W. Jane, S. L. Chen, D. J. Wilkie, Y. C. Lin, S. W. Foreman, R. D. Beaton, J. Y. Fan, M. Y. Lu, Y. Y. Wang, Y. H. Lin, and M. N. Liao, *Pain* 152, 2432 (2011).

[59] E. Bruera, and H. N. Kim, *JAMA* 290, 2476 (2003).

[60] G. W. Hanks, *Cancer Surv.* 7, 87 (1988).

[61] W. Burton, and C. S. Cleeland, *Pain Pract.* 1, 236 (2001).

[62] D. F. Zech, S. Grond, J. Lynch, D. Hertel, and K. A. Lehmann KA, *Pain.* 63, 65 (1995).

[63] Vielhabe, and R. K. Portenoy RK, *Hematol. Oncol. Clin. North Am.* 16, 527 (2002).

[64] Urch, *Palliat. Med.*18, 267 (2004).

[65] J. Estapé, N, Viñolas, B. González, F. Inglés, T.Bofill, M. C. Guzmán, and E. Tarragó, *J. Int. Med. Res.* 18, 298 (1990).

[66] L. M. Fuccella, F. Conti, G. Corvi, V. Mandelli, M. Randelli, and G. Stefanelli, *Clin Pharmacol. Ther.* 17, 277 (1975).

[67] V. Minotti, V. de Angelis, E. Righetti, M. G. Celani, R. Rossetti, M. Lupatelli, M. Tonato, R. Pisati, G. Monza, G. Fumi and A. Del Favero, *Pain.* 74, 133 (1998).

[68] V. Minotti, L. Patoia, F. Roila, C. Basurto, M. Tonato, V. Pasqualucci, V. Maresca, and A. Del Favero, *Pain.* 36, 177 (1989).

[69] J. Stambaugh, and J. Drew, *J. Clin. Pharm.* 28, S34 (1988).

[70] M. J. Staquet MJ, *J. Clin. Pharmacol.* 29, 1031 (1989).

[71] Sunshine, and N. Z. Olson, *J. Clin. Pharm.* 28, S47 (1988).

[72] V. Ventafridda, G. Martino, V. Mandelli, and A. Emanueli, *Clin. Pharmacol. Ther;* 17, 284 (1975).

[73] E. Eisenberg, C. S. Berkey, D. B. Carr, F. Mosteller, and T. C. Chalmers, *J. Clin. Oncol.* 12, 2756 (1994).

[74] S. Levick, C. Jacobs, D. F. Loukas, D. H. Gordon, F. L. Meyskens, and K. Uhm, *Pain.* 35, 253 (1988).

[75] J. E. Stambaugh, and J. Drew, *Clin. Pharmacol. Ther.* 44, 665 (1988).

[76] G. Sacchetti, P. Camera, and A. P. Rossi, *Drug Intell. Clin. Pharm.* 18, 403 (1984).

[77] E. McNicol, S. A. Strassels, L. Goudas, J. Lau, and D. B. Carr, *Cochrane Database Syst. Rev.* Jan 25;(1):CD005180 (2005).

[78] E. McNicol, S. Strassels, L. Goudas, J. Lau, and D. Carr, *J. Clin. Oncol.* 22, 1975 (2004).

[79] H. Sheng, J. Shao, S. C. Kirkland, P. Isakson, R. J. Coffey, J. Morrow, R. D. Beauchanp, and R. N. DuBois, *J. Clin. Invest.* 99, 2254 (1997).

[80] K. Sumitani, R. Kamijo, T. Toyoshima, Y. Nakanishi, K. Takizawa, M. Hatori, and M. Nagumo, *J. Oral Pathol. Med.*; 30, 41 (2001).

[81] M. A. Sabino, J. R. Ghilardi, J. L. Jongen, C. P. Keyser, N. M. Luger, D. B. Mach, C. M. Peters, S. D. Rogers, M. J. Schwei, C. de Felipe, and P. W. Mantyh, *Cancer Res.* 62, 7343 (2002).

[82] M. Isono, T. Suzuki, K. Hosono, I. Hayashi, H. Sakagami, S. Uematsu, S. Akira, Y. A. DeClerck, H. Okamoto, and M. Majima, *Life Sci.* 88, 693 (2011).

[83] E. Bruera, E. Roca, L. Cedaro, S. Carraro, and R. Chacon, *Cancer Treat. Rep.* 69, 751 (1985).

[84] D. M. Cain, P. W. Wacnik, M. Turner, G. Wendelschafer-Crabb, W. R. Kennedy, G. L. Wilcox, and D. A. Simone, *J. Neurosci.* 21, 9367 (2001).

[85] M. Peters, J. R. Ghilardi, C. P. Keyser, K. Kubota, T. H. Lindsay, N. M. Luger, D. B. Mach, M. J. Schwei, M. A. Sevcik, and P. W. Mantyh, *Exp. Neurol.* 193, 85 (2005).

[86] K. G. Halvorson, M. A. Sevcik, J. R. Ghilardi, T. J. Rosol, and P. W. Mantyh, *Clin. J. Pain.* 22, :587 (2006).

[87] J. M. J. Jimeenez-Andrade, and P. Mantyh, Transitional Pain Research: From Mouse to Man. CRC Press, Boca Raton, Fl (2010).

[88] T. Donovan-Rodriguez, A. H. Dickenson, and C. E. Urch, *Anesthesiology.* 102, 132 (2005).

[89] P. Honore, and P. W. Mantyh, *Pain Med.* 1, 303 (2000).

[90] Caraceni, E. Zecca, C. Bonezzi, E. Arcuri, R. Yay Tur, M. Maltoni, M. Visentin, G. Gorni, C. Martini, W. Tirelli, M. Barbieri, and F. De Conno, *J. Clin. Oncol.* 22, 2909 (2004).

[91] Caraceni, E. Zecca, C. Martini, A. Pigni, and P. Bracchi, *Palliat. Med.* 22, 392 (2008).

[92] http://clinicaltrials.gov. NCT00381095.Accessed April 2009.

[93] Kato, K. Minami, H. Ito, T. Tomii, M. Matsumoto, S. Orita, T. Kihara, M. Narita, and T. Suzuki, *Oncology.* 74, 55 (2008).

[94] F. Bailey, and A. Farley, Cancer-related breakthrough pain. Oxford University Press, Oxford (2006).

[95] R. K. Portenoy, D. Payne, and P. Jacobsen, *Pain.* 81, 129 (1999).

[96] L. Costa, and P. P. Major, *Nat. Clin. Pract. Oncol.* 6, 163 (2009).

[97] J. R. Green, *Oncologist.* 9, 3 (2004).

[98] H. Mönkkönen, S. Auriola, P. Lehenkari, M. Kellinsalmi, I. E. Hassinen, J. Vepsäläinen, and J. Mönkkönen, *Br. J. Pharmacol.* 147, 437 (2006).

[99] R. S. Finley, *Semin. Onco.* 129, 32 (2002).

[100] O. P. Purohit, C. Anthony, C. R. Radstone, J. Owen, and R. E. Coleman, *Br. J. Cancer.* 70, 554 (1994).

[101] J. R. Berenson, B. E. Hillner, R. A. Kyle, K. Anderson, A. Lipton, G. C. Yee, and J. S. Biermann; American Society of Clinical Oncology Bisphosphonates Expert Panel, *J. Clin. Oncol.* 20, 3719 (2002).

[102] K. Pistevou-Gombaki, N. Eleftheriadis, I. Sofroniadis, P. Makris, and V. Kouloulias, *J. Exp. Clin. Cancer Res.* 21, 429 (2002).

[103] Santini, M. E. Fratto, B. Vincenzi, S. Galluzzo, and G. Tonini, *Expert Opin. Biol. Ther.* 6:1333 (2006).

[104] M. J. Clemons, G. Dranitsaris, W. S. Ooi, G. Yogendran, T. Sukovic, B. Y. Wong, S. Verma, K. I. Pritchard, M. Trudeau, and D. E. Cole, *J. Clin. Oncol.* 24, 4895 (2006).

[105] Amir, C. Whyne, O. C. Freedman, M. Fralick, R. Kumar, M. Hardisty, and M. Clemons, *Clin. Exp. Metastasis.* 26, 479 (2009).

[106] S. Boissier, M. Ferreras, O. Peyruchaud, S. Magnetto, F. H. Ebetino, M. Colombel, P. Delmas, J. M. Delaissé, and P. Clézardin, *Cancer Res.* 60, 2949 (2000).

[107] T. Hiraga, P. J. Williams, A. Ueda, D. Tamura, and T. Yoneda, *Clin. Cancer Res.* 10, 4559 (2004).

[108] Furlow, *Lancet Oncol.* 7, 894 (2006).

[109] Fulfaro, G. Leto, G. Badalamenti, C. Arcara, G. Cicero, M. R. Valerio, G. Di Fede, A. Russo, A. Vitale, G. B. Rini, A. Casuccio, C. Intrivici, and N. Gebbia, *J. Chemother.* 17, 555 (2005).

[110] T. D. Rachner, S. K. Singh, M. Schoppet, P. Benad, M. Bornhäuser, V. Ellenrieder, R. Ebert, F. Jakob, and L. C. Hofbauer, *Cancer Lett.* 287, 109 (2010).

[111] J. K. Woodward, H. L. Neville-Webbe, R. E. Coleman, and I. Holen, *Anticancer Drugs.* 16:845 (2005).

[112] Santini, B. Vincenzi, S. Galluzzo, F. Battistoni, L. Rocci, O. Venditti, G. Schiavon, S. Angeletti, F. Uzzalli, M. Caraglia, G. Dicuonzo, and G. Tonini, *Clin. Cancer Res.* 13, 4482 (2007).

[113] B. Vincenzi, D. Santini, G. Dicuonzo, F. Battistoni, M. Gavasci, A. La Cesa, C. Grilli, V. Virzì, S. Gasparro, L. Rocci, and G. Tonini, *J. Interferon Cytokine Res.*; 25, 144 (2005).

[114] Tong, L. Gillick, and F. R. Hendrickson, *Cancer* 50, 893 (1982).

[115] Arcangeli, A. Micheli, G. Arcangeli, D. Giannarelli, O. La Pasta, A. Tollis, A. Vitullo, S. Ghera, and M. Benassi, *Radiother. Oncol* . 14, 95 (1989).

[116] K. Dennis, K. Wong, L. Zhang, S. Culleton, J. Nguyen, L. Holden, F. Jon, M. Tsao, C. Danjoux, E. Barnes, A. Sahgal, L. Zeng, K. Koo, and E. Chow, *Clin. Oncol. (R. Coll. Radiol).* Dec;23(10):709 (2011).

[117] C. A. Poulter, D. Cosmatos, P. Rubin, R. Urtasun, J. S. Cooper, R. R. Kuske, N. Hornback, C. Coughlin, I. Weigensberg, and M. Rotman, *Int. J. Radiat. Oncol. Biol. Phys.* 23, 207 (1992).

[118] B. Jeremic, *J. Pain Symptom. Manage.* 22, 1048 (2001).

[119] J. S. Wu, R. Wong, M. Johnston, A. Bezjak, and T. Whelan; Cancer Care Ontario Practice Guidelines Initiative Supportive Care Group, *Int. J. Radiat. Oncol. Biol. Phys.* 55, 594 (2003).

[120] W. M. Sze, M. D. Shelley, I. Held, T. J. Wilt, and M. D. Mason, *Clin. Oncol. (R. Coll. Radiol).* 15, 345 (2003).

[121] Chow, K. Harris, G. Fan, M. Tsao, and W. M. Sze, *J. Clin. Oncol.* 25, 1423 (2007).

[122] D. Rades, S. E. Schild, and J. L. Abrahm, *Nat. Rev. Clin. Oncol.* 7, 220 (2010).

[123] T. Nomiya, K. Teruyama, H. Wada, K. Nemoto. T. Nomiya, K. Teruyama, H. Wada, and K. Nemoto, *Clin. J. .Pain.* 26, 38 (2010).

[124] M. Huisman, M. A. van den Bosch, J. W. Wijlemans, M. van Vulpen, Y. M. van der Linden, and H. M. Verkooijen, *Int. J. Radiat. Oncol. Biol. Phys.* In Press (2012

[125] M. Roqué I Figuls, M. J. Martinez-Zapata, M. Scott-Brown M, and P. Alonso-Coello, *Cochrane Database Syst. Rev.* Jul 6;(7):CD003347 (2011).

[126] M. Paes, and A. N. Serafini. *Semin. Nucl. Med* . 40, 89 (2010).

[127] R. G. Robinson, D. F. Preston, and J. A. Spicer, *Semin Nucl. Med.* 22, 28 (1992).

[128] E. B. Silberstein, and C. Williams, *J. Nucl. Med.* 26, 345 (1985).

[129] G. Finlay, M. D. Mason, and M. Shelley, *Lancet Oncol.* 6, 392 (2005).

[130] Samarium-153-lexidronam. Clinical Pharmacology Web site. Available at *www. cponline.gsm.com*. Accessed 1997

[131] Samarium-153-lexidronam for painful bone metastases. *Med. Lett. Drugs Ther.* 39, 83 (1997).

[132] R. S. Holmes, *Semin. Nucl. Med.* 22, 41 (1992).

[133] J. E. Bayouth, D. J. Macey, L. P. Kasi, and F. V. Fossella, *J. Nucl. Med.* 35, 63 (1994).

[134] C. Collins, J. F. Eary, G. Donaldson, C. Vernon, N. E. Bush, S. Petersdorf, R. B. Livingston, E. E. Gordon, C. R. Chapman, and F. R. Appelbaum, *J. Nucl. Med.* 34, 1839 (1993).

[135] S. Alberts, B. J. Smit, W. K. Louw, A. J. van Rensburg, A. van Beek, V. Kritzinger, and J. S. Nel, *Radioth. Oncol.* 43, 175 (1997).

[136] O. Sartor, R. H. Reid, D. L. Bushnell, D. P. Quick, and P. J. Ell, *Cancer.* 109, 637 (2007).

[137] J. Nazario, J. Hernandez, and A. L. Tam, *Tech. Vasc. Interv. Radiol.* 14, 150 (2001).

[138] M. R. Callstrom, and J. W. Charboneau, *Tech. Vasc. Interv. Radiol.* 10, 120 (2007).

[139] M. Di Staso, L. Zugaro, G. L. Gravina, P. Bonfili, F. Marampon, L. Di Nicola, A. Conchiglia, L. Ventura, P. Franzese, M. Gallucci, C. Masciocchi, and V. Tombolini, *Eur. Radiol.* 21, 2004 (2011).

[140] D. E. Dupuy, R. Hong, B. Oliver, and S. N. Goldberg, *AJR. AM. J. Roentgenal.* 175, 1263 (2000).

[141] D. Dodd, 3rd, M. S. Frank, M. Aribandi, S. Chopra, and K. N. Chintapalli, *AJR. AM. J. Roentgenal.* 177, 777 (2001).

[142] Tancioni, M. A. Lorenzetti, P. Navarria, F. Pessina, R. Draghi, P. Pedrazzoli, M. Scorsetti, M. Alloisio, A. Santoro, and R. Rodriguez y Baena, *J. Support Oncol.* 9, 4 (2011).

[143] W. C. Peh, and A. Gilula, *Br. J. Radiol.* 76, 69 (2003).

[144] B. Lee, I. Franklin, J. S. Lewis, R. C. Coombes, R. Leonard, P. Gishen, and J. Stebbing, *Eur. J. Cancer.* 45, 1597 (2009).

[145] Saliou, M. Kocheida el, P. Lehmann, C. Depriester, G. Paradot, D. LeGars, A. Balut, and H. Deramond, *Radiology.* 254, 882 (2010).

[146] R. H. Kassamali, A. Ganeshan, E. T. Hoey, P. M. Crowe, H. Douis, and J. Henderson, *Ann. Oncol.* 22, 782 (2011).

[147] Z. Qian, Z. Sun, H. Yang, Y. Gu, K. Chen, and G. Wu, *J. Clin. Neurosci.* 18, 763 (2011).

[148] S. Newsome, B. K. Frawley, and C. E. Argoff, *Curr. Pain Headache Rep.* 12, 249 (2008).

[149] S. Smith, T. R. Deer, P. S. Staats, V. Singh, N. Sehgal, and H. Cordner, *Pain Physician.* 11, S89 (2008).

[150] T. J. Smith, P. S. Staats, T. Deer, L. J. Stearns, R. L. Rauck, R. L. Boortz-Marx, E. Buchser, E. Català, D. A. Bryce, P. J. Coyne, G. E. Pool; Implantable Drug Delivery Systems Study Group, *J. Clin. Oncol.* 20, 4040 (2002).

[151] T. Deer, E. S. Krames, S. J. Hassenbusch, A. Burton, D. Caraway, S. Dupen, J. Eisenach, M. Erdek, E. Grigsby, P. Kim, R. Levy, G. McDowell, N. Mekhail, S. Panchal, J. Prager, R. Rauck, M. Saulino, T. Sitzman, P. Staats, M. Stanton-Hicks, L. Stearns, K. D. Willis, W. Witt, K. Follett, M. Huntoon, L. Liem, J. Rathmell, M.

Wallace, E. Buchser, M. Cousins, and A. Ver Donck, *Neuromodulation: Technol. Neural. Interface.* 10, 300 (2007).

[152] T. R. Deer, H. S. Smith, A. W. Burton, J. E. Pope, D. M. Doleys, R. M. Levy, P. S. Staats, M. S. Wallace, L. R. Webster, R. L. Rauck, and M. Cousins; Center For Pain Relief, Inc, *Pain Physician*; 14, E283 (2011).

[153] P. Hawley, E. Beddard-Huber, C. Grose, W. McDonald, D. Lobb, and L. Malysh, *Pain Res. Manag.* 14, 371 (2009).

[154] Y.Y. Kong, U. Feige, I. Sarosi, B. Bolon, A. Tafuri, S. Morony, C. Capparelli, J. Li, R. Elliott, S. McCabe, T. Wong, G. Campagnuolo, E. Moran, E. R. Bogoch, G. Van, L. T. Nguyen, P. S. Ohashi, D. L. Lacey, E. Fish, W. J. Boyle, and J. M. Penninger, *Nature.* 402, 304 (1999).

[155] Hsu, D. L. Lacey, C. R. Dunstan, I. Solovyev, A. Colombero, E. Timms, H. L. Tan, G. Elliott, M. J. Kelley, I. Sarosi, L. Wang, X. Y. Xia, R. Elliott, L. Chiu, T. Black, S. Scully, C. Capparelli, S. Morony, G. Shimamoto, M. B. Bass, and W. J. Boyle, *Proceedings of the Proc. Natl. Acad. Sci. USA.* 96, 3540 (1999).

[156] W. S. Simonet, D. L. Lacey, C. R. Dunstan, M. Kelley, M. S. Chang, R. Lüthy, H. Q. Nguyen, S. Wooden, L. Bennett, T. Boone, G. Shimamoto, M. DeRose, R. Elliott, A. Colombero, H. L. Tan, G. Trail, J. Sullivan, E. Davy, N. Bucay, L. Renshaw-Gegg, T. M. Hughes, D. Hill, W. Pattison, P. Campbell, S. Sander, G. Van, J. Tarpley, P. Derby, R. Lee, and W. J. Boyle, *Cell.* 89, 309 (1997).

[157] S. W. N. Thompson, and D. Tonge, *Nat. Med.* 6, 504 (2000).

[158] J. Body, P. Greipp, R. E. Coleman, T. Facon, F. Geurs, J. P. Fermand, J. L. Harousseau, A. Lipton, X. Mariette, C. D. Williams, A. Nakanishi, D. Holloway, S. W. Martin, C. R. Dunstan, and P. J. Bekker, *Cancer.* 97, 887 (2003).

[159] E. M. Schwarz, and C. T. Ritchlin, *Arthritis Res. Ther.* 9, S7 (2007).

[160] C. S. Cleeland, D. L. Patrick, L. Fallowfield, M. Clemons, A.Lipton, N. Masuda, Y, Qian, A. Braun, and K. Chung, "Comparing the Effects of Denosumab and Zoledronic Acid on Pain Interference with Daily Functioning in a Randomized Phase 3 Trial of Patients With Breast Cancer and Bone Metastases", Presented at 33rd Annual San Antonio Breast Cancer Symposium (SABCS). 12, Dec. 2010 (San Antonio, Texas); Abstract P1-13-01.

[161] T. K. Kaan, P. K. Yip, S. Patel, M. Davies, F. Marchand, D. A. Cockayne, P. A. Nunn, A. H. Dickenson, A. P. Ford, Y. Zhong, M. Malcangio, and S. B. McMahon, *Brain.* 133, 2549 (2010).

[162] Chen, L. Wang, Y. Zhang, and J. Yang, *Acta Biochim. Biophys. Sin. (Shanghai)* 44, 367 (2012).

[163] T. P. Malan Jr, M.M. Ibrahim, J. Lai, T. W. Vanderah, A. Makriyannis, and F. Porreca, *Curr. Opin. Pharmacol.* 3, 62 (2003).

[164] M. Jimenez-Andrade, A. P. Bloom, J. I. Stake, W. G. Mantyh, R. N. Taylor, K. T. Freeman, J. R. Ghilardi, M. A. Kuskowski, and P. W. Mantyh, *J. Neurosci.* 30, 14649 (2010).

[165] D. Cella, D. P. Petrylak, M. Fishman, C. Teigland, J. Young, and P. Mulani, *Eur. Urol.* 49, 781 (2006).

INDEX

N

Q

R

S

T

U